PROLOG

Reproductive Endocrinology and Infertility

FIFTH EDITION

CRITIQUE BOOK

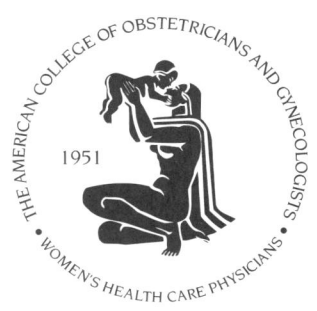

ISBN 1-932328-07-6

Copyright © 2005 by the American College of Obstetricians and Gynecologists. All rights reserved. No part of this publication may be reproduced, stored in a retrieval system, or transmitted, in any form or by any means, electronic, mechanical, photocopying, recording, or otherwise, without prior written permission of the publisher.

12345/98765

The American College of Obstetricians and Gynecologists
409 12th Street, SW
PO Box 96920
Washington, DC 20090-6920

Contributors

PROLOG Editorial and Advisory Committee

CHAIR

Ronald T. Burkman Jr, MD, Chair
   Chair, Department of Obstetrics and
     Gynecology
   Baystate Medical Center
   Springfield, Massachusetts
   Deputy Chair and Professor
   Department of Obstetrics and
     Gynecology
   Tufts University School of Medicine
   Boston, Massachusetts

MEMBERS

Peter E. Nielsen, MD, LTC, MC, USA
   OB/GYN Consultant to the US Surgeon
     General
   Division of Maternal–Fetal Medicine
   Department of Obstetrics and Gynecology
   Madigan Army Medical Center
   Tacoma, Washington

Louis Weinstein, MD
   Paula and Elloise B. Bowers Professor
     and Chair
   Department of Obstetrics and Gynecology
   Thomas Jefferson University
   Philadelphia, Pennsylvania

Sterling B. Williams, MD
   Vice President, Education
   The American College of
     Obstetricians and Gynecologists
   Washington, DC

PROLOG Task Force for *Reproductive Endocrinology and Infertility*, Fifth Edition

COCHAIRS

Robert W. Rebar, MD
   Executive Director
   American Society for Reproductive
     Medicine
   Volunteer Clinical Professor
   Department of Obstetrics and
     Gynecology
   University of Alabama, Birmingham
   Birmingham, Alabama

Craig A. Winkel, MD, MBA
   Professor
   Georgetown University
   School of Nursing
   Washington, DC

MEMBERS

John L. Frattarelli, MD
   Associate Residency Program Director
   Division Chief, Division of Reproductive
     Endocrinology and Infertility
   Department of Obstetrics and
     Gynecology
   Tripler Army Medical Center
   Honolulu, Hawaii

Daniel R. Grow, MD
   Associate Professor
   Chief, Division of Reproductive
     Endocrinology
   Department of Obstetrics and
     Gynecology
   Springfield, Massachusetts

Michael J. Heard, MD
   Reproductive Endocrinology and
     Infertility
   Pediatric/Adolescent Gynecology
   Servy Institute for Reproductive
     Endocrinology
   Augusta, Georgia

Continued on next page

PROLOG Task Force for *Reproductive Endocrinology and Infertility*, Fifth Edition *(continued)*

James H. Liu, MD
   Professor and Arthur H. Bill Chair
   Department of Reproductive Biology
   Case Western Reserve University
   Department of Obstetrics and Gynecology
   University Hospitals of Cleveland
   Cleveland, Ohio

Ricardo Loret de Mola, MD
   Chief, Division of Reproductive Endocrinology and Infertility
   Department of Reproductive Biology
   Case Western Reserve University
   Department of Obstetrics and Gynecology
   University Hospitals of Cleveland
   Cleveland, Ohio

William Meyer, MD
   Associate Professor
   Associate Residency Program Director
   Division of Reproductive Endocrinology and Infertility
   Department of Obstetrics and Gynecology
   University of North Carolina–Chapel Hill
   Chapel Hill, North Carolina

Steven T. Nakajima, MD
   Associate Professor
   Division of Reproductive Endocrinology and Infertility
   Department of Obstetrics, Gynecology, and Women's Health
   University of Iowa Hospitals
   Iowa City, Iowa

Richard H. Reindollar, MD
   Director
   Division of Reproductive Endocrinology and Infertility
   Department of Obstetrics, Gynecology, and Reproductive Biology
   Beth Israel Deaconess Medical Center
   Harvard Medical School
   Boston, Massachusetts

Valerie Montgomery Rice, MD
   Professor and Chair
   Department of Endocrinology and Infertility
   Department of Obstetrics and Gynecology
   Meharry Medical College
   Nashville, Tennessee

Estil Young Strawn Jr, MD
   Associate Professor
   Director, Division of Reproductive Endocrinology and Infertility
   Department of Obstetrics, Gynecology
   Medical College of Wisconsin
   Milwaukee, Wisconsin

ACOG STAFF

Sallye B. Brown, RN, MN
   Director, Educational Development and Testing
   Division of Education

Christopher T. George, MA
   Editor, PROLOG

Note: This PROLOG unit was developed under the direction of the PROLOG Advisory Committee and the Task Force for *Reproductive Endocrinology and Infertility*, Fifth Edition. PROLOG is planned and produced in accordance with the Standards for Enduring Materials of the Accreditation Council for Continuing Medical Education. Any discussion of unapproved uses of products is clearly cited.

Current guidelines state that participants in continuing medical education (CME) activities should be made aware of any affiliation or financial interest by the contributors that may affect the development of the unit. The advisory committee and task force members declare that neither they nor any business associate nor any member of their immediate families has financial interest or other relationships with any manufacturer of any products or any providers of any of the services discussed in this publication except for **Craig A. Winkel, MD**, who is a consultant for and member of the TAP Pharmaceuticals Medical Advisory Board, is a consultant for Ortho-McNeil Pharmaceutical, is a principal in The North Group, is on the Wyeth Pharmaceuticals speakers bureau, and has been an investigator and volunteer intramural co-investigator on intramural studies for the National Institute of Child Health and Human Development (NICHD) and Ortho-McNeil Pharmaceutical; **Ronald T. Burkman Jr, MD**, who is a consultant for Pharmacea, has received lecture support from Ortho-McNeil Pharmaceutical, Wyeth Pharmaceuticals, Berlex Laboratories, Organon Pharmaceuticals USA Inc, and funding for research from NICHD and Ortho-McNeil Pharmaceutical; **Richard H. Reindollar, MD**, who has received research support and honoraria from Organon Pharmaceuticals USA Inc, Serono Laboratories, Wyeth Pharmaceuticals, Genzyme, and Columbia Laboratories; **Steven Nakajima, MD**, who has received research grants from Pfizer Pharmaceuticals and Warner Chilcott Laboratories; **James H. Liu, MD**, who is a member of the advisory boards of Merck US Human Health, Pfizer, Inc, Watson Pharmaceutical, Barr Laboratories, Novartis, and Solvay Pharmaceuticals and has received grants from the National Institutes of Health (NIH), Procter & Gamble Pharmaceuticals, Novartis Pharmaceuticals, Inc, Ortho—Personal Products, Organon Pharmaceuticals USA Inc, and Pfizer Pharmaceuticals; **William R. Meyer, MD**, who was a member of the Merck US Human Health 2003 speaker's bureau; **Valerie Montgomery Rice, MD**, who has received grants and research support from NIH, NICHD, Wyeth Pharmaceuticals, and Eli Lilly and Company; is a consultant for Wyeth Pharmaceuticals and the NICHD Committee; and is on the Advisory Boards of Novo Nordisk and the U.S. Food and Drug Administration Advisory Committee for Reproductive and Urological Health Drugs; **John L. Frattarelli, MD**, who is a speaker for TAP Pharmaceuticals; and **Daniel Grow, MD**, who is a consultant for TAP Pharmaceuticals.

Preface

Purpose

PROLOG (Personal Review of Learning in Obstetrics and Gynecology) is a voluntary, strictly confidential, self-evaluation program. It is designed to enable physicians to assess their current knowledge and to review current concepts within the specialty. The content is carefully selected and presented in multiple-choice questions that are clinically oriented. The questions are designed to stimulate and challenge physicians in areas of medical care that they confront in their practices or when they work as consultant obstetrician–gynecologists.

PROLOG provides the American College of Obstetricians and Gynecologists with a means of identifying the educational needs of the Fellowship. Individual scores are reported only to the participant; however, cumulative performance data obtained for each PROLOG unit help determine the direction for future educational programs offered by the College.

Continuing medical education credits may be earned by participation in the PROLOG self-evaluation process. In addition, PROLOG serves as a valuable study tool, reference guide, and means of attaining up-to-date knowledge in the specialty.

Process

PROLOG offers the most advanced knowledge available in 5 areas of the specialty: 1) obstetrics, 2) gynecology and surgery, 3) reproductive endocrinology and infertility, 4) gynecologic oncology and critical care, and 5) patient management in the office. A new PROLOG unit is produced annually, addressing 1 of those subject areas. *Reproductive Endocrinology and Infertility*, Fifth Edition, is the third unit in the fifth 5-year series of PROLOG.

Each unit of PROLOG represents the efforts of a special task force of subject experts under the supervision of an editorial and advisory committee. PROLOG sets forth current information as viewed by recognized authorities in the field of women's health. This educational resource does not define a standard of care, nor is it intended to dictate an exclusive course of management. It presents recognized methods and techniques of clinical practice for consideration by obstetrician–gynecologists for incorporation into their practices. Variations of practice that take into account the needs of the individual patient, resources, and the limitations that are special to the institution or type of practice may be appropriate.

Each unit of PROLOG is presented as a 2-part set. Performance information and cognate credit are available to those who choose to send their answer sheets for confidential scoring.

The first part of the PROLOG set is the Question Book, which contains educational objectives for the unit, multiple-choice questions, and a computer-scored answer sheet. Participants can work through the book at their own pace, choosing to use PROLOG as a closed- or open-book assessment. Return of the answer sheet for scoring is encouraged but voluntary.

The second part of PROLOG is the Critique Book, which reviews the educational objectives and questions set forth in the Question Book and contains a discussion, or critique, of each question. The critique provides the rationale for correct and incorrect options. Current, accessible references are listed for each question. ACOG Fellows may request additional literature searches as well as information about ACOG publications by contacting the Resource Center, PO Box 96920, Washington, DC 20090-6920, telephone (202) 863-2518.

Participants who return their answer sheets for credit will receive a Performance Report indicating their answers and their correct score percentage. A data package will be sent and will offer participants a means of comparing their scores with the scores of a sample group of other participants. *Please allow 1 month to process answer sheets.*

Fellows who submit their answer sheets for scoring will be credited automatically with 25 cognates of Formal Learning in the ACOG Program for Continuing Professional Development. For the Physician's Recognition Award of the American Medical Association, 25 category 1 credit hours may be reported.

Credit for PROLOG *Reproductive Endocrinology and Infertility*, Fifth Edition, is initially available through December 2007. During that year, the unit will be reevaluated. If it is determined that content in the unit remains current, credit will be extended for an additional 3 years. PROLOG is planned and produced in accordance with the Standards for Enduring Materials of the Accreditation Council for Continuing Medical Education.

Conclusion

PROLOG was developed specifically as a personal study resource for the practicing obstetrician–gynecologist. It is presented as a self-assessment mechanism that, with its accompanying performance information, should assist the physician in designing a personal, self-directed learning program. The many quality resources developed by the College, as detailed each year in the ACOG *Publications and Educational Materials Catalog*, are available to help fulfill the educational interests and needs that have been identified. PROLOG is not intended as a substitute for the certification or recertification programs of the American Board of Obstetrics and Gynecology.

PROLOG Objectives

PROLOG is a voluntary, strictly confidential, personal continuing education resource that is designed to be both stimulating and enjoyable. By participating in PROLOG, obstetrician–gynecologists will be able to do the following:

- Review and update clinical knowledge
- Recognize areas of knowledge and practice in which they excel, be stimulated to explore other areas of the specialty, and identify areas requiring further study
- Plan continuing education activities in light of identified strengths and deficiencies
- Compare and relate present knowledge and skills with those of other participants
- Obtain continuing medical education credit, if desired
- Have complete personal control of the setting and of the pace of the experience

The obstetrician–gynecologist who completes *Reproductive Endocrinology and Infertility*, Fifth Edition, will be able to do the following:

- Associate history as well as signs and symptoms with clinical diagnoses of specific gynecologic, obstetric, and general medical conditions
- Select appropriate laboratory tests and procedures and then analyze the results to make specific diagnoses
- Use an efficacious and cost-effective program of office management for each selected diagnosis
- Understand fundamental concepts of physiology and pathophysiology
- Apply epidemiologic principles to the health care of women
- Counsel patients regarding the extent of their medical problems, including benefits and risks of treatment as well as alternatives
- Apply professional medical ethics to the practice of obstetrics and gynecology
- Incorporate appropriate legal, risk management, and office management guidelines and techniques into clinical practice

Reproductive Endocrinology and Infertility, Fifth Edition, includes the following topics:

SCREENING AND DIAGNOSIS
Amenorrhea diagnosis
Biochemical hyperthyroidism and osteoporosis
Bone density studies
Bone markers for osteoporosis
Breast cancer in *BRCA*-positive patients
Chromosomal abnormalities in couples with recurrent abortion
Chronic labial agglutination
Chronic pelvic pain
Cushing's syndrome diagnosis
Ectopic pregnancy
Environmental toxicity and sperm counts
Evaluation of bleeding with hormone therapy
Fallopian tube occlusion
Gonadotropin-secreting tumors
Hereditary cancer syndromes
Hypogonadism as a cause of male infertility
Hypothyroidism diagnosis
Hysterosalpingogram versus sonohysterogram
Imperforate hymen versus transverse vaginal septum
Indicators for future fractures

Insulin resistance in polycystic ovary syndrome
Menopausal transition
Metabolic syndrome
Minimal endometriosis and infertility
Occlusion of the fallopian tubes
Oral contraceptives and venous thromboembolism
Osteoporosis markers
Ovarian androgen-secreting tumors
Ovarian hyperstimulation syndrome
Postpartum thyroiditis
Precocious thelarche
Premature ovarian failure
Prolactinemia
Salpingitis isthmica nodosa
Screening before hormone therapy
Secondary amenorrhea
Serum human chorionic gonadotropin levels
Sheehan's syndrome
Testing for thyroid dysfunction
Uterosacral ligament transection

MEDICAL MANAGEMENT
Abnormal uterine bleeding
Add-back therapy with analogs
Alternative therapies for the treatment of hot flushes
Androgen–estrogen use for increasing bone mineral density
Androgen insensitivity syndrome
Antiandrogen usage
Blastocysts and twinning
Bone loss with or following hormone therapy
Bulimia versus anorexia
Cardiovascular disease and hormone therapy
Chemotherapy, irradiation, and premature ovarian failure
Choice of agent in ovulation induction
Chronic labial agglutination
Contraception in menopausal transition
Craniopharyngioma
Depot medroxyprogesterone and abnormal bleeding
Depot medroxyprogesterone acetate and appetite
Dysmenorrhea
Emergency contraception
Fertility drugs and ovarian cancer
Fibroids in infertile women
Glucocorticoid-induced osteoporosis
Gonadotropin-releasing hormone agonist and antagonist
Hormonal contraception and weight gain
Hormonal contraceptive method choices
Hormone therapy and risk of breast cancer
Hyperprolactinemia
Hysterosalpingogram complications
Hyperthyroidism
Impotence
Intrauterine insemination complications
Late-onset adrenal hyperplasia and nonclassic congenital adrenal hyperplasia
Levonorgestrel intrauterine system

Lipids and hormone therapy
Luteal phase support
Macroadenoma
Male infertility and hypergonadotropic hypogonadism
Male infertility and retrograde ejaculation
Management of delayed puberty
Metabolic syndrome
Mifepristone (Mifeprex) and pregnancy termination
Migraines and hormonal contraception
Oligospermic males and assisted reproductive technologies
Oral contraceptives and preexisting conditions
Ovarian cyst management during ovulation induction
Ovarian hyperstimulation syndrome
Ovulation induction selection of appropriate patients
Perimenopausal changes
Postpartum thyroiditis
Precocious adrenarche
Primary amenorrhea
Recurrent pregnancy loss
Risk of in vitro fertilization in Turner's syndrome
Selective estrogen receptor modulators and breast cancer
Selective estrogen receptor modulators in osteoporosis
Sheehan's syndrome
Transdermal patch versus vaginal ring
Treatment-related complications of uterine arterial embolization
Use of antiestrogens
Use of bisphosphonates and other agents in osteoporosis
Use of oral contraceptives to treat acne
Uterine and associated anomalies
Vaginoplasty versus Frank method for müllerian aplasia

SURGICAL MANAGEMENT
Bicornuate uterus
Bilateral tubal ligation and future fertility
Bowel injury during endoscopy
Chronic pelvic pain
Endometrial ablation complications
Endoscopic surgery risks
Hydrosalpinges and success of in vitro fertilization
Hysteroscopic endometrial ablation
In vitro fertilization versus surgery
Laser characteristics and safety
Management of weight reduction
Nonhysteroscopic endometrial ablation
Prevention of adhesions
Ruptured endometrioma
Septate uterus
Tubal anastamosis
Vascular injury with laparoscopy

PHYSIOLOGY AND PATHOPHYSIOLOGY
Diethylstilbestrol exposure
Hypothyroidism and hyperprolactinemia
Mechanism of action of oral contraceptives
Normal bone physiology

Normal pubertal development
Premature ovarian failure
Premature thelarche
Primary amenorrhea
Prolactin-secreting pituitary microadenoma
Sheehan's syndrome
Sperm physiology
Uterine and associated anomalies

COUNSELING
Achieving fertility with premature ovarian failure
Blastocysts and twinning
Bone loss with or following hormone therapy
Cardiovascular disease and hormone therapy
Congenital adrenal hyperplasia
Donor oocyte in the older patient
Hormone therapy and risk of breast cancer
Intracycloplastic sperm injection for male infertility
Lifestyle factors and fertility
Mifepristone (Mifeprex) and pregnancy termination
Risks of intracytoplasmic sperm injection

ETHICAL AND LEGAL ISSUES
Informed consent for donor eggs
Reproduction in individuals with acquired immunodeficiency disease syndrome (AIDS)
Use of donor sperm

A subject matter index appears at the end of the Critique Book.

1
Premature ovarian failure

A 25-year-old woman received a diagnosis of premature ovarian failure. Her karyotype is 46,XX. Which of the following laboratory studies is most likely to be abnormal in this patient?

    (A) Fasting glucose
    (B) Calcium
    (C) Cortisol
* (D) Thyroid-stimulating hormone (TSH)
    (E) Vitamin B_{12}

Premature ovarian failure, commonly defined as the loss of ovarian function before age 40 years, affects 1% of women and is associated with symptoms of amenorrhea, estrogen deficiency, and elevated gonadotropin levels. A common cause of premature ovarian failure is an abnormal karyotype, which leads to decreased ovarian function. In women with a normal karyotype, viral infections, genetic etiologies, prior injury to the ovaries (eg, irradiation, chemotherapy, or surgery), or an autoimmune etiology often are suspected. Women with a normal 46,XX karyotype and idiopathic premature ovarian failure associated with autoimmunity are at increased risk for developing other autoimmune diseases (eg, hypothyroidism, diabetes mellitus, adrenal failure, hypoparathyroidism, and pernicious anemia).

The incidence of these other autoimmune diseases has been recently clarified in a study of 119 women with spontaneous premature ovarian failure, a normal karyotype, and a negative history of other causes of ovarian failure. The investigators measured the women's levels of serum free thyroxine, TSH, fasting serum glucose, serum electrolytes, total calcium, and serum vitamin B_{12}. The women also received an adrenocorticotropic hormone (ACTH) stimulation test and a 3-hour glucose tolerance test. After the screening tests were performed, 10 new cases of hypothyroidism and 3 new cases of diabetes mellitus were diagnosed. No new cases of adrenal failure, hypoparathyroidism, or pernicious anemia were detected. Of the 3 new cases of diabetes mellitus, 3 had abnormal fasting glucose levels (greater than 105 mg/dL), and 1 had an abnormal 3-hour glucose tolerance test result (2-hour glucose level greater than 200 mg/dL). The individual with the abnormal 3-hour evaluation also had a positive family history for diabetes mellitus.

These findings suggest that women with spontaneous premature ovarian failure and a normal karyotype need to be alert to possible development of other autoimmune diseases. The incidence of hypothyroidism was 26.9% (32/119); adrenal failure, 2.5% (3/119); and diabetes mellitus, 2.5% (3/119). The results indicate that a serum TSH level is the best screening test to detect the most common associated autoimmune disease with premature ovarian failure. The authors recommend that serum-free thyroxine levels should be obtained to confirm the diagnosis and a fasting glucose level to detect the less common development of diabetes mellitus. Before instituting thyroid therapy, screening for adrenal insufficiency should be performed. Because adrenal insufficiency usually is insidious in onset before it becomes life threatening, the clinician should look for symptoms and screen for its development. A random cortisol level less than 5 µg/dL suggests adrenal insufficiency whereas cortisol levels greater than 17 µg/dL suggest normal adrenal reserve. Random values of 5–17 µg/dL do not rule out adrenal insufficiency. Without symptoms of hypoparathyroidism or pernicious anemia, routine screening for these diseases appears to be of low yield. Annual surveillance of patients with premature ovarian failure may include serum calcium, cortisol, TSH, and antithyroid antibody panel and a screening test for diabetes mellitus.

American College of Obstetricians and Gynecologists. Premature ovarian failure. In: Precis: An update in obstetrics and gynecology. Reproductive endocrinology. 2nd ed. Washington, DC: ACOG; 2002. p. 93–6.

Kim TJ, Anasti JN, Flack MR, Kimzey LM, Defensor RA, Nelson LM. Routine screening for patients with karyotypically normal spontaneous premature ovarian failure. Obstet Gynecol 1997;89:777–9.

Speroff L, Glass RH, Kase NG. Clinical gynecologic endocrinology and infertility. 6th ed. Baltimore (MD): Lippincott Williams & Wilkins; 1999. p. 432–5.

Yen SS, Jaffe RB, Barbieri RL. Reproductive endocrinology. 4th ed. Philadelphia (PA): WB Saunders; 1999. p. 313–4.

* Indicates correct answer.
Note: See Appendix A for a table of normal values for laboratory tests.

2
Surgery for chronic pelvic pain

A 38-year-old multiparous woman with a history of 2 previous laparoscopic procedures for moderate to severe endometriosis desires long-term relief of symptoms. The most appropriate next surgical procedure is

* (A) total abdominal hysterectomy and bilateral salpingo-oophorectomy
* (B) laparoscopy and destruction of all identified lesions
* (C) hysterectomy alone
* (D) laparoscopic presacral neurectomy

The surgical treatment of women with chronic pelvic pain must be based primarily on 2 factors: 1) the likely etiology of the pain, and 2) the patient's desires regarding her future fertility potential. Chronic pelvic pain usually is defined as pain of greater than 6 months' duration. It is important to distinguish between pain of acute, or recent, onset and pain that has existed for an extended period because the differential diagnosis of the former is likely quite different from that of the latter.

Gynecologic causes of chronic pelvic pain commonly include endometriosis, adenomyosis, chronic pelvic inflammatory disease, and abdominopelvic adhesive disease, whereas nongynecologic causes may include interstitial cystitis, irritable bowel syndrome, and fibromyalgia. It is critical to the successful management of women with chronic pelvic pain to tailor the treatment to the cause of pain. Surgical treatment, for example, is unlikely to improve symptoms in a woman with chronic pelvic pain secondary to fibromyalgia. It also is important to remember that pain is a matter of perception, and that perception may be modified significantly in women who have been the subject of physical or sexual abuse. Up to one third of women with chronic pelvic pain are found to have a history of physical or sexual abuse when questioned closely.

The practitioner should discuss surgical treatment options with the patient. In addition, the physician should review the likely outcomes of the various surgical procedures.

For the woman with severe and recurrent symptoms believed to result from endometriosis who has completed her childbearing, a discussion of total abdominal hysterectomy and bilateral salpingo-oophorectomy is appropriate. One study confirmed the superiority of hysterectomy and bilateral salpingo-oophorectomy over hysterectomy alone or hysterectomy and unilateral oophorectomy for long-term relief of pain symptoms and reduction in the chance of pain recurrence. In addition, the same authors demonstrated reduced risk of the need for further surgery with removal of the uterus, fallopian tubes, and ovaries (Table 2-1). Importantly, women younger than 30 years are more likely than women older than 40 years to experience residual symptoms, feel a sense of loss, and report that pain disrupts different aspects of their lives. It has been reported that removal of the uterus, fallopian tubes, and ovaries is associated with up to a 15% risk of recurrence of endometriosis and that the most common site for recurrence involves the intestines.

Laparoscopically directed ablation, or excision, of endometriotic lesions for pain relief has been the subject

TABLE 2-1. Recurrence of Symptoms and Need for Reoperation Among Women With Endometriosis Managed by Hysterectomy With or Without Ovarian Conservation

Procedure	No. of Women	Incidence of Pain Recurrence	Incidence of Reoperation	Relative Risk (95% Confidence Interval) With Ovarian Conservation vs Without Ovarian Conservation
Hysterectomy without ovarian conservation	109	11/109 (10%)	4/109 (3.7%)	6.9 (2.5–14.6)
Hysterectomy with ovarian conservation	29	18/29 (62%)	9/29 (31%)	8.1 (2.1–31.3)

Modified and reprinted from Fertility & Sterility, Vol 64, Namnoum AB, Hickman TN, Goodman SB, Gehlbach DL, Rock JA, Incidence of symptom recurrence after hysterectomy for endometriosis, 898–902, Copyright 1995, with permission from Elsevier.

of significant controversy in recent years. To date, there is only 1 prospective, randomized, controlled trial in which women with endometriosis underwent either diagnostic laparoscopy and visualization of lesions alone or laser ablation of lesions and uterosacral nerve ablation. This study found that 56% of women experienced pain relief after surgical treatment 6 months after surgery whereas only 23% of women who underwent diagnostic laparoscopy alone experienced pain relief. The results are confounded, however, by the fact that the surgeons performed lesion ablation and uterosacral nerve ablation. Thus, it is not possible to know what the impact of lesion ablation alone might have been. The study also demonstrates a significant placebo effect of diagnostic laparoscopy.

A major difficulty with surgical treatment of endometriosis by lesion destruction is the difficulty with visualization of lesions as a technique for identification of disease. Two recent reports demonstrated that the positive predictive value of visualization of lesions for histologic confirmation of disease was approximately 43–45%. Moreover, endometriosis may be present even in pelvic peritoneum that appears to be normal. Thus, visualization of lesions during laparoscopy does not mean that the cause of the pain has been found. Conversely, the inability to visualize lesions does not mean that endometriosis is not present.

Adenomyosis is defined as the finding of endometrial glands and stroma insinuated into the myometrium. A condition that often is associated with dysmenorrhea, adenomyosis may be diffuse or, less commonly, focal with the formation of an adenomyoma. The treatment of adenomyosis, which is most easily diagnosed by magnetic resonance imaging, can be medical or surgical. Medical treatment modalities involve hormonal suppression with medications similar to those used for suppressive therapy for endometriosis. Surgical treatment should be based on the patient's desire for future childbearing. For the woman who does not desire future childbearing, hysterectomy provides definitive therapy.

Presacral neurectomy, as well as uterosacral nerve ablation, has been shown to be of some value for the management of midline pain, especially that associated with dysmenorrhea. These procedures are based on the concept that the nociceptive, efferent nerves from the uterus may be interrupted as they traverse the uterosacral ligaments or enter the Frankenhäuser's plexus just anterior to the sacral promontory. Neither procedure has been shown to increase the relief of pain associated with destruction of endometriotic lesions. However, based on the results of a recent systematic review of the available medical evidence, it appears that presacral neurectomy has been found to be effective for the relief of dysmenorrhea.

MacDonald SR, Klock SC, Milad MP. Long-term outcome of nonconservative surgery (hysterectomy) for endometriosis-associated pain in women <30 years old. Am J Obstet Gynecol 1999;180:1360–3.

Namnoum AB, Hickman TN, Goodman SB, Gehlbach DL, Rock JA. Incidence of symptom recurrence after hysterectomy for endometriosis. Fertil Steril 1995;64:898–902.

Proctor ML, Farquhar CM, Sinclair OJ, Johnson NP. Surgical interruption of pelvic nerve pathways for primary and secondary dysmenorrhoea (Cochrane Review). In: The Cochrane Library, Issue 2, 2004. Chichester, UK: John Wiley & Sons, Ltd.

Redwine DB. Endometriosis persisting after castration: clinical characteristics and results of surgical management. Obstet Gynecol 1994; 83:405–13.

Stratton P, Winkel CA, Sinaii N, Merino MJ, Zimmer C, Nieman LK. Location, color, size, depth, and volume may predict endometriosis in lesions resected at surgery. Fertil Steril 2002;78:743–9.

Sutton CJ, Ewen SP, Whitelaw N, Haines P. Prospective, randomized, double blind, controlled trial of laser laparoscopy in the treatment of pelvic pain associated with minimal, mild, and moderate endometriosis. Fertil Steril 1994;62:696–700.

Walter AJ, Hentz JG, Magtibay PM, Cornella JL, Magrina JF. Endometriosis: correlation between histologic and visual findings at laparoscopy. Am J Obstet Gynecol 2001;184:1407–11; discussion 1411–3.

3
Primary amenorrhea

A 16-year-old adolescent (Fig. 3-1) is referred with primary amenorrhea. She has a normal cervix and vagina. The best explanation for these findings is

     (A) androgen insensitivity
* (B) pituitary insufficiency
     (C) *DAX-1* gene mutation
     (D) luteinizing hormone (LH) receptor gene mutation
     (E) 21-hydroxylase deficiency

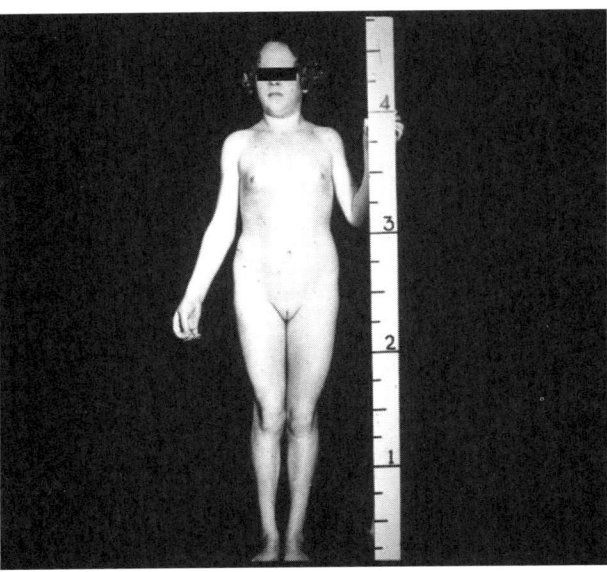

FIG. 3-1. Patient with primary amenorrhea.

Both primary and secondary amenorrhea may be caused by common etiologies. Evaluation of patients with amenorrhea provides the opportunity to identify problems specific to these patients. Most of the etiologies found only in patients with primary amenorrhea are genetic in origin or associated with congenital malformations. Although a thorough history will begin to identify some of these disorders, the physical examination will be revealing for others.

This patient has absence of breast and pubic and axillary hair development. The lack of breast development is not uncommon in such patients; many disorders responsible for primary amenorrhea are associated with absent thelarche because of hypergonadotropinism or hypogonadotropinism and subsequent ovarian hypofunction. The total absence of pubic hair, however, is particularly abnormal in any patient older than 13 years. Pubic hair development is the result of androgen secretion from the ovaries and adrenal glands in females combined with the effect of these androgens at the target tissue (ie, the hair follicles). Therefore, the appearance of pubic hair requires presence of androgen production from either the ovaries or adrenal glands and functional androgen receptors. Its absence suggests that androgen production from one of these sites is missing. If the androgen receptors are intact, patients with ovarian failure or hypogonadotropic hypogonadism will still have adrenal androgen production and pubic hair, if only sparse.

For the patient in Fig. 3-1, the findings of a normal vagina and cervix in association with absent pubic hair provide the most important clinical clues to the etiology of her primary amenorrhea. Such findings rule out androgen insensitivity syndrome and 46,XY 17-hydroxylase deficiency, both disorders which are associated with testes, müllerian inhibiting substance production, and blind vaginas. Absence of pubic hair and axillary hair and breast development as seen in this patient with primary amenorrhea and a normal müllerian system suggests that she has ovaries, not testes, and that sex steroidogenesis is absent from her ovaries as well as her adrenal glands. Until shown otherwise, she should be considered to have pituitary insufficiency, either complete or fractional. Another cause, which is less common and less life threatening, is 46,XX 17-hydroxylase deficiency, an enzyme defect that prevents sex steroid production in the ovaries and adrenal glands.

Pituitary insufficiency is caused by a number of congenital and acquired etiologies. It is now thought that all congenital forms of hypopituitarism are the result of specific mutations, most of which are present in developmental or transcription factor genes. Mutations in *DAX-1* cause hypogonadotropic hypogonadism and congenital adrenal hypoplasia in males but not females. Although a number of gene mutations cause isolated pituitary hormone deficiency (eg, LH receptor gene mutations), only a few are known to cause congenital multiple pituitary hormone deficiencies. Mutations in *RPX/HESX-1*, *PROP-1*, and *PIT-1* genes cause various degrees of hypopituitarism but are separately unlikely in this patient because of varying phenotypes not exhibited by her. Given the rarity of these disorders, further discussion of them is unnecessary here.

Acquired pituitary insufficiency may be the result of nonfunctional tumors within the sella or suprasellar regions (eg, pituitary adenomas and craniopharyngiomas) and from infarction or hemorrhage within a preexisting adenoma or postpartum (eg, Sheehan's syndrome). In addition, inflammatory lesions (eg, lymphocytic hypophysitis, sarcoidosis, Langerhans cell histiocytosis), Rathke's cysts, and infections (eg, bacterial abscess, fungal infection, or toxoplasmosis) also may cause hypopituitarism. Finally, pituitary insufficiency may follow surgery or radiation for primary lesions and result from head trauma. For a number of patients, the etiology of hypopituitarism is unknown.

As stated previously, the steroid enzyme deficient disorder associated with this patient's phenotype is 46,XX 17-hydroxylase deficiency (not 21-hydroxylase deficiency). Such patients will similarly have absent pubic hair and breast development and a normal müllerian system. As with 46,XY 17-hydroxylase-deficient women, they also may have hypokalemic hypertension and adrenal cachexia. Both, however, are very rare disorders. Unlike patients with pituitary insufficiency, they should have normal to tall stature because of normal growth and thyroid hormone production as well as unclosed epiphyses in the absence of estrogen production.

Given the presumed diagnosis of pituitary insufficiency in this patient, further evaluation will be needed to understand the specific endocrine systems adversely affected. This will require baseline hormone testing as well as provocative pituitary stimulation with hypothalamic–pituitary releasing factors and other stimuli, such as insulin. Head imaging also should be performed.

Deladoey J, Fluck C, Buyukgebiz A, Kuhlmann BV, Eble A, Hindmarsh PC, et al. "Hot spot" in the PROP-1 gene responsible for combined pituitary hormone deficiency. J Clin Endocrinol Metab 1999;84: 1645–50.

Fofanova O, Takamura N, Kinoshita E, Parks JS, Brown MR, Peterkova VA, et al. Compound heterozygous deletion of the PROP-1 gene in children with combined pituitary hormone deficiency. J Clin Endocrinol Metab 1998;83:2601–4.

Reindollar RH, Byrd JR, McDonough PG. Delayed sexual development: a study of 252 patients. Am J Obstet Gynecol 1981;140: 371–80.

Sedlmeyer IL, Palmert MR. Delayed puberty: analysis of a large case series from an academic center. J Clin Endocrinol Metab 2002;87: 1613–20.

4

Bulimia versus anorexia

A 22-year-old woman who desires pregnancy presents with a 4-year history of amenorrhea. She is 1.6 m (5 ft 4 in.) tall and weighs 55.3 kg (122 lb). She lost 9.1 kg (20 lb) about the time her menses ceased. Her weight gradually increased with a total weight gain of more than 6.8 kg (15 lb) over the next 2 years, but menses did not resume. She admits to vomiting several times each week. The treatment most likely to effect resumption of menses is

      (A) phenothiazine
      (B) nutritional counseling
      (C) selective serotonin reuptake inhibitors (SSRIs)
*   (D) cognitive–behavioral therapy
      (E) monoamine oxidase inhibitors

Eating disorders are common in adolescents and young adult women. They generally are divided into 3 diagnostic categories: 1) anorexia nervosa, 2) bulimia nervosa, and 3) atypical eating disorders; binge eating disorder has been proposed as a fourth group.

All eating disorders are characterized by altered eating habits or weight-control behavior. Poor nutrition can result in a clinically significant impairment in physical health or psychosocial functioning. In addition, disturbed behavior in bulimia and anorexia is not secondary to any general medical disorder or to any other psychiatric condition.

The characteristic that distinguishes bulimia nervosa from anorexia nervosa is that efforts in bulimia to restrict food intake are interrupted by repeated binges during which there is loss of self-control, and an usually large amount of food is eaten. In most cases, binge eating is followed by compensatory self-induced vomiting or laxative abuse. Together, the combination of binge eating and undereating results in body weight that is altered very little from ideal. Thus, body weight is the most obvious difference that distinguishes bulimia nervosa from anorexia nervosa. Many women with bulimia are distressed and ashamed by their loss of control over eating, making it easier for women with bulimia than those with anorexia nervosa to accept treatment. Symptoms of depression and anxiety disorders often are prominent.

Anorexia nervosa typically starts in the mid-adolescent years. Self-induced dietary restriction quickly gets out of control. In some cases, the disorder is self-limiting and short-lived, whereas in others the disorder becomes more entrenched or even intractable.

Bulimia nervosa usually begins in later adolescence. Most often, bulimia starts similarly to anorexia. Eventually, however, episodes of binge eating interrupt the dietary restriction, and body weight increases to near normal or normal levels. Bulimia tends to perpetuate itself, and women commonly seek treatment more than 5 years after onset.

The woman in this case has features typical of bulimia nervosa. Although clinicians have documented that it is possible to successfully induce ovulation in women with eating disorders, this is not the prudent medical course. It is more rational to treat the underlying disorder first. In this regard, several approaches to the treatment of eating disorders have been proposed.

A Cochrane review, evaluating more than 100 trials, supports the efficacy of cognitive–behavioral therapy in the treatment of individuals with bulimia nervosa. The most effective therapy is cognitive–behavioral therapy that focuses on modification of the specific behaviors and ways of thinking that support the patient's eating disorder. Generally, 20 individual sessions over 4–5 months are needed, and between one third and one half of patients make a complete and lasting recovery. The remaining patients have results that range from greatly improved to not improved. It is important to remember that the patient's menses may not resume even if her eating disorder is successfully treated. She may require ovulation induction following treatment for the eating disorder.

A lack of data exists about the effect of antipsychotic drugs, such as phenothiazine, in the treatment of bulimia. In contrast, there is good evidence that antidepressant drugs, especially SSRIs, are effective in treating bulimia nervosa. They result in a rapid decrease in the frequency of binge eating and purging and an improvement in mood, but the effect is not as great as with cognitive–behavioral therapy. Moreover, limited data suggest that the effects of antidepressants often are not sustained. Adding cognitive–behavioral therapy to antidepressant therapy appears to confer no additional benefit. Nutritional counseling without the addition of cognitive–behavioral therapy is unlikely to be effective.

Fairburn CG, Harrison PJ. Eating disorders. Lancet 2003;361:407–16.

Hay PJ, Bacaltchuk J. Psychotherapy for bulimia nervosa and binging (Cochrane Review). In: The Cochrane Library, Issue 2, 2004. Chichester, UK: John Wiley & Sons, Ltd.

Mehler PS. Clinical practice. Bulimia nervosa. N Engl J Med 2003;349:875–81.

5
Lipids and hormone therapy

A 53-year-old woman, para 2, presents with hot flushes, trouble concentrating, and problems sleeping. Her menstrual cycle length has increased from 32 days to more than 45 days, and her last menstrual period was approximately 2 months ago. Her physical examination is unremarkable. The results of a Pap test, thyroid-stimulating hormone test, and mammogram are normal. Her baseline lipid profile before starting hormone therapy shows total cholesterol level of 236 mg/dL, high density lipoprotein (HDL) cholesterol level of 35 mg/dL, low density lipoprotein (LDL) cholesterol level of 156 mg/dL, very LDL cholesterol level of 45 mg/dL, and triglyceride level of 378 mg/dL. She is started on cyclic micronized estradiol and medroxyprogesterone acetate. She returns 8 weeks later for follow-up. She reports relief of hot flushes and an improvement in her sleep pattern. She has noted intermittent "heartburn" 1–2 hours after she eats. The most appropriate next step in management is

    (A) ultrasonography of the gallbladder
    (B) liver function test
* (C) repeat lipid profile
    (D) stool hemoccult

Findings from the Women's Health Initiative (WHI) trial have demonstrated that use of oral conjugated estrogen, 0.625 mg, with medroxyprogesterone acetate, 2.5 mg, daily is associated with an increased risk of myocardial infarction in the hormone therapy group. An excess risk of 7 additional events per 10,000 person-years was observed in the treatment group compared with the placebo group. Despite these findings, the WHI trial demonstrated a more favorable lipid profile in the hormone treatment group. Oral estrogen therapy has been associated with favorable changes in lipoprotein profiles: total cholesterol levels will decrease 10–15%; LDL cholesterol levels will decrease 10–15%; HDL cholesterol levels will increase 4–7%; and triglyceride levels will increase by variable amounts up to 34%.

By contrast, transdermal, transcutaneous, subcutaneous, or vaginal administration of estrogen leads to relatively modest changes in lipoprotein profiles: total cholesterol levels will decrease 3–5%, LDL cholesterol levels will decrease 3–5%, HDL cholesterol levels will increase slightly, and triglyceride levels will remain relatively stable. These differences in lipoprotein levels between the oral and transdermal routes mainly reflect the direct effect of oral estrogen on liver lipoprotein metabolism because of the first-pass effect, whereas the nonoral routes of administration lead to relatively modest effects on lipoprotein concentrations.

In this patient, the baseline lipid profile is abnormal based on National Cholesterol Education Program Adult Treatment Panel III (NCEP ATP III) criteria. Her elevated triglyceride levels are of particular concern, and her total cholesterol and LDL cholesterol levels are higher than the acceptable range (Table 5-1). If triglyceride lev-

TABLE 5-1. National Cholesterol Education Program Adult Treatment Panel III (NCEP ATP III) Guidelines for Classification of Lipid Profiles

Lipid	Comment
Total cholesterol level (mg/dL)	
<200	Desirable
200–239	Borderline high
≥240	High
Low-density lipoprotein cholesterol level (mg/dL)	
<100	Optimal
100–129	Near optimal/above optimal
130–159	Borderline high
160–189	High
≥190	Very high
High-density lipoprotein cholesterol level (mg/dL)	
<40	Low
≥60	High
Triglyceride level (mg/dL)	
<150	Normal
150–199	Borderline high
200–499	High
≥500	Very high

From ATP III At A Glance: Quick Desk Reference. Available at: http://www.nhlbi.nih.gov/guidelines/cholesterol/atglance.htm

els exceed 500 mg/dL, the patient will be at increased risk for pancreatitis.

Because this patient started using oral estrogen therapy before her baseline lipid profile results were available, the lipid profile should be repeated promptly. The anticipated 30% increase in triglyceride levels caused by oral estrogens and her elevated baseline triglyceride level may increase her risk of pancreatitis.

Although her "heartburn" symptoms could be an early sign of gallbladder disease, the symptoms are not sufficiently severe or persistent to suggest cholecystitis or to justify evaluation for gallstones with ultrasonography. A trial of antacids may be more appropriate for this patient who has heartburn. If her symptoms persist or become more severe, referral to a gastroenterologist may be warranted. A routine liver panel usually is not necessary for a patient taking hormone therapy unless there has been a past history of hepatitis, jaundice, or other underlying liver disease. The stool hemoccult test is a routine test that should be performed as part of the routine preventive health visit. It may be helpful in detecting ulcers in the upper gastrointestinal tract but is not the best choice in this patient.

ATP III At A Glance: Quick Desk Reference. Available at: http://www.nhlbi.nih.gov/guidelines/cholesterol/atglance.htm

Beral V, Banks E, Reeves G. Evidence from randomized trials on the long-term effects of hormone replacement therapy. Lancet 2002;360: 942–4.

Hodis HN, Mack WJ, Lobo RA, Shoupe D, Sevanian A, Mahrer PR, et al. Estrogen in the prevention of atherosclerosis. A randomized, double-blind, placebo-controlled trial. Estrogen in the prevention of Atherosclerosis Trial Research Group. Ann Intern Med 2001;135: 939–53.

Moorjani S, Dupont A, Labrie F, De Lignieres B, Cusan L, Dupont P, et al. Changes in plasma lipoprotein and apolipoprotein composition in relation to oral versus percutaneous administration of estrogen alone or in cyclic association with utrogestan in menopausal women. J Clin Endocrinol Metab 1991;73:373–9.

Rossouw E, Anderson GL, Prentice RL, LaCroix AZ, Kooperberg C, Stefanick ML, et al. Risks and benefits of estrogen plus progestin in healthy postmenopausal women: principal results from the Women's Health Initiative randomized controlled trial. Writing Group for the Women's Health Initiative Investigators. JAMA 2002;288:321–33.

6

Selective estrogen receptor modulators and breast cancer

A 48-year-old woman, gravida 1, para 0, underwent a simple mastectomy 5 years ago secondary to stage I breast cancer. She recently completed 5 years of tamoxifen citrate (Nolvadex) therapy for prevention of contralateral breast cancer. She has been amenorrheic for 6 months and is having occasional night sweats. She is interested in knowing whether she should consider taking raloxifene hydrochloride (Evista) to further decrease her risk of recurrent breast cancer and to reduce her vasomotor symptoms. You advise that at this time, the clinical indication for taking raloxifene is for

(A) cardiovascular disease
(B) endometrial hyperplasia
(C) recurrent breast cancer
* (D) osteoporosis
(E) vasomotor symptoms

A considerable number of women who have had breast cancer are prematurely menopausal as a result of long-term chemotherapy. The role of estrogen therapy or combined hormone therapy in women with a history of breast cancer is controversial. Clinical evidence does not contraindicate the use of combined hormone therapy in breast cancer survivors who are symptomatic. Given the data from the Women's Health Initiative (WHI) trial, in which 8 additional breast cancers were found for every 10,000 women who took combined hormone therapy, many providers are hesitant to recommend such therapy. Data from women enrolled in the WHI trial and the Postmenopausal Estrogen/Progestin Interventions Trial have found that at 1 year of therapy, combined hormone therapy was associated with greater mammographic density, an independent risk factor for breast cancer, when compared with estrogen alone.

Selective estrogen receptor modulators (SERMs) are estrogenlike compounds that act as weak estrogen agonists in some organs and as estrogen antagonists in others. One SERM, tamoxifen citrate (Nolvadex), is approved for breast cancer therapy and also has been shown to reduce the risk of breast cancer in women at high risk. Studies are ongoing to determine its ability to increase bone mineral density (BMD). Preliminary findings suggest it may reduce fractures by as much as 35%.

Another SERM, raloxifene hydrochloride (Evista), became available in the United States and Canada during the late 1990s for the prevention and treatment of osteoporosis. In postmenopausal women, it increases BMD in the spine, hip, and wrist in the range of 1–3% over 3 years. Raloxifene may offer protection against some types of breast cancer; however, raloxifene is not FDA approved for any breast health indication. An osteoporosis prevention trial found that after 2 years of treatment, raloxifene did not increase breast density compared with estrogen or placebo.

Raloxifene has been shown to increase the incidence of hot flushes, and, therefore, cannot be used to treat vasomotor symptoms associated with menopause. Long-term symptom data also are needed. Raloxifene decreases total and low-density lipoprotein cholesterol concentrations but does not increase high-density lipoprotein cholesterol levels, as estrogen does. Conversely, raloxifene does not have the unfavorable effect of increasing triglyceride levels that is seen with oral estrogens. The overall effect of raloxifene on cardiovascular disease risk is unknown but may carry the same risk as combined hormone therapy, which has been associated with thromboembolic events, such as deep vein thrombosis. Raloxifene does not appear to have any adverse effects on the endometrium, and, therefore, does not impose any increased risk of endometrial hyperplasia.

The U.S. Preventive Services Task Force found that both tamoxifen and raloxifene reduce the incidence of estrogen receptor-positive breast cancer in women. The absolute risk reduction was found to vary by risk factors for breast cancer, which must be balanced against potential harms in judging the appropriateness of treatment for individual women. Results of the ongoing Study of Tamoxifen and Raloxifene trial, which is comparing the effectiveness of the 2 drugs in preventing or slowing the development of breast cancer, will provide some insight as to the role raloxifene may play in breast cancer prevention. There are no clinical data on the effects of raloxifene on the breast and endometrium following treatment with tamoxifen. Ultimately, newer compounds, such as aromatase inhibitors, may replace tamoxifen and raloxifene for prevention and treatment of breast cancer.

Cummings SR, Eckert S, Krueger KA, Grady D, Powles TJ, Cauley JA, et al. The effect of raloxifene on risk of breast cancer in postmenopausal women: results from the MORE randomized trial. Multiple Outcomes of Raloxifene Evaluation. JAMA 1999;281:2189–97.

Delmas PD, Bjarnason NH, Mitlak BH, Ravoux AC, Shah AS, Huster WJ, et al. Effects of raloxifene on bone mineral density, serum cholesterol concentrations, and uterine endometrium in postmenopausal women. N Engl J Med 1997;337:1641–7.

Freedman M, San Martin J, O'Gorman J, Eckert S, Lippman ME, Lo SC, et al. Digitized mammography: a clinical trial of postmenopausal women randomly assigned to receive raloxifene, estrogen, or placebo. J Natl Cancer Inst 2001;93:51–6.

Greendale GA, Reboussin BA, Slone S, Wasilauskas C, Pike MC, Ursin G. Postmenopausal hormone therapy and change in mammographic density. J Natl Cancer Inst 2003;95:30–7.

Heaney RP, Draper MW. Raloxifene and estrogen: comparative bone-remodeling kinetics. J Clin Endocrinol Metab 1997;82:3425–9.

Kinsinger LS, Harris R, Woolf SH, Sox HC, Lohr KN. Chemoprevention of breast cancer: a summary of the evidence for the U.S. Preventive Services Task Force. Ann Intern Med 2002;137:59–69.

Rossouw JE, Anderson GL, Prentice RL, LaCroix AZ, Kooperberg C, Stefanick ML, et al. Risks and benefits of estrogen plus progestin in healthy postmenopausal women: principal results from the Women's Health Initiative randomized controlled trial. Writing Group for the Women's Health Initiative Investigators. JAMA 2002;288:321–33.

Walsh BW, Kuller LH, Wild RA, Paul S, Farmer M, Lawrence JB, et al. Effects of raloxifene on serum lipids and coagulation factors in healthy postmenopausal women. JAMA 1998;279:1445–51.

7
Minimal endometriosis and infertility

A 33-year-old nulliparous woman, who has regular menstrual periods, presents with a 1-year history of infertility. A recent workup, including hysterosalpingography, semen analysis, and prenatal laboratory values, was normal. She and her husband have been timing intercourse appropriately. Laparoscopy performed 2 years ago for suspected appendicitis showed minimal endometriosis, which was ablated. The next step in the management of this patient's infertility is

* (A) laparoscopy for repeat coagulation of the endometriotic implants
* (B) gonadotropin-releasing hormone (GnRH) agonist for 3 months
* (C) empiric clomiphene citrate with intrauterine insemination (IUI)
* (D) expectant management and stress reduction
* (E) in vitro fertilization

The mechanism by which minimal endometriosis causes infertility remains elusive. The theories are so numerous that a detailed summary of even the most common ones in this short space is not possible. Contemporary clinical practice protocols consider infertility associated with mild endometriosis to be idiopathic.

In the past 15–20 years, there has been a marked increase in the use of superovulation, with or without IUI, in the treatment of unexplained infertility. Both clomiphene citrate and gonadotropins have been used for superovulation. These medicines may overcome a subtle defect in ovulatory function not uncovered by conventional testing, or they may increase the number of eggs available for fertilization. Intrauterine insemination increases the sperm density in the fallopian tubes by placing a concentrated aliquot of sperm directly into the uterus. Thus, ovarian stimulation and IUI may improve the monthly pregnancy rate by simply increasing the number of gametes in the reproductive tract, leading to an increased number of embryos available for implantation.

A meta-analysis of 45 published reports for the treatment of idiopathic infertility documents monthly fertility rates for various therapies (Fig. 7-1).

Women with minimal and mild endometriosis do have decreased monthly fecundity (the probability of conceiving in any 1 cycle), with most studies finding a rate of 4–5% if no treatment is provided. When endometriosis is detected at laparoscopy, surgical ablation or resection of the lesions is warranted. This likely produces a small increase in the monthly fertility rate, although this concept is controversial, because some studies reveal no benefit to surgery. One study that compared laparoscopy with and without treatment of the lesions showed a small difference at 36 months of follow-up. The no treatment group had a monthly fertility rate of 2.4%, whereas the treatment group had a monthly fertility rate of 4.7%. Another study, similarly designed, had a 1-year follow-up period. There was no difference in pregnancy rate 1 year after surgery for the treatment versus no treatment groups (20% versus 22%). In the case cited here, repeat laparoscopy is not warranted.

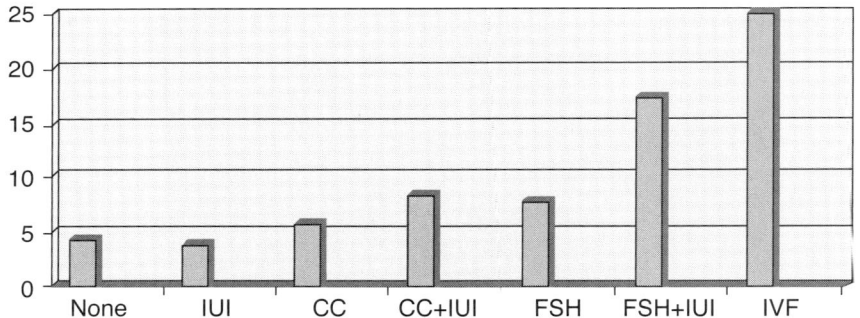

FIG. 7-1. Results of a meta-analysis of 45 published reports for the treatment of idiopathic infertility showing monthly fertility rates by intervention. Abbreviations: CC, clomiphene citrate; FSH, follicle-stimulating hormone; IUI, intrauterine insemination; IVF, in vitro fertilization. (Data from Guzick DS, Sullivan MW, Adamson GD, Cedars MI, Falk RJ, Peterson EP, et al. Efficacy of treatment for unexplained infertility. Fertil Steril 1998;70:207–13.)

Medical suppression of ovarian steroids for the treatment of endometriosis does not produce benefit but simply delays treatment of infertility. In a randomized trial of endometriosis suppression with danazol (Danocrine) compared with a control group with no treatment, the controls had a higher monthly fertility rate than the danazol-treated group after treatment was completed. A similar effect is expected after suppression with GnRH analogs. Thus, in the described case, medical suppression of minimal endometriosis is not justified.

Expectant management and stress reduction may be valuable, but results to date have been inconsistent. Examples of stress reduction include exercise, massage, yoga, and acupuncture. Although in vitro fertilization is effective in this situation, it should be considered only after less expensive and time consuming methods are tried.

Adamson GD. Treatment of endometriosis-associated infertility. Semin Reprod Endocrinol 1997;15:263–71.

Barbieri RL. Infertility. In: Yen SS, Jaffe RB, Barbieri RL, eds. Reproductive endocrinology: physiology, pathophysiology, and clinical management. 4th ed. Philadelphia (PA): WB Saunders; 1999, p. 562–93.

Guzick DS, Sullivan MW, Adamson GD, Cedars MI, Falk RJ, Peterson EP, et al. Efficacy of treatment for unexplained infertility. Fertil Steril 1998;70:207–13.

Marcoux S, Maheux R, Berube S. Laparoscopic surgery in infertile women with minimal or mild endometriosis. Canadian Collaborative Group on Endometriosis. N Engl J Med 1997;337:217–22.

Oehninger S, Coddington CC, Hodgen CD, Seppala M. Factors affecting fertilization: endometrial placental protein 14 reduces the capacity of human spermatozoa to bind to the human zona pelucida. Fertil Steril 1995;65:377–83.

Parazzini F. Ablation of lesions or no treatment in minimal–mild endometriosis in infertile women: a randomized trial. Gruppo Italiano per lo Studio dell'Endometriosi. Hum Reprod 1999;14:1332–4.

Seibel MM, Berger MJ, Weinstein FG, Taymor ML. The effectiveness of danazol on subsequent fertility in minimal endometriosis. Fertil Steril 1982;38:534–7.

8

Treatment for impotence

Your patient's spouse is a 45-year-old male with a history of oligospermia who goes to the emergency room with chest pains. He is presently taking L-carnitine (Proxeed) and sildenafil citrate (Viagra) to help improve sperm quality as well as duration of erection and sexual response during timed intercourse. The medication that would most likely precipitate chest pains in the presence of sildenafil or other erection-enhancing drugs, such as tadalafil (Cialis) or vardenafil (Levitra), is

    (A) tissue plasminogen activator
    (B) nifedipine (Procardia)
* (C) sublingual nitroglycerin
    (D) lidocaine
    (E) cimetidine (Tagamet)

Phosphodiesterase inhibitors, such as sildenafil, are oral medications approved for the treatment of erectile dysfunction. Sildenafil is commonly used in daily clinical practice, and its effectiveness to treat erectile dysfunction has been proved in clinical trials with up to 82% of men who have taken the drug having improved erections versus 24% taking placebo. Sildenafil is effective in most patients and has a safety profile that has been evaluated in clinical practice over many years. The drug should be used with caution in patients with a cardiac history, especially those who take nitrate antianginal agents.

During sexual stimulation, nitric oxide that is released into the corpus cavernosum is responsible for the physiologic mechanism of penile erection. Sildenafil enhances the effect of nitric oxide by inhibiting phosphodiesterase type 5. This results in increased levels of cyclic guanine monophosphate into the corpus cavernosum, which results in smooth muscle relaxation and an inflow of blood into this area. The onset of action is within 30 minutes and has a lasting effect up to 4 hours. In the absence of erectile dysfunction or sexual stimulation, sildenafil has no effect.

Despite its physiologic mechanism of action, sildenafil has been shown to work with organic or psychogenic erectile dysfunction in numerous randomized trials. It is prescribed in doses of 25–100 mg taken no more than once per day. Sildenafil is only indicated for the treatment of erectile dysfunction in men. Although research studies are lacking with regard to sildenafil and its affect on fertility, there is no evidence that its use has an adverse effect on semen parameters.

Adverse effects of sildenafil occur in 2.5% of patients, a rate that does not differ significantly from placebo. The most common side effects are related to the vasodilatory effects and include flushing, headache, and dyspepsia. With the effect of vasodilation and venous pooling, there is a potential for cardiac risk in patients with a history of cardiovascular disease, especially if organic nitrates are taken concomitantly with the drug. Acute cardiac events (eg, ischemia, myocardial infarction, and arrhythmia) have been reported, and deaths have occurred. For this reason, the use of antianginal nitrates is contraindicated with the use of sildenafil. Patients who have a history of cardiac conditions, kidney or liver disease, or who are taking medications that may prolong the half-life of the drug, such as cimetidine (Tagamet) or erythromycin prescriptions, should be prescribed with caution according to the American College of Cardiology/American Heart Association. Medications such as magnesium sulfate or nifedipine are not contraindicated when used with sildenafil and can be used safely.

Couples, such as the one described, are becoming more common in infertility practice as women delay childbearing or develop relationships with older men. The use of sildenafil is common practice in urology and can benefit a couple that is trying to conceive. Because nitrates are contraindicated with sildenafil, sublingual nitroglycerin should not be offered to this patient and may precipitate a severe cardiac event because of its vasodilatory effects. Although high cholesterol is a contributing factor in erectile dysfunction, it is not the cause of the symptoms. In addition, stress and anxiety or the medication dosage most likely would not be responsible for the symptoms either.

A careful evaluation of male factor infertility is important for couples who are unable to conceive. Recognizing risk factors related to the medical history along with the use of medications, such as sildenafil, will help prevent potential problems in clinical practice. Contact with referral providers (eg, urologists), who prescribe the drug, would improve overall patient care.

Kloner RA, Zusman RM. Cardiovascular effects of sildenafil citrate and recommendations for its use. Am J Cardiol 1999;84(5B):11N–17N.

Lim PH, Moorthy P, Benton KG. The clinical safety of viagra. Ann N Y Acad Sci 2002;962:378–88.

Marwick TH. Safe sex for men with coronary artery disease: exercise, sildenafil, and risk of cardiac events. JAMA 2002;287:766–7.

Mitka M. Studies of Viagra offer some reassurance to men with concerns about cardiac effects. JAMA 2001;285:1950–1.

9

Normal pubertal development

A 7½-year-old African-American girl is referred for evaluation of precocious puberty. The appearance of pubic hair was noted at 6 years 11 months and breast budding 1 month ago. She is otherwise in excellent health and without any additional symptoms. Examination reveals Tanner stage III pubic hair and Tanner stage II breast development. Longitudinal growth has increased from the 55th to the 60th percentile. Her growth velocity chart demonstrates that she has moved from 4-cm to 5.5-cm growth per year. The most appropriate initial management is

* (A) observation only
  (B) bone age X-ray of the hand only
  (C) magnetic resonance imaging (MRI) of the head only
  (D) adrenocorticotropic hormone (ACTH) challenge test

The definition of precocious puberty has previously been the appearance of secondary sexual development before age 8 years. Although the evaluation of precocious puberty has not changed, not all patients younger than 8 years need to be evaluated. Many young girls with early pubertal development, such as this patient, need only close observation. Recent evidence has demonstrated that puberty appears to be occurring much earlier than was previously thought and that there are significant racial differences in the time of onset of pubertal landmarks.

Fig. 9-1 (see color plate) demonstrates a pubertal development chart that is based on the norms for pubertal landmarks collected from British white girls shortly after World War II and published in the classic report of Marshall and Tanner. It demonstrates that the first event of puberty in girls is an acceleration of growth velocity. During the acceleration of limb growth, between ages 9 and 11 years, secondary sexual characteristics appeared for this study population. Thelarche preceded adrenarche 85% of the time. The adolescent growth spurt follows thelarche and adrenarche, with growth velocity increasing from 4 cm to 9 cm in height per year. The first menstrual period occurs as the epiphyses begin to close and growth velocity decelerates at a mean age of 12.8 years.

A cross-sectional study of 17,077 U.S. girls in the 1990's suggests that puberty is occurring earlier than previously thought. It also appears that the timing of pubertal events is different for a heterogeneous U.S. society than it was for the British population studied nearly 40–50 years earlier. The Pediatric Research in Office Settings Network Study reported that the onset of breast or pubic hair growth or both was noted in 27.2% and 48.3% of African-American girls by ages 7 and 8 years, respectively, and that 7% and 14.5% of Caucasian girls had initiated puberty by ages 7 and 8 years, respectively. Menarche was reported in 27.9% and 62.1% of African-American girls and in 13.4% and 35.2% of Caucasian girls at ages 11 and 12 years, respectively. The mean ages of initiation of each of the pubertal events are shown in Table 9-1. These data demonstrate that sexual maturation occurs earlier than was previously thought and that girls mature differently based on race: African-American girls initiate puberty on average between ages 8 and 9 years, and Caucasian girls initiate puberty closer to age 10 years. The different timing and sequence for adrenarche and thelarche in the African-American population is not a new observation. A study of African girls in the 1980s demonstrated that adrenarche preceded thelarche in most of the girls studied in Nairobi, Kenya.

The definitions of precocious and delayed puberty have been based on the time of onset of secondary sexual characteristic appearance that is 2.5 standard deviations removed from the mean. The ages that define precocious and delayed puberty based on post-World War II standards have been 8 and 13 years, respectively. Published recommendations have been made for modifying the definition of precocious but not delayed puberty based on the Pediatric Research Network in Office Settings data. New guidelines suggest that evaluation be initiated if secondary sexual characteristics appear before age 6 years in African-American girls and age 7 years in white girls unless there are other central nervous system (CNS) findings or behavioral changes that warrant evaluation and possible treatment.

TABLE 9-1. Mean Age of Appearance of Pubertal Landmarks in the Pediatric Research in Office Settings Network Study, 1997

Race of Child	Breast	Pubic Hair	Menses
African American	8.87 y	8.78 y	12.16 y
Caucasian	9.96 y	10.51 y	12.88 y

Data from Herman-Giddens ME, Slora EJ, Wasserman RC, Bourdony CJ, Bhapkar MV, Koch GG, et al. Secondary sexual characteristics and menses in young girls seen in office practice: a study from the Pediatric Research in Office Settings Network. Pediatrics 1997;99:505–12.

The Pediatric Research Network in Office Settings study and the associated recommendations for modifying the definition of precocious puberty are not without considerable controversy. Some investigators oppose these recommendations. They believe that the method for determining Tanner stages II and III breast development was flawed and could have misinterpreted "chubby" chests for true breast maturation. The examiners based their findings on visual and not palpatory inspection; although pubic hair staging was likely accurate, breast staging may have been subject to normal prepubertal variations that are based on weight. In addition, several recent reports have identified significant pathology as etiologic for pubertal signs that appeared after the age limits of the new definition for precocious puberty. These reports and conflicting opinions underscore the need to use the new recommendations as guidelines only and to initiate an evaluation in any girl who begins puberty before age 8 years with any hint of CNS, behavioral, or other systemic symptomatology.

This patient is African American and began puberty between ages 6 and 7 years without any other systemic signs or symptoms, which emphasizes the fact that it is wrong to place children of different races under the same expectations and guidelines for defining normal and abnormal puberty. It emphasizes the need to individualize care and, in the absence of physical or psychosocial evidence of pathology, that treatment during this previously thought premature period may not be warranted. In the absence of treatment, it should be remembered that CNS tumors could rarely exist and that the early appearance of pubic hair may signify the presence of the carrier state for 21-hydroxylase deficiency and, especially in populations such as African Americans and Caribbean Hispanics, early manifestations of insulin resistance. Further testing of this patient by means of a bone age X-ray of her hand, an MRI of her head, or an ACTH test are, therefore, not necessary.

Chalumeau M, Chemaitilly W, Trivin C, Adan L, Breart G, Brauner R. Central precocious puberty in girls: an evidence-based diagnosis tree to predict central nervous system abnormalities. Pediatr 2002;109: 61–7.

Herman-Giddens ME, Slora EJ, Wasserman RC, Bourdony CJ, Bhapkar MV, Koch GG, et al. Secondary sexual characteristics and menses in young girls seen in office practice: a study from the Pediatric Research in Office Settings Network. Pediatrics 1997;99:505–12.

Kaplowitz PB. Precocious puberty in girls and the risk of a central nervous system abnormality: the elusive search for diagnostic certainty. Pediatr 2002;109:139–41.

Kaplowitz PB, Oberfield SE, and the Drug and Therapeutics and Executive Committees of the Lawson Wilkins Pediatric Endocrine Society. Pediatr 1999;104:936–41.

Marshall WA, Tanner JM. Variations in the pattern of pubertal changes in girls. J Adolesc Health Care 1969;44:291–303.

10
Treatment of acne with oral contraceptives

A 21-year-old nulligravid college student comes to the student health center to request treatment for acne that significantly worsens the week before her menses and is associated with dysmenorrhea. The most cost-effective treatment for this patient is

    (A) depot medroxyprogesterone acetate
    (B) transdermal patch
    (C) levonorgestrel intrauterine system
*   (D) monophasic combined oral contraceptive
    (E) progestin-only pill

Compelling evidence exists that oral contraceptives are effective in the management of mild to moderate acne vulgaris. Patients with acne have elevated androgen levels when compared with appropriate controls, and such elevations constitute an underlying pathophysiologic factor that increases the risk for acne. The antiandrogenic effects of oral contraceptives improve acne by several mechanisms. First, there is an increase in sex-hormone binding globulin levels, which decreases free testosterone levels and suppresses androgen production by reducing luteinizing hormone (LH) secretion. In addition, the progestins in oral contraceptives compete with testosterone for binding sites. Oral contraceptives also inhibit the enzyme 5α-reductase, which converts free testosterone in target tissues to dihydrotestosterone, the active androgen in skin and hair follicles. Because acne is an androgen-related disorder, and all oral contraceptives are antiandrogenic, all commonly used types have the potential to improve acne. Therefore, the lowest dose (20–30 mg of ethinyl estradiol) and least expensive oral contraceptive should be used.

A prospective placebo-controlled study of 200 subjects showed a significant reduction in acne inflammatory lesions after 6 cycles of monophasic low-dose oral contraceptives. Women who received oral contraceptives had significant reductions in inflammatory acne lesions (mean reduction of 51% versus 35% against placebo) and total lesions (mean reduction of 46% versus 34% for placebo). Decreases in inflammatory lesions and total lesions were observed in most studies of oral contraceptives when used as therapy for acne and, in some cases, the acne completely disappeared.

Unlike oral contraceptives, the transdermal patch may not alter sex-hormone binding globulin production and, therefore, may not be as effective in improving acne. However, no data are available in regard to the effect of the patch on acne. Another consideration is that the patch is more costly than generic oral contraceptives.

The levonorgestrel intrauterine system releases 15 µg of levonorgestrel per day and, therefore, will not change LH-stimulated androgen levels or cause significant changes in the skin. Thus, the levonorgestrel intrauterine system should not be used in the treatment of acne.

Progestin-only pills may cause a decrease in sex-hormone binding globulin levels, leading to an increase in free testosterone levels, which is likely to worsen acne. This is in contrast to combined oral contraceptives that contain levonorgestrel, where the estrogen increases sex-hormone binding globulin levels and produces a decrease in unbound free androgen levels.

Lemay A, Archer DF, Roberts JL, Harrison DD. The efficacy of an oral contraceptive containing 20-microgram ethinyl estradiol and 100-microgram of levonorgestrel for the treatment of moderate acne. Gynecol Endocrinol 2000;14:RT61.

Lemay A, Langley RG. The use of low-dose oral contraceptives for the management of acne. Skin Therapy Lett 2002;7(10):1–5.

Thiboutot D, Archer DF, Lemay A, Washenik K, Roberts J, Harrison D. A randomized, controlled trial of a low-dose contraceptive containing 20 microg of ethinyl estradiol and 100 microg of levonorgestrel for acne treatment. Fert Steril 2001;76:461–8.

11
Emergency contraception

A 29-year-old woman comes to your office with a history of unprotected intercourse within the past 24 hours. She requests emergency contraception therapy. The oral steroid hormone treatment that would provide her best option for emergency contraception is

    (A) ethinyl estradiol and norgestrel
    (B) mestranol
    (C) desogestrel
*   (D) levonorgestrel
    (E) norgestimate

The goal of emergency contraception is to prevent conception after a contraceptive failure or after unprotected sexual intercourse. The U.S. Food and Drug Administration has approved 2 products for emergency contraception: the Preven emergency contraceptive kit (a combination estrogen- and progestin-containing medication) and Plan B (a progestin-containing medication) (Table 11-1). The steroid hormones in Preven are ethinyl estradiol and levonorgestrel, the components of a combination oral contraceptive (OC). In contrast, the steroid hormone in Plan B is only levonorgestrel. In a randomized controlled trial of the progestin medication levonorgestrel versus a combination OC, levonorgestrel was more effective and better tolerated than the combination OC method. The study was conducted in 1,955 women, and the crude pregnancy rate was 1.1% (11/976) in the levonorgestrel group versus 3.2% (31/979) in the combination OC group. It was estimated that the percentage of pregnancies prevented using the levonorgestrel method was 85% versus 57% for the combination OC method. Significant

TABLE 11-1. Examples of Emergency Contraception Pills Available in the United States*

Trade Name	Formulation	Pills per Dose†
Dedicated products		
Plan B	0.75 mg levonorgestrel	1 white
Preven	0.25 mg levonorgestrel, 0.05 mg ethinyl estradiol	1 blue
Progestin-only contraceptives		
Ovrette	0.075 mg norgestrel	20 yellow
Combination contraceptives		
Alesse	0.1 mg levonorgestrel, 0.02 mg ethinyl estradiol	5 pink
Levlen	0.15 mg levonorgestrel, 0.03 mg ethinyl estradiol	4 light orange
Lo/Ovral‡	0.30 mg norgestrel, 0.03 mg ethinyl estradiol	4 white
Nordette	0.15 mg levonorgestrel, 0.03 mg ethinyl estradiol	4 light orange

*Other contraceptive preparations containing equivalent doses of synthetic estrogens and progestins also may be used.

†Treatment consists of 2 doses taken 12 hours apart. Use of an antiemetic agent before taking the medication will decrease the risk of nausea, a common adverse effect.

‡When compared with products containing levonorgestrel, norgestrel was associated with higher rates of adverse effects (Sanchez-Borrego R, Balasch J. Ethinyl oestradiol plus dinorgestrel or levonorgestrel in the Yuzpe method for post-coital contraception: results of an obsevational study. Hum Reprod 1996;11:2449–53.).

Modified from American College of Obstetricians and Gynecologists. Emergency oral contraception. ACOG Practice Bulletin 25. Washington, DC: ACOG; 2001.

reductions in the side effects of nausea and vomiting were observed, ie, 23.1% versus 50.5% and 5.6% versus 18.8% for the levonorgestrel group versus the combination OC group, respectively (P <.01). The decrease in these 2 side effects was attributed to the absence of estrogen in the levonorgestrel-only method. The addition of an antiemetic 1 hour before the use of the combination OC method, however, reduced the incidence of nausea and vomiting. The concept of using combination OCs for emergency contraception can be extended to the use of other prescription OC formulations. Similarly, progestin-only pills containing norgestrel have been used for emergency contraception. Because of the lower dose of progestin contained in progestin-only OCs (0.075 mg norgestrel per pill), more pills are used in each course of medication.

Investigators have examined whether the 2 doses of 0.75 mg levonorgestrel used in Plan B taken 12 hours apart could be combined into a single 1.5 mg dose without loss of effectiveness. The study was a randomized, double-blind trial in 15 family-planning clinics in 10 countries. Each arm of the study had 1,356 subjects included in the efficacy analysis. The pregnancy rates were 1.5% and 1.8% in the individuals assigned single-dose and 2-dose levonorgestrel, respectively. No significant difference was observed between pregnancy rates and side effects between the 2 methods.

In combination OCs, 2 estrogen formulations have been consistently used: 1) ethinyl estradiol, the predominant estrogen used in current low-dose combination OCs; and 2) mestranol (ethinyl estradiol 3-methyl ether), an estrogen found in older high-dose combination OCs. Once mestranol is ingested, it is metabolized to ethinyl estradiol. Both desogestrel and norgestimate are progestins used in combination OCs. Their use as single agents for emergency contraception has not been studied to date.

Currently, available evidence indicates that major mechanisms of action involve delay of ovulation and prevention of fertilization. Most pregnancies that occur in patients who have been given emergency contraception occur when coitus coincided with ovulation. Thus, it appears that emergency contraception is unlikely to interrupt implantation of an otherwise normal embryo. It is much more likely to prevent fertilization. The emergency contraception method widely used in European countries, mifepristone, is not currently approved for this use in the United States.

American College of Obstetricians and Gynecologists. Emergency oral contraception. ACOG Practice Bulletin 25. Washington, DC: ACOG; 2001.

Randomised controlled trial of levonorgestrel versus the Yuzpe regimen of combined oral contraceptives for emergency contraception. Task Force on Postovulatory Methods of Fertility Regulation. Lancet 1998;352:428–33.

Raymond EG, Creinin MD, Barnhart KT, Lovvorn AE, Rountree RW, Trussell J. Meclizine for prevention of nausea associated with use of emergency contraceptive pills: a randomized trial. Obstet Gynecol 2000;95:271–7.

Von Hertzen H, Piaggio G, Ding J, Chen J, Song S, Bartfai G, et al. Low dose mifepristone and two regimens of levonorgestrel for emergency contraception: a WHO multicentre randomised trial. WHO Research Group on Post-ovulatory Methods of Fertility Regulation. Lancet 2002;360:1803–10.

12

Reproduction in individuals with acquired immunodeficiency syndrome

A 33-year-old nulligravid woman who is human immunodeficiency virus (HIV) negative requests information on how to eliminate her risks of becoming HIV positive when conceiving with sperm from her HIV-positive partner. They currently use condoms for all acts of sexual intercourse. You inform her that the only way to eliminate her risk is

      (A) in vitro fertilization with the partner's sperm
*   (B) not to use her partner's sperm
      (C) intrauterine insemination with her partner's sperm
      (D) high-dose antiretroviral therapy for her partner
      (E) use of antiretroviral therapy by the patient

An increasing number of couples desire pregnancy when the man is HIV positive and the woman is HIV negative. In counseling these couples, it is important to emphasize that there is no completely risk-free method of pursuing conception using the partner's sperm. However, there are several strategies that can minimize the risk of transmission to the woman, although these procedures are performed in specialized centers.

Decreasing the male partner's viral load to undetectable levels with an effective antiretroviral agent can potentially reduce the risk of sexual transmission, which has been correlated with HIV-RNA levels. Condoms should be used for all coital activity except during the ovulatory period. An alternative strategy has been proposed using a combination of periexposure prophylaxis with antiretroviral agents for the HIV-negative woman, which is similar to the strategy used in exposed health care workers. Because of the number of variables that can effect transmission, it is difficult to estimate the HIV transmission risk with each act of coitus. A specific technique of sperm washing using a combination of Percoll gradient and swim up technique for intrauterine insemination has been developed to decrease viral load in the semen and the risk of HIV transmission. In a study of 350 couples using this technique, there was no evidence of seroconversion in the HIV-negative women. In vitro fertilization will not limit the risk of transmission unless the semen is prepared with this specific technique.

Rates of perinatally acquired acquired immunodeficiency syndrome (AIDS) have steeply decreased following introduction of zidovudine (AZT) as a means of reducing perinatal transmission. It has become standard practice to offer HIV-infected pregnant women antiretroviral therapy to reduce the likelihood of perinatal transmission. When HIV infection is more advanced in the pregnant woman, there is an increased risk of certain pregnancy complications, including preterm delivery, low birth weight, and intrauterine growth restriction. Use of antiretroviral therapy during pregnancy has not been shown to have an adverse impact on pregnancy. In this patient, the only way to completely eliminate the risk of HIV transmission is with the use of donor sperm.

Chrystie IL, Mullen JE, Braude PR, Rowell P, Williams E, Elkington N, et al. Assisted conception in HIV discordant couples: evaluation of semen processing techniques in reducing HIV viral load. J Reprod Immunol 1998;41:301–6.

Drapkin Lyerly A, Anderson J. Human immunodeficiency virus and assisted reproduction: reconsidering evidence, reframing ethics. Fertil Steril 2001;75:843–57.

Public Health Service Task Force recommendations for the use of antiretroviral drugs in pregnant women infected with HIV-1 for maternal health and for reducing perinatal HIV-1 transmission in the United States. Centers for Disease Control and Prevention. MMWR 1998;47 (RR-2):1–30.

Quinn TC, Wawer MJ, Sewankambo N, Serwadda D, Li C, Wabwire-Mangen F, et al. Viral load and heterosexual transmission of human immunodeficiency virus type-I. Rakai Project Study Group. N Engl J Med 2000;342:921–9.

Semprini AE, Fiore S, Pardi G. Reproductive counselling for HIV discordant couples [letter]. Lancet 1997;349:1401–2.

13
Breast cancer in *BRCA*-positive patients.

The occurrence of breast cancer in 2 first-degree relatives prompts genetic evaluation in a 38-year-old woman, gravida 2, para 2. Testing reveals the presence of a *BRCA1* gene mutation. The treatment option that would result in the lowest risk of breast cancer in this patient is

      (A) progestin-only contraceptive
      (B) a selective progesterone receptor modulator
*   (C) bilateral mastectomy
      (D) bilateral oophorectomy
      (E) a selective estrogen receptor modulator

The genes *BRCA1* and *BRCA2* encode for proteins that participate in the cellular response to DNA damage. Inactivating mutations in these genes increase a woman's susceptibility to both breast and ovarian cancer. The susceptibility is a consequence of inheritance of one mutant allele of either *BRCA1* or *BRCA2* followed by loss of the second allele in the epithelial cells of the breast or ovary, loss of heterozygosity, or complete inactivation of the second allele. Such mutations contribute to a small fraction of the total number of cases of breast cancer but as many as 40% of breast cancer cases diagnosed before age 40 years and up to 75% of familial cases. Approximately 10% of ovarian cancer cases are attributable to *BRCA* mutations.

Studies have demonstrated that breast tissue proliferation (ie, peak mitotic activity), unlike the endometrium, primarily occurs during the luteal phase. This observation, coupled with the results of the Women's Health Initiative trial and the Million Women Study, suggests that combination hormone therapy may increase the risk of breast cancer. Therefore, high doses of progestins would not be the treatment of choice in a woman with a genetic predisposition for breast cancer.

Selective progesterone receptor modulators are mixed progesterone agonist-antagonist compounds that have numerous proven and potential therapeutic applications in women's health care. Several small studies using selective progesterone receptor modulators have been performed in women with breast carcinoma. Results of the studies have been disappointing, and to date no such study has been specifically performed in *BRCA* patients. It is likely that combined therapy of selective progesterone receptor modulators with antiestrogens or aromatase inhibitors may improve the results in the endocrine therapy of breast cancer.

Carriers of a *BRCA1* mutation have a 50–85% lifetime risk of breast cancer and a 20–40% lifetime risk of ovarian cancer. The efficacy of bilateral prophylactic mastectomy in carriers of *BRCA* mutations is well documented. During a 3-year study period, breast cancer developed in 8 of 63 carriers of *BRCA* mutations who declined mastectomy but in only 1 of the 76 carriers who chose surgery. Even with improvements in postoperative reconstructive cosmetic surgery, chest disfigurement and sexual impairment may occur in women who may never have actually needed the surgery. Others argue that early cancer detected by intensive surveillance, including magnetic resonance imaging, obviates the need for this aggressive management protocol.

Although not as effective as prophylactic mastectomy in the limited and not directly comparable studies published to date, prophylactic bilateral oophorectomy has decreased the risk of breast cancer in *BRCA*-positive women. The risk of ovarian cancer compared with breast cancer is much lower in *BRCA*-positive women, and the absence of an early means of detection and the lethality of ovarian cancer have prompted oncologists to recommend oophorectomy. In women who underwent this procedure in 2 studies, the risk of breast cancer was reduced from 12.6% to 4.4% in one study and from 42% to 21% in the second study. Prophylactic oophorectomy would not be desirable in cases where the patient wishes to bear children but may be performed when childbearing is completed.

The protective effect of selective estrogen receptor modulators, such as tamoxifen citrate (Nolvadex), against breast cancer in women of moderate risk has been demonstrated. However, the data specific to carriers of *BRCA* remain unclear. Of 288 women with breast cancer, a protective effect of tamoxifen citrate was found among carriers of only the *BRCA2* mutations but not in carriers of the *BRCA1* mutations. This may reflect the fact that *BRCA2* mutations are more commonly estrogen receptor-positive, which suggests that tamoxifen may be more effective for certain genotypes.

Beral V. Breast cancer and hormone-replacement therapy in the Million Women Study. Million Women Study Collaborators. Lancet 2003;362: 419–27.

Kauff ND, Satagopan JM, Robson ME, Scheuer L, Hensley M, Hudis CA, et al. Risk-reducing salpingo-oophorectomy in women with a BRCA1 or BRCA2 mutation. N Engl J Med 2002;346:1609–15.

King MC, Wieand S, Hale K, Lee M, Walsh T, Owens K, et al. Tamoxifen and breast cancer incidence among women with inherited mutations in BRCA1 and BRCA2: National Surgical Adjuvant Breast and Bowel Project (NSABP-P1) Breast Cancer Prevention Trial. JAMA 2001;286:2251–6.

Klijn JG, Setyono-Han B, Foekens JA. Progesterone antagonists and progesterone receptor modulators in the treatment of breast cancer. Steriods 2000;65:825–30.

Meijers-Heijboer H, van Geel B, van Putten WJ, Henzen-Logmans SC, Seynaeve C, Menke-Pluymers MB, et al. Breast cancer after prophylactic bilateral mastectomy in women with a BRCA1 or BRCA2 mutation. N Engl J Med 2001;345:159–64.

Rebbeck TR, Lynch HT, Neuhausen SL, Narod SA, Van't Veer L, Garber JE, et al. Prophylactic oophorectomy in carriers of BRCA1 or BRCA2 mutations. Prevention and Observation of Surgical End Points Study Group. N Engl J Med 2002;346:1616–22.

Rossouw E, Anderson GL, Prentice RL, LaCroix AZ, Kooperberg C, Stefanick ML, et al. Risks and benefits of estrogen plus progestin in healthy postmenopausal women: principal results from the Women's Health Initiative randomized controlled trial. Writing Group for the Women's Health Initiative Investigators. JAMA 2002;288:321–33.

14
Uterine and associated anomalies

A 15-year-old adolescent comes in for evaluation. During corrective surgery for an imperforate anus identified at birth, she was found to have an ectopic kidney and anomalous ureters, which were repaired. She now experiences cyclic bloating and pain that has been labeled mittelschmerz, but she has amenorrhea. She has normal secondary sexual characteristics. A magnetic resonance imaging (MRI) study is suggestive of a bicornuate uterus. On examination under anesthesia, she is found to have a blind vaginal pouch and no evidence of a cervix. The study most likely to yield additional relevant clinical information about this patient is

* (A) X-ray of the spine
  (B) barium enema
  (C) molecular evaluation for fragile X syndrome
  (D) renal ultrasonography

In the absence of müllerian inhibitory factor, the müllerian ducts develop into the upper vagina, uterus, and fallopian tubes. During this same period, and in the absence of testosterone produced by the male gonads, the Wolffian ducts regress spontaneously. By 17–18 weeks of gestation, the vagina is formed.

Congenital anomalies of the müllerian system are relatively common and the prevalence of these phenomena, based on findings during postnatal examination of female infants, has been reported to be 2–3%. Anomalies of the uterus are the most common form of müllerian abnormality, and they occur in 1 in 200–600 women of childbearing age. Because many women with these abnormalities may be relatively symptom-free, the actual incidence may be considerably higher considering that up to 57% of women with uterine defects experience successful fertility and pregnancy.

A significant percentage of women with reproductive difficulty are found to have a uterine abnormality, and, therefore, the focus of most clinicians often is directed solely at the reproductive tract. If a müllerian anomaly is suspected, hysterosalpingography, MRI, and even hysteroscopy and laparoscopy often lead to diagnosis and development of a plan for management. Müllerian system abnormalities, however, are seen commonly in association with a number of other developmental and anatomic defects that may have significant health consequences. Thus, when a müllerian abnormality is suspected or identified, a thorough and complete investigation to identify other related abnormalities is required.

Urinary tract abnormalities are frequently associated with defects in müllerian system development. The most common associated abnormalities are renal agenesis and ureteral anomalies, such as duplication. In a recent review of a large number of women with different types of müllerian developmental defects, the authors used MRI studies to evaluate women with different müllerian abnormalities. Renal agenesis was found in 29.8% of the women studied. Among women with unilateral obstructed uterus didelphys, renal agenesis, present in virtually all of these patients, was observed ipsilateral to the obstructed hemiuterus. In the patient described, exploration and correction of anomalous ureters has been accomplished, and further evaluation of the kidneys is not required.

Imperforate anus occurs when the membrane that separates the endodermal hindgut from the ectodermal anal dimple fails to perforate. This anomaly is said to occur in 1 in 5,000 newborns. Imperforate anus is associated with renal anomalies in approximately 48% of cases. Although anal abnormalities have been reported in patients with vertebral, anal, cardiac, tracheal, esophageal, renal, and limb bud deformities, they usually are not associated with müllerian abnormalities. In this patient, repair as a newborn has resulted in normal bowel function and further evaluation via barium enema is not indicated.

A 1979 study reported a series of women with uterine hypoplasia or aplasia, renal agenesis or ectopy, vertebral anomalies, and short stature. This particular group of findings was designated the müllerian, renal, cervical spine association. Since that time, there has been increasing recognition of the common association of these abnormalities. Primary amenorrhea is the most common symptom in females with normal secondary sexual characteristics and a blind ending vagina, as observed in this patient. Scoliosis is commonly seen in these patients, and fusion of the cervical and upper thoracic vertebrae is occasionally observed. Thus, in a woman with müllerian developmental defects, radiographic evaluations of the urinary tract and the cervical spine commonly demonstrate associated abnormality. The mode of inheritance of müllerian, renal, cervical spine association is not known.

Fragile X syndrome is the most common cause of mental retardation and is second only to Down syndrome. It is estimated to cause 1 case of mental retardation in every 1,000–1,500 males and 1 case of generally milder mental handicap in every 2,000–2,500 females. It is believed to be caused by mutation in the fragile X gene located on the X chromosome. Affected females generally have less severe mental impairment than affected males; approximately 8% of females have mental retardation, 81% demonstrate developmental delay, and 11% show no evidence of mental impairment. Importantly, although the carrier state for fragile X is associated with mental deficiencies, this syndrome is not associated with müllerian or other anatomic abnormalities. Thus, molecular testing for fragile X is not indicated in the patient presented.

Duncan PA, Shapiro LR, Stangel JJ, Klein RM, Addonizio JC. The MURCS association: Mullerian duct aplasia, renal aplasia, and cervicothoracic somite dysplasia. J Pediatr 1979;95:399–402.

Gilliam ML, Shulman LP. Tetralogy of Fallot, imperforate anus, and Mullerian, renal, and cervical spine (MURCS) anomalies in a 15-year-old girl. J Pediatr Adolesc Gynecol 2002;15:231–3.

Li S, Qayyum A, Coakley FV, Hricak H. Association of renal agenesis and mullerian duct anomalies. J Comput Assist Tomogr 2000;24:829–34.

Nonsurgical diagnosis and management of vaginal agenesis. ACOG Committee Opinion No. 274. American College of Obstetricians and Gynecologists. Obstet Gynecol 2002;100:213–6.

Rock JA, Markham SM. Developmental anomalies of the reproductive tract. In: Keye WR Jr, Chang RJ, Rebar RW, Soules MR, eds. Infertility evaluation and treatment. Philadelphia (PA): WB Saunders; 1995. p. 387–411.

15
Bone markers for osteoporosis

A 65-year-old woman, who has had amenorrhea for 10 years and is not taking hormone therapy, comes in to discuss the results of her recent dual-energy X-ray absorptiometry (DXA) study. The DXA reveals decreases in the patient's lumbar and hip bone densities with T-scores of -2.7 and -2.4, respectively. You prescribe calcium, vitamin D, and a bisphosphonate and decide to check bone biomarkers after 3 months. The test result that would most likely represent evidence of compliance and drug efficacy is

    (A) a decrease in bone-specific serum alkaline phosphatase
    (B) an increase in urinary hydroxyproline
*   (C) a decrease in urinary N-telopeptide
    (D) an increase in urinary deoxypyridinoline
    (E) a decrease in serum osteocalcin

Serum and urinary markers of bone turnover are not useful in making a diagnosis of osteopenia or osteoporosis. The criterion standard for measurement of bone mineral density remains the DXA scan. However, these markers may be useful for monitoring the response to antiresorptive therapy in patients with osteoporosis (see Appendix B). Human bone is continuously remodeled through a coupled process of bone resorption by osteoclasts followed by bone formation by osteoblasts. This process is necessary for normal development and bone growth as well as skeletal integrity. Measurement of specific degradation products of bone matrix allows analysis of the rate of bone remodeling. Rapid progress is being made in the development of easily performed and reliable assays for bone markers.

Controversy exists with regard to which markers provide the most useful information about the subsequent risk of bone loss and the response to therapy directed at preventing or treating osteoporosis. Some studies have demonstrated that markers of bone turnover may be useful in the prediction of rates of future bone loss and may, therefore, provide information about fracture risk beyond measurements of bone mineral density. The mean values for biochemical markers of bone turnover are higher in patients with osteoporosis than in matched normal subjects. In most studies, there is a highly significant correlation between markers of bone turnover and subsequent rates of bone loss.

Alkaline phosphatase is a ubiquitously distributed enzyme produced by a variety of cells from different tissues. More than 95% of the total serum activity of alkaline phosphatase is derived from liver cells and osteoblasts. As a result, the quantification of alkaline phosphatase as a biochemical index can be used in the diagnosis and follow-up of liver and metabolic bone disease. In subjects with normal liver function, serum alkaline phosphatase has been shown to be a useful index of bone formation. Approximately 90% of hydroxyproline is liberated during the degradation of bone collagen and is primarily metabolized in the liver. However, hydroxyproline is relatively nonspecific for bone in that it can be found in other tissues, such as the skin.

Of all the bone markers discussed, urinary N-telopeptide is the most widely available commercially. The N-telopeptide molecule is specific to bone. The N-telopeptide peptide is a direct product of osteoclastic proteolysis and is found in the urine as a stable end product of degradation. Low levels of N-telopeptide in urine, therefore, have been proposed as a marker of bone stabilization. In this patient, low levels of N-telopeptide would document compliance with antiresorptive therapy.

Pyridinoline and deoxypyridinoline, which are derivatives of 3-hydroxypyridinium, are formed during the extracellular maturation of collagens. Urinary values show a high specificity for skeletal tissues. Pyridinoline is derived from cartilage and bone but also from other tissues, including ligaments and blood vessels. In contrast, deoxypyridinoline is present almost exclusively in bone. It should not increase in a compliant patient with biphosphonate.

Osteocalcin is one of the major components of the noncollagenous bone matrix. The quantification of osteocalcin in serum is considered to be a sensitive measure of osteoblast function. High serum levels of immunoreactive osteocalcin have been shown to correlate with the bone formation rate; however, the protein is relatively unstable and is rapidly metabolized on release into the circulation. Because concentrations vary widely from moment to moment, measurement of osteocalcin would not be the best test to document compliance.

16
Oral contraceptives and deep vein thrombosis

Three months after she began taking low-dose oral contraceptives, a previously healthy 21-year-old woman has a "red, swollen, painful leg." Evaluation is consistent with deep vein thrombosis (DVT). Further evaluation is most likely to show which one of the following genetic abnormalities?

(A) Protein S deficiency
(B) Antithrombin III deficiency
(C) Protein C deficiency
(D) 20210A prothrombin mutation
* (E) Factor V Leiden mutation

Deep vein thrombosis is an uncommon disorder in a young woman, even one who is taking combination oral contraceptives. Although certain risk factors, including use of oral contraceptives, increase the risk of DVT by inducing a hypercoagulable state (Box 16-1), a genetic predisposition for DVT should be considered in any young woman with a history and symptoms such as those of the present patient. An inherited thrombophilia or coagulopathy may serve to trigger DVT where none may otherwise develop. On the basis of level I evidence, a College of American Pathologists consensus conference has recommended that testing for an inherited thrombophilia be carried out in women who experience DVT during oral contraceptive use. Thus, coagulation evaluation is warranted in this patient. Physicians who are inexperienced with evaluation of such patients should refer them to an appropriate specialist.

Many different opinions exist as to what constitutes an appropriate laboratory workup for a patient who has had any thromboembolic episode. Generally, laboratory diagnosis of primary hypercoagulable states requires testing for each of the possible disorders individually because no general screening test is available to determine whether a patient may have such a condition. At this time, functional, immunologic, or DNA-based assays are available to test for antithrombin deficiency, protein C deficiency, protein S deficiency, activated protein C (APC) resistance (factor V Leiden mutation), the prothrombin gene mutation, and hyperhomocysteinemia. Fig. 16-1 (see color plate) illustrates the role of these tests in the clotting cascade.

See Box 16-2 for suggested tests for a woman, such as the described patient, who develops a spontaneous DVT

BOX 16-1

Conditions Associated With a "Hypercoagulable" State

- Autoimmune disorders
- Corticosteroid use
- Dehydration
- Immobilization
- Infection
- Malignancy
- Obesity
- Oral contraceptive use
- Personal or family history of deep venous thromboembolism
- Pregnancy
- Polycythemia
- Postpartum period
- Renal disease
- Sepsis
- Surgery
- Trauma

> **BOX 16-2**
>
> **Suggested Tests for Spontaneous Deep Vein Thrombosis (DVT)**
>
> If DVT is not triggered by surgery, trauma, or immobilization:
> - Activated protein C (APC) test (followed by polymerase chain reaction [PCR] test for factor V Leiden if positive)
> - Prothrombin 20210 mutation genetic test
> - Protein S activity
> - Protein C activity
> - Antithrombin III activity
> - Antiphospholipid antibodies, consisting of lupus anticoagulant and anticardiolipin immunoglobulin G and immunoglobulin M antibodies
> - Homocysteine level (fasting)
> - Complete blood count
>
> If there is a strong family history of DVT or pulmonary embolism, add:
> - Thrombin clot time
> - Fibrinogen activity
> - Fibrinogen electrophoresis
> - Plasminogen activity

(or pulmonary embolus) that was not caused by trauma, surgery, or immobilization. Additional tests should be added if there is a strong family history of DVT or pulmonary embolus. Generally, there is no need to obtain the thermolabile methylene–tetrahydrofolate reductase genetic test because studies do not show this mutation to be a risk factor for venous thromboembolism. It is important to remember that both protein C and protein S activity are low in patients who take warfarin (Coumadin). Individuals must be off this medication for at least 10 days before these activities are determined.

The factor V Leiden mutation (ie, APC resistance) is the most common of the inherited thrombophilias, affecting as many as 40% of women with DVT. In a large cross-sectional study in the United States, prevalence varied widely by race, with the heterozygous condition found in 5.3% of Caucasians, 2.2% of Hispanic Americans, 1.2% of African Americans, 0.45% of Asian Americans, and 1.25% of Native Americans. It has been estimated that more than 11.3 million Americans carry this mutation. The disorder is inherited in an autosomal dominant manner and is caused by an adenine for guanine point mutation, which results in replacement of glutamine with arginine at position 506 on the factor V molecule.

The risk for DVT increases approximately 4-fold for normal women with oral contraceptive use (over a baseline rate of 1 case per 10,000 women-years), 8-fold with heterozygous factor V Leiden mutation alone, and more than 30-fold in women with heterozygous factor V Leiden mutation who also use oral contraceptives. Even with such increased odds, the incidence of DVT among women with factor V Leiden mutation is low. However, the risk is such that individuals with this disorder should not be given oral contraceptives. The American College of Obstetricians and Gynecologists (ACOG) recommends that women with a documented history of unexplained DVT or DVT associated with pregnancy or exogenous estrogen use should not use combination oral contraceptives unless they are taking anticoagulants.

The incidence of fatal DVT in oral contraceptive users is even lower, approximately 0.7 in 100,000. Because the absolute risk of DVT in the United States is estimated at 1 in 200–500 in heterozygotes for the factor V Leiden mutation, wide screening of the population has been viewed as impractical and not cost-effective for the U.S. population at large. It has been estimated by ACOG that screening more than 1 million combination oral contraceptive candidates would, at best, prevent 2 oral contraceptive-associated deaths.

Laboratory testing for this mutation begins with the APC test. This test was developed to investigate the anticoagulant response to APC and can be performed on anticoagulated blood. The patient's plasma is prediluted with factor V-deficient plasma. A carefully standardized amount of APC is added in an activated partial thromboplastin time (aPTT) reaction. An aPTT test without APC also is performed, and results are expressed as the quotient (APC ratio) of the former clotting time divided by the latter clotting time. Individuals with APC resistance usually have a ratio less than 2.0 compared with a ratio of greater than 2.0 for patients without APC resistance. This test is rapid, relatively inexpensive, and highly reproducible. However, APC resistance may arise as an acquired coagulation disorder, and some cases may fall into a zone that is borderline for diagnosis. Patients who screen positive or have a borderline result can be analyzed with direct genotyping to confirm the presence of the factor V Leiden allele.

Protein S deficiency is inherited as an autosomal dominant trait in which heterozygotes have an increased risk for DVT. Its incidence is approximately 0.5%, but it is found in up to 4% of individuals with a history of DVT. Protein S is a co-factor for APC, is vitamin K-dependent, and facilitates prevention of excessive clot formation. As much as 50% of protein S circulates in an inactive form bound to C4b-binding protein (see Fig. 16-1). Levels of this binding protein increase in hypercoagulable states. This in turn decreases the levels of free (unbound) protein S, which subsequently increases the risk of DVT. Heterozygotes have a 15–50% reduction in protein S levels that may be as much as 95% lower than normal.

Antithrombin III deficiency also is an autosomal dominant disorder and has been noted in 1 of 5,000 healthy blood donors. Antithrombin III inactivates thrombin and other serine proteases. In individuals with the disorder, antithrombin III is either absent, reduced, or dysfunctional. The risk of DVT is increased approximately 8-fold in women with this disorder.

Protein C deficiency also is inherited in incidence similar to protein S deficiency. Protein C is a vitamin K-dependent anticoagulant plasma protein, with levels reduced by 60% in affected heterozygotes. Homozygotes do not survive, and they typically die from neonatal purpura fulminans characterized by generalized microvascular thrombosis.

Protein C becomes "activated" as thrombin binds to its endothelial cell surface receptor. Activated protein C prevents clot formation at the surface of endothelium or platelets by inhibiting the effects of factors V and VII in the clotting cascade (see Fig. 16-1).

The G20210A prothrombin mutation involves a guanine to adenine substitution at nucleotide position 20210 in the 3′ untranslated region of the prothrombin gene. In the United States, its prevalence is estimated to be 1–2%, and it is highly dependent on race. The mutation is uncommon in African Americans (approximately 0.2%) and also is rare in Asian Americans and Native Americans. The G20210A prothrombin mutation appears to increase the risk for DVT only modestly, in the range of 2- to 3-fold. However, accumulating data show an increased risk when this mutation occurs together with factor V Leiden mutation or with protein C or S deficiency.

American College of Obstetricians and Gynecologists. The use of hormonal contraception in women with coexisting medical conditions. ACOG Practice Bulletin 18. Washington, DC: ACOG; 2000.

Brenner BR, Nowak-Göttl U, Kosch A, Manco-Johnson M, Laposata M. Diagnostic studies for thrombophilia in women on hormonal therapy and during pregnancy, and in children. Arch Pathol Lab Med 2002;126:1296–303.

McGlennen RC, Key NS. Clinical and laboratory management of the prothrombin G20210A mutation. Arch Pathol Lab Med 2002;126:1319–25.

Ninia JG. Inherited coagulopathies in OB/GYN. Prim Care Update Ob Gyns 2000;7:70–3.

Ridker PM, Miletich JP, Hennekens CH, Buring JE. Ethnic distribution of factor V Leiden in 4047 men and women. Implications for venous thromboembolism screening. JAMA 1997;277:1305–7.

Sheppard DR. Activated protein C resistance: the most common risk factor for venous thromboembolism. J Am Board Fam Pract 2000;13:111–5.

Thomas RH. Hypercoagulability syndromes. Arch Intern Med 2001;161:2433–9.

17

Alternative therapies for the treatment of hot flushes

A 42-year-old woman, gravida 1, para 1, presents with severe hot flushes, trouble sleeping, fatigue, severe headaches, and increasing irritability for the past 2 months. One year ago, she received a diagnosis of breast cancer and was treated with wide local excision and chemotherapy. One lymph node was positive, and the tumor was estrogen and progestin receptor negative. After undergoing multiple courses of chemotherapy, her menstrual cycles became irregular. Her physical examination is unremarkable. Laboratory results showed normal thyroid stimulating hormone, elevated follicle-stimulating hormone, and low estradiol levels. Her complete blood count was within normal limits. The most appropriate next step in her management is

  (A) clonidine
  (B) progesterone
* (C) selective serotonin reuptake inhibitor (SSRI)
  (D) conjugated equine estrogen
  (E) black cohosh

This patient with a diagnosis of breast cancer has severe vasomotor symptoms. In her assessment, it is apparent that her chemotherapeutic treatment may have induced an early reduction in her ovarian reserve resulting in a perimenopausal pattern of uterine bleeding and severe hot flushes that have disrupted her life. Although estrogen therapy is the most effective treatment for hot flushes with approximately a 90% response rate, this is not the best option in a patient with a prior history of breast cancer. Progestins, such as megestrol acetate, also have been shown to be effective (response rate, 80–85%); however, progestins are contraindicated in patients with breast cancer because of their reported proliferative stimulatory effects.

A variety of nonhormonal approaches have been proposed for treatment of menopausal symptoms. The best clinical trial data have been derived from studies of premenopausal women with a prior history of breast cancer who, similar to the patient described, are severely affected by vasomotor symptoms. Nonhormonal approaches that have been evaluated include vitamin E, phytoestrogens, dong quai, ginseng, black cohosh, clonidine, and SSRIs. Because of a significant placebo response in subjective rating of vasomotor symptoms, double-blinded randomized trials are needed to evaluate the efficacy of these compounds. Examples of the relative effectiveness of these compounds for the treatment of vasomotor symptoms are shown in Fig. 17-1 (see color plate).

Generally, the placebo response during a 12-week hot flush study have ranged from 20% to 40%. As shown in Fig. 17-1 (see color plate), the impact of soy or phytoestrogens on hot flushes is similar to placebo alone. Clonidine appears to reduce hot flushes by approximately 30% with an onset of action observed after 1 week of treatment. Of the nonhormonal therapies, venlafaxine (Effexor) and paroxetine (Paxil) were shown to achieve approximately a 50% reduction in vasomotor flushes in randomized placebo-controlled trials. Other SSRIs, such as fluoxetine, are less effective. Vitamin E appears to be less effective than the SSRIs. In a recent randomized trial, black cohosh (Remifemin) appeared to be similar in efficacy to placebo. Thus, in choosing a nonestrogen treatment option for women with severe vasomotor symptoms, the latest data from randomized placebo-controlled clinical trials should be considered because of the high placebo response rates. At this time, an SSRI would appear to provide the most appropriate next step in management of this patient.

Barton DL, Loprinzi CL, Quella SK, Sloan JA, Veeder MH, Egner JR, et al. Prospective evaluation of vitamin E for hot flashes in breast cancer survivors. J Clin Oncol 1998;16:495–500.

Goldberg RM, Loprinzi CL, O'Fallon JR, Veeder MH, Miser AW, Mailard JA, et al. Transdermal clonidine for ameliorating tamoxifen-induced hot flashes. J Clin Oncol 1994;12:155–8.

Jacobson JS, Troxel AB, Evans J, Klaus L, Vahdat L, Kinne D, et al. Randomized trial of black cohosh for the treatment of hot flashes among women with a history of breast cancer. J Clin Oncol 2001;19: 2739–45.

Loprinzi CL, Kugler JW, Sloan JA, Malliard JA, LaVasseur BI, Barton DL, et al. Venlaxfaxine in management of hot flashes in survivors of breast cancer: a randomized controlled trial. Lancet 2000;356: 2059–63.

Loprinzi CL, Michalak JC, Quella SK, O'Fallon JR, Hatfield AK, Nelimark RA, et al. Megestrol acetate for the prevention of hot flashes. N Engl J Med 1994;331:347–52.

Newton KM, Buist DS, Keenan NL, Anderson LA, LaCroix AZ. Use of alternative therapies for menopause symptoms: results of a population-based survey. Obstet Gynecol 2002;100:18–25.

Stearns V, Beebe KL, Iyengar M, Dube E. Paroxetine controlled release in the treatment of menopausal hot flashes: a randomized controlled trial. JAMA 2003;289:2827–34.

Tice JA, Ettinger B, Ensrud K, Wallace R, Blackwell T, Cummings SR. Phytoestrogen supplements for the treatment of hot flashes: the Isoflavone Clover Extract (ICE) Study: a randomized controlled trial. JAMA 2003;290:207–14.

18

Cardiovascular disease and hormone therapy

A 52-year-old woman, gravida 2, para 2, is referred for management of severe vasomotor symptoms. Her last regular menstrual period occurred 2 years ago. She has kept a diary and has documented more than 7 hot flushes per day and 4–5 periods of awakenings per night. On examination, she is of normal weight with a body mass index of 26 kg/m². She has an initial blood pressure reading of 140/90 mm Hg; however, following a rest period, her reading is 130/80 mm Hg. She occasionally exercises and smokes one half pack of cigarettes per day. Although she desires treatment for her vasomotor symptoms, she is concerned that taking hormone therapy (HT) may increase her risk for cardiovascular disease (CVD). In counseling her, you explain that the best intervention to decrease her risk for CVD is

    (A) weight loss
    (B) combination HT
*   (C) smoking cessation
    (D) 30 minutes of exercise per day
    (E) antihypertensive therapy

Despite widespread belief that breast cancer is the leading cause of death among U.S. women, cardiovascular disease continues to be the leading cause of death. Since the mid-1980s, a greater proportion of women (52%) have died from CVD than have men (46%), and although there is a trend toward a reduction in CVD mortality among men, no reduction has been observed among women.

Cigarette smoking is among the modifiable CVD risk factors. In women, cigarette smoking is directly responsible for 21% of all mortality from CVD and 50% of all acute coronary heart disease events before age 55 years. Although smoking in recent decades in the United States has decreased at a rate of 0.3% per year, smoking initiation has increased by 1% per year (Table 18-1). Cigarette smoking exerts its effects through multiple mechanisms. The major chemical component in cigarette smoke, nicotine, stimulates the sympathetic nervous system and increases plasma levels of free fatty acids and low-density lipoprotein cholesterol. Cessation of smoking is associated with an estimated reduction of 50–70% in the risk of coronary heart disease and, therefore, would be appropriate for this patient to stop smoking to reduce her risk for CVD.

It has been estimated that 70% of all coronary heart disease can be attributed to obesity. Being more than 30% overweight places a woman at risk for coronary heart disease, even if she has no other risk factors. Based on the World Health Organization definitions, this patient has normal weight and is not considered at risk based on her current weight.

Although a large number of observational studies demonstrated that HT was associated with a lower incidence of coronary heart disease in those who used estrogen therapy or HT compared with nonusers, data from the Women's Health Initiative trial, which evaluated HT in the primary prevention of coronary heart disease, did not support these findings. Therefore, the decision to use HT must be based on established noncoronary risks and benefits. The use of HT in this patient might be indicated for prevention and treatment of her severe vasomotor symptoms, but not for reduction in her risk of coronary heart disease.

The effect of physical exercise on the risk of CVD in women is not as clearly defined as it is for men. In men with an active lifestyle, the estimated reduction of acute coronary heart disease is 35–55%. In women, studies have been variable in the risk reduction associated with increasing activity. However, conventional thinking would suggest that active individuals would have lower weight, which would subsequently decrease their risk of CVD.

Hypertension is defined as an arm cuff reading of 140/90 mm Hg and has been reported to have a greater impact on CVD in women than men. Elevated diastolic and systolic blood pressure levels are both independent risk factors for CVD. Postmenopausal women are at greatest risk with more than 50% affected beyond age 55 years. In women, reducing the diastolic blood pressure level is associated with reductions in acute coronary heart disease events. In this patient, her repeat blood pressure reading would be considered prehypertensive under the Seventh Report of the Joint National Committee on Prevention, Detection, Evaluation, and Treatment of High Blood Pressure (JNC 7) guidelines (ie, systolic blood pressure level of 120–139 mm Hg or diastolic blood pressure level of 80–89 mm Hg), requiring her to adopt health-promoting lifestyle modifications to prevent CVD. These include weight reduction, adopting a Dietary Approaches to Stop Hypertension eating plan that is rich in potassium and calcium, reducing dietary sodium, increasing physical activity, and moderating alcohol consumption. If she had other "compelling indications," such as heart failure, postmyocardial infarction, high coronary heart disease risk, diabetes mellitus, chronic kidney disease, or needed to prevent recurrent stroke, medical therapy also would be indicated.

In the JNC 7 report, blood pressure classification is based on the mean of 2 or more properly measured seated blood pressure readings on each of 2 or more office visits. Stage 1 hypertension (140–159 mm Hg systolic or 90–99 mm Hg diastolic blood pressure levels) and stage 2 hypertension ($\geq$160 mm Hg systolic or $\geq$100 mm Hg diastolic blood pressure levels) should be treated with both lifestyle modification and drug therapy. Most patients would receive a thiazide-type diuretic for stage 1 hypertension and a 2-drug combination (thiazide-type diuretic and angiotensin converting enzyme inhibitor or angiotensin-receptor blocker, β-blocker, or calcium channel blocker) for stage 2 hypertension. Hormone therapy has not been associated with increasing blood pressure levels.

TABLE 18-1. Prevalence (%) of Common Risk Factors of Coronary Atherosclerotic Heart Disease in Adult Women

Factor	Age		
	19 y	25–34 y	35–44 y
Obesity	25	20	27
Cigarette smoking	27	33	34
Total cholesterol*	37	18	13
Hypertension†	—	4	11

*Measurements are: $\geq$170 mg/dL at age 19 years; $\geq$220 mg/dL at age 20–25 years; $\geq$240 mg/dL at age 30–39 years; and $\geq$260 mg/dL at age >40 years.

†Blood pressure level $\geq$160/95 mm Hg.

Data from Lobo RA, ed. Treatment of postmenopausal woman: basic and clinical aspects. 2nd ed. Philadelphia (PA): Lippincott Williams & Wilkins; 1999. p. 216. National Institutes of Health. Chartbook on cardiovascular, lung and blood diseases. Washington, DC: U.S. Department of Health and Human Services; 1992. Manson JE, Tosteson H, Ridker PM, Satterfield S, Hebert P, O'Connor GT, et al. The primary prevention of myocardial infarction. N Engl J Med 1992;326:1406–16. American Heart Association. 1993 Heart and stroke facts. Dallas, Texas: American Heart Association National Center; 1993.

American Heart Association. 2003 Heart and stroke facts. Dallas (TX): American Heart Association National Center; 2003.

Chobanian AV, Bakris GL, Black HR, Cushman WC, Green LA, Izzo JL Jr, et al. The Seventh Report of the Joint National Committee on Prevention, Detection, Evaluation, and Treatment of High Blood Pressure. The JNC 7 Report. JAMA 2003;289:2560–72.

LaCroix AZ, Lang J, Scherr P, Wallace RB, Cornoni-Huntley J, Berkman L, et al. Smoking and mortality among older men and women in three communities. N Engl J Med 1991;324:1619–25.

MacMahon S, Peto R, Cutler J, Collins R, Sorlie P, Neaton J, et al. Blood pressure, stroke, and coronary heart disease. Part 1, Prolonged differences in blood pressure: prospective observational studies corrected for the regression dilution bias. Lancet 1990;335:765–74.

Mjos OD. Lipid effects of smoking. Am Heart J 1988;115:272–5.

Powell KE, Thompson PD, Caspersen CJ, Kendrick JS. Physical activity and the incidence of coronary heart disease. Annu Rev Public Health 1987;8:253–87.

Rossouw JE, Anderson GL, Prentice RL, LaCroix AZ, Kooperberg C, Stefanick ML, et al. Risks and benefits of estrogen plus progestin in healthy postmenopausal women: principal results from the Women's Health Initiative randomized controlled trial. Writing Group for the Women's Health Initiative Investigators. JAMA 2002;288:321–33.

Willett WC, Green A, Stampfer MJ, Speizer FE, Colditz GA, Rosner B, et al. Relative and absolute excess risks of coronary heart disease among women who smoke cigarettes. N Engl J Med 1987;317:1303–9.

19
Cushing's syndrome

The patient in Fig. 19-1 (see color plate) presents with a 6-month history of amenorrhea, 9.1 kg (20 lb) weight gain, fatigue, and occasional headaches. Based on this patient's presentation, the best screening test for her condition is

    (A) 24-hour urinary free cortisol excretion test
    (B) high-dose dexamethasone (8 mg) suppression test
* (C) overnight dexamethasone (1 mg) suppression test
    (D) plasma adrenocorticotropic hormone (ACTH) concentration
    (E) 4:00 PM serum cortisol concentration

The patient in this case should be suspected of having Cushing's syndrome. Overproduction of cortisol in the disorder can be related to overproduction of pituitary corticotropin (Cushing's disease), overproduction by tumors secreting corticotropin (eg, especially in the lungs), secretion of corticotropin-releasing hormone (CRH) by a hypothalamic tumor, or autonomous cortisol secretion by the adrenal gland hyperplasia or neoplasms.

The most useful test for evaluating cortisol secretion is the 24-hour urinary free cortisol excretion test. Typically, normal basal excretion is less than 100 µg per day. Values greater than 250 µg per day are virtually diagnostic of Cushing's syndrome. Values greater than 100 µg per day unfortunately sometimes occur in patients with obesity, depression, alcoholism, or chronic stress. Thus, some endocrinologists suggest obtaining at least 3 24-hour measurements.

A more simple screening suppression test may be conducted on an outpatient basis. The patient is instructed to take 1 mg of dexamethasone by mouth between 11:00 PM and midnight. A specimen for plasma cortisol is then obtained the following morning at 8:00 AM. In normal individuals, plasma cortisol levels decrease to less than 5 µg/dL after taking dexamethasone, whereas they commonly remain higher than 10 µg/dL in patients with Cushing's syndrome. Once again, abnormal values are common and can occur in patients with obesity, depression, alcoholism, or chronic stress. This test does not appear to be as sensitive as a measurement of 24-hour urinary free cortisol.

If the screening tests either strongly suggest or confirm the diagnosis of Cushing's syndrome, further evaluation is warranted to verify the diagnosis and determine the etiology. Although practice is changing, low-dose and high-dose dexamethasone is commonly used in such additional evaluation. Normal individuals, but not individuals with Cushing's syndrome, generally will be suppressed (ie, with cortisol value of less than 5 µg/dL) with 2 mg of dexamethasone (0.5 mg 4 times per day) daily for 2 days (the low-dose test).

Measurement of plasma corticotropin concentrations offers the most reliable means of making the differential diagnosis and is the most logical step in the assessment of hypercortisolism. Values are high in patients without adrenal tumors, undetectable in patients with adrenal tumors, and normal or elevated in patients with pituitary neoplasms or the ectopic ACTH syndrome. Thus, low values of corticotropin indicate adrenal disease, whereas normal or elevated values indicate that the hypercortisolism is ACTH dependent. If plasma corticotropin levels are low or undetectable, primary adrenal disease should be sought by computed tomography scan of the adrenal glands. Plasma ACTH values are sufficiently variable that they should not be used as a screening test. Although it is true that very high values indicate a disorder, there are many false-positive and false-negative test results.

If ACTH levels are normal or elevated, CRH (1 µg/kg body weight intravenously over 1 minute) can be administered. Approximately 90% of ACTH-secreting tumors release increased quantities of corticotropin in response to CRH. In contrast, individuals with extrapituitary ACTH-secreting tumors rarely respond to CRH.

If reliable measurements of corticotropin are unavailable, the high-dose dexamethasone suppression test (2 mg 4 times per day for 2 days immediately after the low-dose test) should be used in an effort to differentiate among the various causes for increased cortisol levels. Most patients with pituitary-dependent corticotropin oversecretion will have at least a 50% suppression of plasma cortisol or urinary-free cortisol or both. Patients with adrenal tumors do not suppress adequately even with this high dose, and patients with ACTH-producing tumors of nonendocrine organs have unpredictable responses. High-dose dexamethasone suppression should not be used as a screening test.

Findling JW, Raff H. Diagnosis and differential diagnosis of Cushing's syndrome. Endocrinol Metab Clin North Am 2001;30:729–47.

Puig J, Wagner A, Caballero A, Rodriguez-Espinosa J, Webb SM. Cost-effectiveness and accuracy of the tests used in the differential diagnosis of Cushing's syndrome. Pituitary 1999;1:125–32.

20

Nonhysteroscopic endometrial ablation

A 37-year-old woman presents with menorrhagia. She has a history of chronic renal failure, type 1 diabetes mellitus, and controlled hypertension. Her hematocrit concentration is 30%. Management of her condition with cyclic progestins has caused weight gain, mastalgia, bloating, and depression. Endometrial biopsy demonstrates secretory endometrium and sonohysterography is normal. Her partner has had a vasectomy, and she has no interest in fertility. The next step in management is

    (A) laparoscopically assisted vaginal hysterectomy
* (B) nonhysteroscopic endometrial ablation
    (C) hysteroscopically directed endometrial resection
    (D) levonorgestrel intrauterine system

Approximately 20% of women worldwide are affected by menorrhagia. More than one third of hysterectomies performed each year in the United States are for menorrhagia, and 35–50% of the uterine specimens demonstrate no histologic abnormality that explains the abnormal bleeding. Consequently, it has been suggested that many hysterectomies may be unnecessary and that perhaps less than extirpative surgery may suffice. A number of technologies have been developed that selectively destroy the endometrial lining while preserving the uterus. These procedures are intended to provide long-term treatment for abnormal uterine bleeding and are termed endometrial ablation.

The criterion standard for endometrial ablation is to perform the procedure through direct visualization using the hysteroscope. Hysteroscopic procedures involve continuous flow of a distension medium that contains sorbitol or glycine. Often, a fluid collection system will be used to ensure optimal fluid management. Distension medium can escape into a patient's vascular system. If infused distension medium exceeds that collected by greater than the safe range of 500–1,000 cc, serious electrolyte disturbances may occur, especially if they go undetected by the operating team. This explains why less skill-intensive technologies are necessary. In this patient with chronic renal failure, hysteroscopic ablation would not be the procedure of choice.

Nonhysteroscopic devices have been developed to provide ablation of nearly the entire endometrial cavity without the need for direct visualization. Proper patient selection is necessary, with a uterine cavity evaluation performed before the procedure. An endometrial biopsy is always necessary before an ablative procedure to rule out endometrial cancer.

Several nonhysteroscopic methods for endometrial ablation have been approved by the U.S. Food and Drug Administration. NovaSure is a disposable, fan shaped, expandable bipolar electrode with a porous metallic membrane draped over a metallic skeleton. It is introduced into the uterine cavity and deployed from its protective sheath. Uterine depth and width measurements are taken, and when these are entered into the device, the power necessary to ablate the uterine lining is calculated. Suction then draws the uterine lining close to the device during the procedure to facilitate steam and moisture release and to allow extensive desiccation of the tissue. Treatment times average 90 seconds. Postprocedure hysterectomy specimens reveal depth of ablation at 4 mm in the uterine corpus and 2–3 mm in the cornu. Serosal surface temperatures are not significantly elevated. Rates of amenorrhea following the procedure are approximately 40%. Patient satisfaction ranges near 90%. No endometrial preparation seems to be necessary for high patient satisfaction.

Thermal balloons allow nearly complete endometrial ablation without operative hysteroscopy. A specialized balloon catheter wand is inserted through the cervix to touch the uterine fundus. The balloon is filled with enough 5% dextrose in water to allow balloon pressure between 90 and 190 mm Hg. After stabilization at 180 mm Hg, a controller unit is activated, which heats the water in the balloon to 87° C for 8 minutes. An impeller circulates the fluid so that uniform endometrial temperature results. The endometrial temperatures achieved allow tissue destruction to a depth that reaches the shallow myometrium. Uterine serosal temperatures stay below 45° C. The device constantly monitors pressure and terminates heating if the pressure decreases, which could signal poor balloon placement. Other modalities for endometrial destruction include microwave and laser.

Success with endometrial ablation, generally defined as reduction of menstrual flow to eumenorrhea or less, is reported in nearly 90% of patients. In a 2-year follow-up report in which balloon ablation was compared with rollerball ablation, the success rates were 89.1% and 90.4%, respectively, with patient satisfaction rates being nearly identical. Amenorrhea is typically achieved in approximately one third of patients, with higher rates of amenorrhea perhaps possible with medical preparation of the endometrium with danazol (Danocrine) or gonadotropin-releasing hormone agonist. Medical pretreatment does not seem to be necessary for high patient satisfaction. Complications from the procedure are infrequent. Perforation is less common than with hysteroscopy, and the potential for distention media problems are nonexistent. Postprocedural cramping pain can last for 1 day. Patients are discharged within 2 hours with ibuprofen or mild narcotic analgesia. Only approximately 10% of patients require a subsequent procedure, repeat ablation, or hysterectomy.

The levonorgestrel intrauterine system is a useful device for contraception and can effect a decrease of menstrual flow in many patients. Satisfaction and reduction of menses is comparable to the endometrial ablation procedures. This device remains effective for 5 years. During the first 3 months after placement, there often is some vaginal spotting. Progestin is released from the device at a slightly accelerated rate during the first 2 months, and side effects typical of progestins are sometimes experienced during this time frame. The levonorgestrel intrauterine system may not be appropriate for this patient because of the symptoms she experiences with cyclic progestins.

A laparoscopic hysterectomy would certainly cure this patient's menorrhagia. However, the perioperative morbidity associated with hysterectomy for a patient with a normal uterine cavity and preexisting chronic disease are not warranted.

Cooper JM, Erickson ML. Global endometrial ablation technologies. Obstet Gynecol Clin North Am 2000;27:385–96, viii.

Cooper J, Gimpelson R, Laberge P, Galen D, Garza-Leal JG, Scott J, et al. A randomized, multicenter trial of safety and efficacy of the NovaSure system in the treatment of menorrhagia. J Am Assoc Gynecol Laparosc 2002;9:418–28.

Gambon JC, Mittman BS, Munro MG, Scialli AR, Winkel CA; Chronic Pelvic Pain/Endometriosis Working Group. Consensus statement for the management of chronic pelvic pain and endometriosis: proceedings of an expert-panel consensus process. Fertil Steril 2002; 78:961–72.

Grainger DA, Tjaden BL, Rowland C, Meyer WR. Thermal balloon and rollerball ablation to treat menorrhagia: two-year results of a multicenter, prospective, randomized, clinical trial. J Am Assoc Gynecol Laparosc 2000;7:175–9.

Lethaby A, Hickey M. Endometrial destruction techniques for heavy menstrual bleeding: a Cochrane review. Hum Reprod 2002;17: 2795–806.

Meyer WR, Walsh BW, Grainger DA, Peacock LM, Loffer FD, Steege J. Thermal balloon and rollerball ablation to treat menorrhagia: a multicenter comparison. Obstet Gynecol 1998;92:98–103.

Teirney R, Arachchi GJ, Fraser IS. Menstrual blood loss measured 5–6 years after endometrial ablation. Obstet Gynecol 2000;95:251–4.

Winkel CA. Evaluation and management of women with endometriosis. Obstet Gynecol 2003;102:397–408.

21
Management of weight reduction by bariatric surgery

A 42-year-old obese woman, who is 1.63 m (5 ft 4 in.) tall, weighs 111 kg (245 lb), and has a body mass index (BMI) of 42 kg/m², comes in to be evaluated for bariatric surgery. She has a long-term history of obesity and is being treated for diabetes mellitus and hypertension. Her previous attempts at weight loss with diet, exercise, and medical therapy have failed. The most important criterion in recommending bariatric surgery is

    (A) medical co-morbidities
    (B) failed diet and exercise therapy
    (C) long-term obesity
*   (D) BMI
    (E) age

Obesity has become the second leading cause of death in the United States, second only to medical conditions related to smoking. According to statistics from the National Institute of Health, among U.S. adults, 55% or 97 million are overweight or obese. This chronic disease is steadily increasing in prevalence and can be debilitating and ultimately fatal. Estimated medical costs to treat complications of this disorder, such as diabetes mellitus, hypertension, and cardiovascular disease, totaled more than $51.5 billion dollars in 1995.

Obesity is defined as BMI higher than 30 kg/m² whereas morbid obesity is defined as BMI higher than 40 kg/m². Generally, an obese individual is 22.7 kg (50 lb) overweight whereas a morbidly obese individual is 45.4 kg (100 lb) or more overweight.

Treatment options for obesity include diet, exercise, medical therapy, and bariatric surgery. Studies have shown that the nonoperative methods are not successful in achieving long-term weight loss in severely obese adults. This includes the use of anorectic medications, such as phentermine hydrochloride (Adipex), sibutramine hydrochloride (Meridia), and phendimetrazine tartrate (Bontril). Surgical treatment is preferred for the morbidly obese patient because it currently is the only method that can achieve weight control on a more long-term basis.

Bariatric surgery involves decreasing the size of the stomach to a size that will affect eating behavior by causing early satiety with a component of malabsorption. This results in reduced caloric intake with small portions with the potential for more permanent weight loss over time.

A BMI higher than 40 kg/m² is the most common indication for obesity surgery. Individuals with BMIs higher than 35–40 kg/m² often exhibit existing co-morbidities, such as cardiovascular problems and diabetes mellitus, which may interfere with daily activities (eg, ambulation, exercise, and difficulties in the work place).

When patients have failed more conservative therapies, surgical treatment may be considered. Two of the most common operative procedures performed by trained bariatric surgeons are: 1) gastric bypass ("stomach stapling") and 2) laparoscopic gastric banding (Lap-Band). The gastric bypass is an open procedure, which involves operative reduction of the stomach, leaving a small reservoir for food. The laparoscopic band procedure, a newer procedure also performed in select patients, involves the placement of a band around the stomach to decrease its size (Figs. 21-1 and 21-2; see color plates). No incision is made on the stomach or gastrointestinal tract, and the device is adjustable and can be removed at any time. The gastric bypass remains the standard for management of morbid obesity. Studies have shown a significant decrease in BMI with long-term weight loss in excess of 50% over 10 years. The Lap-Band procedure is approved by the U.S. Food and Drug Administration and is gaining more acceptance because of the decrease in operative risks along with faster recovery. The Lap-Band method has been shown to decrease 50% of excess body weight over an 18-month period, although results are not available from any long-term weight loss studies.

Patients who are selected to undergo surgical treatment for obesity must be counseled appropriately about the risks of the procedure. In addition to receiving a full medical evaluation, they should receive a preoperative psychologic evaluation to identify any contraindications to surgery. All patients pose a higher operative risk because of morbid obesity. Existing co-morbidities may increase this risk but usually are not the most common reason for surgery. Surgical risks for the gastric bypass include infection, wound problems, thromboembolism, and a gastric leak around the anastomosis created. In addition, because a portion of the stomach is removed, important medical conditions that need to be addressed are long-term need for vitamin B_{12} supplementation as well as a dietary-induced "dumping syndrome" causing gastrointestinal side effects. The Lap-Band procedure has become more attractive because the placement of an inert constricting device can be removed and does not cause medically related problems as does the gastric bypass. Other than injury to the stomach from placement of the device, the risk associated with Lap-Band is similar to that of a laparoscopic cholecystectomy.

Surgical treatment should be offered to patients who are morbidly obese, highly motivated, and well informed about the possible operative risks and long-term medical benefits. This patient has several indications for bariatric surgery, the most common of which is her BMI. Other factors, such as preexisting medical conditions and failure of conservative therapy, also may be considered. Age and long-term obesity are not major factors when selecting candidates for these bariatric procedures.

Calle EE, Thun MJ, Petrelli JM, Rodriguez C, Heath CW Jr. Body-mass index and mortality in a prospective cohort of US adults. N Engl J Med 1999;341:1097–105.

Flegal KM, Carroll MD, Kuezmarski RJ, Johnson CL. Overweight and obesity in the United State: prevalence and trends, 1960–1994. Int J Obes Relat Metab Disord 1998;22:39–47.

Rand CS, Macgregor AM, Hankins GC. Eating behavior after gastric bypass surgery for obesity. South Med J 1987;80:961–4.

Weintraub M, Sundaresen PR, Schuster B, Averbuch M, Stein EC, Cox C, et al. Long-term weight control study. IV (weeks 156–190). The second double-blind phase. Clin Pharmacol Ther 1992;51:608–14.

22

Evaluation of hyperprolactinemia

A 32-year-old woman, gravida 2, para, 2, presents with amenorrhea of 1-year duration. Initial laboratory studies reveal follicle-stimulating hormone level of 3 mIU/mL, thyroid-stimulating hormone (TSH) level of 2.1 µU/mL, and serum prolactin level of 55 ng/mL. As you consider additional laboratory testing, you perform a directed physical examination to look specifically for

    (A) reduced body hair
    (B) increased generalized adiposity
    (C) skin hypopigmentation
*   (D) acral changes
    (E) exophthalmos

The causes of hyperprolactinemia are diverse and can be categorized into physiologic, pharmacologic, and pathologic groups. The evaluation of hyperprolactinemia is ultimately directed toward determining whether or not a prolactinoma is present. Generally, a linear relationship exists between the prolactin level and presence and size of prolactinomas. Although most prolactinomas are identified in patients with prolactin levels greater than 100 ng/mL, imaging studies should be considered for patients with prolactin levels that are persistently higher than normal and cannot be explained by physiologic processes or pharmacologic agents. The goal for imaging studies is not only to identify the prolactinoma but also to rule out other potential central nervous system (CNS) causes of hyperprolactinemia.

The evaluation of women with hyperprolactinemia includes a comprehensive history to rule out potential physiologic or pharmacologic etiologies and a physical examination to discover specific pathologic processes associated with hyperprolactinemia. The physical examination is particularly important for patients with elevations of prolactin that are less than 100 ng/mL because it is in this range that most of the other causes of hyperprolactinemia will be identified. Physiologic processes and states and pharmacologic agents associated with hyperprolactinemia are shown in Box 22-1. Apart from pregnancy and the early stages of breastfeeding, most other physiologic processes are associated with only mild to (in rare instances) moderate temporary elevations of prolactin. An even more common cause of persistent hyperprolactinemia is a pharmacologic agent, such as those listed in the box.

A number of pathologic causes, other than prolactinomas, are associated with hyperprolactinemia. A directed physical examination after a complete history also may provide clues for these disease processes. Causes of hirsutism, not hair loss, are variably associated with prolactin excess and include polycystic ovary syndrome (PCOS) and Cushing's syndrome. Although most patients with PCOS have increased generalized obesity, it would be unlikely for them to present with a prolactin level of 55 ng/mL because less than 20% of them have hyperprolactinemia, and the prolactin level usually is just higher than the upper limit of normal. The obesity of Cushing's syndrome is centripetal, not generalized. Patients with Cushing's syndrome also may exhibit the physical find-

> **BOX 22-1**
>
> **Physiologic Processes and States and Pharmacologic Agents Associated With Hyperprolactinemia**
>
> **Physiologic Processes and States**
> - Pregnancy
> - Breastfeeding
> - Sleep
> - Hypoglycemia
> - Stress
> - Exercise
> - Orgasm
> - Nipple stimulation
>
> **Pharmacologic Causes**
> - Dopamine antagonists, eg, the phenothiazines, haloperidol, risperidone, metoclopramide, reserpine, methyldopa, amoxapine, and opioids.
> - Monoamine oxidase inhibitors, eg, cimetidine, verapamil, vasoactive intestinal peptide, cocaine, and, rarely, estrogen.

ings of facial (moon facies), supraclavicular, and dorsocervical (buffalo hump) fat pad accumulation; plethora; acne; epidermal atrophy with ecchymoses; and mucocutaneous fungal infections (eg, tinea versicolor). Hyperpigmentation, not hypopigmentation, is rare with Cushing's syndrome but common in individuals with the very rare ectopic adrenocorticotropic hormone syndrome. The fact that up to 85% of patients with Cushing's syndrome have hypertension is a reminder of the importance of obtaining vital signs in any patient with a potential systemic condition.

A number of CNS lesions other than prolactinomas are associated with hyperprolactinemia (ie, empty sella syndrome, meningiomas, gliomas, lymphoma, tuberculosis, sarcoidosis, and eosinophilic granuloma), but most are extremely rare. The most problematic are the nonprolactin secreting tumors, notably the craniopharyngioma and the growth hormone (GH) secreting tumor. The craniopharyngioma causes hyperprolactinemia infrequently and usually by pituitary stalk compression. It has a bimodal distribution of occurrence, in children and adolescents and then in adults after age 50–60 years, and, thus, would be rarely found in a 32-year-old woman.

Nevertheless, GH-secreting tumors can occur at any age and usually present in their fourth decade as in this patient. Approximately 15% of these tumors co-secrete excessive GH and prolactin, with prolactin levels usually being less than 100 ng/mL. These plurihormonal tumors present special treatment considerations compared with tumors that secrete GH alone. Patients may exhibit a number of features related to GH excess. A directed physical examination may identify the acral changes of acromegaly and other signs of bone, cartilage, or soft tissue overgrowth. Although acral specifically refers to those changes of the "peripheral parts," such as hands and fingers (Fig. 22-1; see color plate), feet, toes, and ears, periosteal new bone formation also is associated with the hypertrophy and enlargement of a number of other body structures, including the mandible, maxilla, frontal, and nasal bones. The coarsening of acral and facial features may result from soft tissue hypertrophy as much as bone changes. Oily skin and hyperhidrosis may be evident. A careful clinician may make the diagnosis of acromegaly by observing a very sweaty and enlarged hand on the initial handshake.

Although the most common tumor besides the prolactinoma that may be identified in a patient as presented here is the GH secreting adenoma, the most common endocrinopathy found in a patient who has hyperprolactinemia without tumor is hypothyroidism. This patient had a normal TSH level. Patients with hypothyroidism may be first identified with prolactin levels elevated in the 40–50 ng/mL range, although higher values may be present. A directed physical examination may identify features of hypothyroidism (ie, dry, cool, and rough skin; edematous face and hands; and slow pulse and reflexes). Many of these are soft findings that make the diagnosis one that often is missed by physical examination. Puffy eyes, not exophthalmos, and other signs of myxedema are late findings and are not seen in most patients who present with hypothyroidism.

Biller BM, Luciano A, Crosignani PG, Molitch M, Olive D, Rebar R, et al. Guidelines for the diagnosis and treatment of hyperprolactinemia. J Reprod Med 1999;44(suppl):1075–84.

De Marinis L, Zuppi P, Valle D, Mancini A, Bianchi A, Lauriola L, et al. A retrospective hormonal and immunohistochemical evaluation of 47 acromegalic patients: prognostic value of preoperative plasma prolactin. Horm Metab Res 2002;34:137–43.

Klibanski A, Zervas NT. Diagnosis and management of hormone-secreting pituitary adenomas. N Engl J Med 1991;324:822–31.

Kunwar S, Wilson CB. Pediatric pituitary adenomas. J Clin Endocrinol Metab 1999;845:4385–9.

Ross F, Nusynowitz ML. A syndrome of primary hypothyroidism, amenorrhea and galactorrhea. J Clin Endocrinol Metab 1968;28:591–5.

Teramoto A, Hirakawa K, Sanno N, Osamura Y. Incidental pituitary lesions in 1,000 unselected autopsy specimens. Radiology 1994;193:161–4.

23
Contraception in menopausal transition

A 41-year-old woman with symptoms of irregular vaginal bleeding, hot flushes, and dyspareunia is concerned about her risk for an unplanned pregnancy. She smokes 15 cigarettes per day and has a history of depression. She is self-conscious about her weight and is following a low-fat diet. The most convenient contraceptive method with the lowest failure rate for this woman is the

    (A) combination estrogen and progestin oral contraceptive
    (B) progestin-only oral contraceptives
    (C) intermittent injection of progestin, depot medroxyprogesterone acetate
* (D) progestin-releasing intrauterine device (IUD)
    (E) use of a diaphragm

During the menopausal transition, a woman must still use a reliable contraceptive method to prevent pregnancy because of her intermittent ovulatory cycles. For women who do not smoke cigarettes, the use of low-dose oral contraceptives prevents ovulation and vasomotor symptoms and provides cycle control. In one study, a 20 µg ethinyl estradiol oral contraceptive formulation not only prevented ovulation and vasomotor symptoms but further decreased bleeding severity and improved the patient's quality of life. The use of low-dose oral contraceptives is not an option for individuals who smoke cigarettes and are older than 35 years. These women are at increased risk for myocardial infarction and stroke.

The barrier method or progestin-only medication provide reasonable options for women who smoke cigarettes, but both methods have disadvantages. Among women who use a diaphragm with spermicide, approximately 16% experience an unintended pregnancy within the first year of use. When using progestin-only oral contraceptives, the failure rate is 8%, which is higher than any other progestin-only method, because the dose of medication fails to consistently inhibit ovulation. Progestin-only oral contraceptive use also is accompanied by the side effect of irregular vaginal bleeding. Use of depot medroxyprogesterone acetate is more convenient because it is administered every 12 weeks and inhibits ovulation, but it is associated with some depression and weight gain. It is associated with a failure rate of 3% in the first year of use.

The best option for this patient would be a progestin-releasing IUD. The progestin-releasing IUD appears to minimize side effects while providing the lowest failure rate. In typical use, approximately 0.1% of women experience an unintended pregnancy during the first year of use with the progestin-releasing IUD. In one study of 165 reproductive-aged women who used the levonorgestrel-releasing intrauterine system for a period of 3 years, 98% had a change in their menstrual bleeding pattern. Cessation or transient absence of menses occurred in 47% and 9% of the women, respectively. In this study, 33% of the women were aged 41 years or older.

American College of Obstetricians and Gynecologists. The use of hormonal contraception in women with coexisting medical conditions. ACOG Practice Bulletin 18. Washington, DC: ACOG; 2000.

Baldaszti E, Wimmer-Puchinger B, Loschke K. Acceptability of the long-term contraceptive levonorgestrel-releasing intraterine system (Mirena[R]): a 3-year follow-up study. Contraception 2003;67:87–91.

Casper RF, Dodin S, Reid RL. The effect of 20 µg ethinyl estradiol/1 mg norethindrone acetate (Minestrin[TM]), a low-dose oral contraceptive, on vaginal bleeding patterns, hot flashes, and quality of life in symptomatic perimenopausal women. Menopause 1997;4:139–47.

Hatcher RA, Nelson AL, Zieman M, Darney PD, Creinin MD, Stosur HR, et al. A pocket guide to managing contraception. Tiger (GA): Bridging the Gap Foundation; 2002. p. 36.

Schiff I, Bell WR, Davis V, Kessler CM, Meyers C, Nakajima S, et al. Oral contraceptives and smoking, current considerations: recommendations of a consensus panel. Am J Obstet Gynecol 1999;180: S383–4.

24

Surgical therapy for the bicornuate uterus

A 38-year-old woman, gravida 2, comes in for evaluation. She has had 2 first-trimester pregnancy losses that occurred at 6 and 8 weeks of gestation. The patient's family history is negative for thromboembolic events and infertility. Her lupus anticoagulant and anticardiolipin test results are negative. A hysterosalpingogram performed after her last pregnancy loss is as shown (Fig. 24-1). You recommend a laparoscopy and possible hysteroscopy and inform her that if a bicornuate uterus is discovered, you will

(A) perform a hysterectomy
(B) perform a uterine unification procedure
(C) remove one of the uterine horns
* (D) perform a laparoscopy only

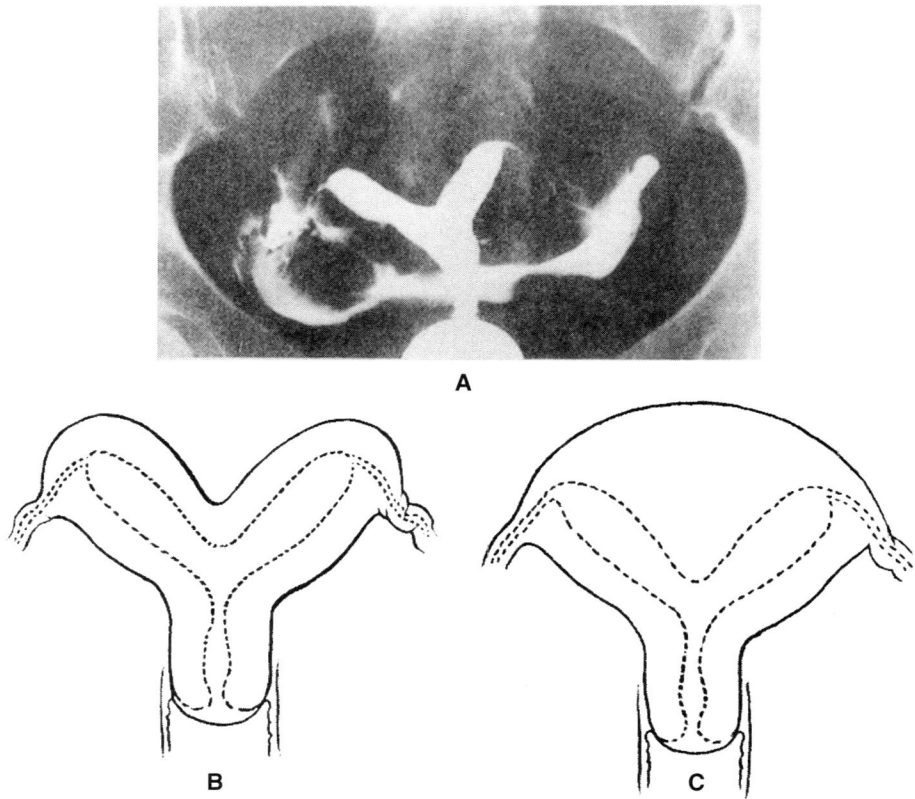

FIG. 24-1. A. Hysterosalpingogram of a uterine cavity consistent with either a septate uterus (class V) or a bicornuate uterus (class V). **B.** Drawing of a bicornuate uterus. **C.** Drawing of a septate uterus. Direct visualization is required to distinguish them. (Adeshi EY, Rock JA, Rozenwaks Z, eds. Reproductive endocrinology, surgery, and technology. Vol. 2. Philadelphia [PA]: Lippincott-Raven; 1996. p. 2152.)

Recurrent first-trimester pregnancy loss occurs in approximately 1% of reproductive-aged women. A definitive cause for such losses can be established in approximately 50% of these couples. A generally accepted definition of recurrent pregnancy loss is 2 or more consecutive pregnancy losses.

Congenital uterine anomalies are associated with second-trimester pregnancy loss and fetal malpresentation and have been demonstrated in 10–15% of women with recurrent pregnancy loss, with the predominant finding of a septate uterus. A bicornuate uterus is most commonly associated with late second-trimester or early third-trimester delivery as well as fetal malpresentation. First-trimester miscarriage is more common with bicornuate uteri, but it is an uncommon cause for repeated first-trimester pregnancy loss.

Hysterectomy can be considered in the patient with rudimentary fibrotic uteri that typically do not support menstruation or when there is obstructive symptomatology. It would not be appropriate in this patient.

Uterine unification procedures are typically performed via laparotomy and have the potential side effects of significant blood loss and postoperative infection (Fig. 24-2). Historically, these procedures (Strassman metroplasty, Tompkins metroplasty) were performed in women with uterine anomalies and poor reproductive histories. However, such procedures are rarely indicated in cases of first-trimester pregnancy loss. Women must undergo cesarean delivery following these procedures.

Removal of a rudimentary horn is indicated if the horn is obstructed and the patient is symptomatic or in cases of rupture associated with a pregnancy. Removal of one of this patient's horns would not be appropriate.

In cases where the only finding is that of a bicornuate uterus, the recommendation is to defer surgical correction. All other possible etiologies for a poor reproductive history must be ruled out (ie, balanced translocation in the parents, maternal age, antiphospholipid syndrome).

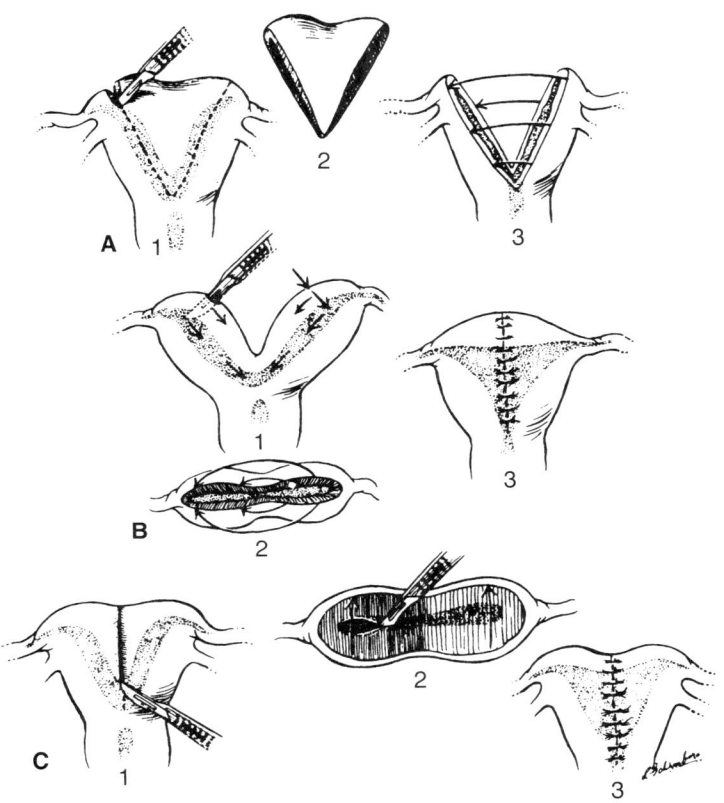

FIG. 24-2. A. Diagram of wedge resection method of repair of a septate uterus. **B.** Strassmann technique for repair of a bicornuate uterus. **C.** Tompkins metroplasty repair of a septate uterus. (Adeshi EY, Rock JA, Rozenwaks Z, eds. Reproductive endocrinology, surgery, and technology. Vol. 2. Philadelphia (PA): Lippincott-Raven; 1996. p. 2158.)

Acien P. Reproductive performance of women with uterine malformations. Hum Reprod 1993;8:122–6.

American College of Obstetricians and Gynecologists. Management of recurrent pregnancy early pregnancy loss. American College of Obstetricians and Gynecologists Practice Bulletin 24. Washington, DC: ACOG; 2001.

Centers for Disease Control and Prevention, American Society for Reproductive Medicine, Society for Assisted Reproductive Technology, RESOLVE 1999 Assisted Reproductive Technology Success Rates. Atlanta (GA): Centers for Disease Control and Prevention; 2001.

Empson M, Lassere M, Craig JC, Scott JR. Recurrent pregnancy loss with antiphospholipid antibody: a systematic review of therapeutic trials. Obstet Gynecol 2002;99:135–44.

Ogasawara M, Kajiura S, Katano K, Aoyama T, Aoki K. Are serum progesterone levels predictive of recurrent miscarriage in future pregnancies? Fertil Steril 1997;68:806–9.

Strassman EO. Fertility and unification of double uterus. Fertil Steril 1966;17:165–76.

25

Treatment-related complications of uterine arterial embolization

A 39-year-old woman undergoes uterine artery embolization for a 16-week gestation size uterus with intramural myomas. Several hours after the procedure, she develops severe pelvic pain, cramping, and a low-grade fever. The next best step in her management is

    (A) blood cultures
* (B) hospital observation with analgesia
    (C) pelvic magnetic resonance imaging (MRI) study
    (D) dilation and curettage
    (E) total abdominal hysterectomy

The value of vascular embolization in uncontrollable hemorrhage in obstetric emergencies and gynecologic oncology is well recognized. Non-emergent selective uterine arterial embolization for myomas is an extension of this technique. Absolute and relative contraindications to uterine arterial embolization have evolved as familiarity and long-term follow-up with the procedure is continually updated and evaluated. Active genital infection, undiagnosed vaginal bleeding, and iodine contrast allergy are considered absolute contraindications to uterine arterial embolization. Some practitioners who perform uterine arterial embolization consider as contraindications uterine size greater than 20 cm, submucosal and pedunculated subserosal myomas, multiple myomas, and desire for future conception.

Patient satisfaction scores are high after the procedure. However, some patients experience "postembolization syndrome" characterized by general malaise, low-grade fever, pelvic pain, nausea, and leukocytosis. The syndrome, which is pronounced during the first 24 hours postprocedure and regresses over the next several days, is presumed to result from transient fibroid and uterine ischemia.

Severe ischemic injury to the uterus, a potential outcome of the procedure, occurs in only 1–2% of patients. Postprocedure overnight in-hospital observation of patients with intravenous analgesia often is required. Clinical differentiation from septic uterine necrosis may be difficult. Pelvic MRI may demonstrate air bubbles within the uterine abscess, but this is not an immediate finding. Although a dilation and curettage would be of little value, exploratory laparotomy with hysterectomy may be prudent if the pain persists in duration and intensity. Two other complications of the procedure include premature ovarian failure, possibly the result of compromised arterial blood supply to the ovaries, and spontaneous passage of a necrotic fibroid.

Comparative complication rates from women who have undergone uterine arterial embolization, myomectomy, and hysterectomy appear to be similar. Women who have uterine arterial embolization are more likely to need further invasive treatment (repeat uterine arterial embolization or surgery) in the 3–5 years after the index procedure than women who undergo myomectomy.

Broder MS, Goodwin S, Chen G, Tang LJ, Costantino MM, Nguyen MH, et al. Comparison of long-term outcomes of myomectomy and uterine artery embolization. Obstet Gynecol 2002;100:864–8.

Hutchins F, Worthinton-Kinsch R, Berkowitz R. Selective uterine artery embolization as primary treatment for symptomatic leiomyomata uteri. J Am Assoc Gynecol Laparosc 1999;6:279–84.

Schwartz ML, Klein A, McLucas B. Uterine artery embolization to treat fibroids. Contemporary Ob/Gyn 2001;8:14–37.

Spies JB, Roth AR, Jha RC, Gomez-Jorge J, Levy EB, Chang TC, et al. Leiomyomata treated with uterine artery embolization: factors associated with successful symptoms and imaging outcome. Radiology 2002;222:45–52.

Spies JB, Spector A, Roth AR, Baker CM, Mauro L, Murphy-Skrynarz K. Complications after uterine artery embolization for leiomyomas. Obstet Gynecol 2002;100:873–80.

Vashisht A, Studd J, Carey A, Burn P. Fatal septicaemia after fibroid embolisation. Lancet 1999;354:307–8.

26

Migraines and hormone contraception

A 33-year-old woman comes in for advice regarding her current oral contraceptive therapy. She has a medical history significant for type 2 diabetes mellitus, migraines with focal neurologic signs, hypertension, and menorrhagia. Recently, she had a breast biopsy, which revealed a fibroadenoma. She tells you that she has a family history of breast cancer. Her diabetes and hypertension are well controlled. Her physical examination is remarkable for a 14-week irregular uterus consistent with leiomyomata. In this patient's medical history, the most compelling reason to discontinue oral contraceptive use is

    (A) diabetes mellitus
* (B) migraine headaches with focal neurologic signs
    (C) hypertension
    (D) leiomyomata
    (E) breast disease and family history of breast cancer

For women with co-existing medical conditions or other special circumstances, the risks and benefits of oral contraceptive therapy must be carefully evaluated before use. There are a number of absolute and relative contraindications to the use of oral contraceptives (Box 26-1 and 26-2). Decisions regarding the use of oral contraceptives in the presence of co-existing medical conditions are difficult. Contraceptive researchers have established the increased safety and benefits of various contraceptive choices in women with medical conditions that until recently were contraindications for their use.

Diabetes mellitus is not a contraindication to oral contraceptive treatment, but some women with diabetes may need a small increase in insulin dose. In theory, oral contraceptives may impair carbohydrate metabolism and accelerate the occurrence of vascular disease in women with diabetes mellitus. The current low-dose oral contraceptives do not seem to have this effect. However, the use of oral contraceptives in women with diabetes mellitus should be limited to women who are nonsmokers; younger than 35 years; and in good health without evidence of diabetic sequelae, such as cardiovascular disease, retinopathy, and vascular disease.

Evidence is growing that migraines increase ischemic stroke risk but not the risk of hemorrhagic stroke and that this risk is higher in migraines with aura than in migraines without aura. Oral contraceptives also increase stroke risk. The increased stroke risk attributable to migraines and oral contraceptive therapy may be additive. The risk of ischemic stroke in young women is very low and likely remains acceptably low in young women with migraines without aura or focal neurologic signs when oral contraceptives are prescribed. The presence of a

---

BOX 26-1

Absolute Contraindications to Oral Contraceptive Therapy*

- Previous thromboembolic event or stroke
- Active liver disease
- History of cholestatic jaundice
- Uncontrolled hypertension
- History of an estrogen-dependent tumor
- Breast cancer
- Undiagnosed uterine bleeding
- Pregnancy

*Patients with contraindications to oral contraceptive therapy should be counseled. An alternative form of contraception should be offered to patients with these medical conditions.

BOX 26-2

Relative Contraindications to Oral Contraceptive Therapy*

- Cardiovascular disease
- Hypertension
- Dyslipidemia
- Tobacco use if older than 35 years
- Active gallbladder disease
- Sickle cell anemia
- Migraine headaches
- Diabetes mellitus
- Systemic lupus erythematosus
- Hypertriglyceridemia
- Diabetic neuropathy or retinopathy

*The risks and benefits of hormonal contraception must be weighed before starting oral contraceptive therapy. Many patients with relative contraindications may use the current low-dose oral contraceptives. Patients must be carefully monitored for disease progression.

complex or prolonged migraine aura, or of additional stroke risk factors (eg, increased age, smoking, and hypertension), likely increases the ischemic stroke risk further in patients with migraines when oral contraceptives are prescribed. Thus, the presence of migraine with focal neurologic signs in this woman would be the most compelling reason that would preclude her from taking oral contraceptives.

The use of oral contraceptives should be carefully considered in women with poorly controlled hypertension. The appropriate candidate for such use would be a woman younger than 35 years with well-controlled hypertension who is otherwise healthy. If the woman's blood pressure remains well controlled, the use of oral contraceptives can be continued.

Oral contraceptives have several well-established benefits. Menorrhagia and dysmenorrhea are both ameliorated with use of oral contraceptives. Several large epidemiologic studies have observed that oral contraceptive use does not induce the growth or worsen the symptoms of leiomyomata. In fact, oral contraceptives have been found to reduce menorrhagia associated with a leiomyomatous uterus.

In general population samples, oral contraceptives have been observed to be weakly associated with the risk of breast cancer up to 10 years after a woman discontinues use. Much less is known, however, regarding the association between oral contraceptives and breast neoplasms among women with a familial predisposition to breast cancer. There is little or no evidence associating a family history of breast cancer with increased risks for use of oral contraceptives. Likewise, there is no evidence for an increased risk of breast cancer associated with use of oral contraceptives after 1975 in first-degree relatives or second-degree relatives. No data have shown that women with benign breast disease who take oral contraceptives are at an increased risk for malignancy. Therefore, a positive family history of breast cancer or a history of benign breast disease should not be considered a contraindication to taking oral contraceptives. In fact, oral contraceptives decrease the incidence of benign breast and ovarian disease as well as endometrial and ovarian cancer.

American College of Obstetricians and Gynecologists. The use of hormonal contraception in women with coexisting medical conditions. ACOG Practice Bulletin 18. Washington, DC: ACOG; 2000.

Breast cancer and hormonal contraceptives: collaborative reanalysis of individual data on 53,297 women with breast cancer and 100,239 women without breast cancer from 54 epidemiological studies. Collaborative Group on Hormonal Factors in Breast Cancer. Lancet 1996;347:1713–27.

Chang CL, Donaghy M, Poulter N. Migraine and stroke in young women: case-control study. The World Health Organisation Collaborative Study of Cardiovascular Disease and Steroid Hormone Contraception. BMJ 1999;318:13–8.

Grabrick DM, Hartmann LC, Cerhan JR, Vierkant RA, Therneau TM, Vachon CM, et al. Risk of breast cancer with oral contraceptive use in women with a family history of breast cancer. JAMA 2000;284:1791–8.

Marshall LM, Spiegelman D, Goldman MB, Manson JE, Colditz GA, Barbieri RL, et al. A prospective study of reproductive factors and oral contraceptive use in relation to the risk of uterine leiomyomata. Fertil Steril 1998;70:432–9.

27
Selective estrogen receptor modulators in osteoporosis

A 65-year-old woman comes in for her annual examination. She has vaginal dryness and burning during and after intercourse. Her pelvic examination shows a pale, pink, thinned vulva and absence of rugation of the vaginal mucosa. The remainder of her physical examination is normal. She had a normal mammogram and Pap test result 1 year ago. A cholesterol profile performed this year revealed a total cholesterol level of 236 mg/dL, high-density lipoprotein (HDL) cholesterol level of 35 mg/dL, low-density lipoprotein (LDL) cholesterol level of 156 mg/dL, very LDL cholesterol level of 45 mg/dL, and triglyceride level of 278 mg/dL. Her thyroid-stimulating hormone level was 3.3 µU/mL and thyroxine level was 9.8 mg/dL. A dual-energy X-ray absorptiometry (DXA) screening test showed T-scores of -1.2 at the spine and -1.3 at the hip. She takes a multivitamin, 1,500 mg of calcium, and 800 IU of vitamin D daily. The most appropriate management of this patient is

  (A) vaginal lubricant
  (B) alendronate sodium (Fosamax)
  (C) oral estrogen-progestin therapy
  (D) raloxifene hydrochloride (Evista)
* (E) low-dose vaginal estrogen

This patient is approximately 15 years postmenopausal and is not taking estrogen therapy. She reports symptoms related to long-term hypoestrogenic changes in the vulvar and vaginal tissues. She appears to be a compliant patient, and her preventive screening tests indicate normal mammogram, Pap test, and bone density test results. Her lipoprotein profile is abnormal with an increase in total cholesterol level, low HDL cholesterol level, high LDL cholesterol level, and high triglyceride level. These values indicate that she is at increased risk for cardiovascular disease.

Her most immediate concern is the vaginal dryness and burning associated with intercourse and continued sexual activity. The use of vaginal lubricants may reduce the vaginal dryness but may not significantly alter the vaginal burning. This latter symptom may be related to microabrasions and microtears that can arise following intercourse in women with thin vaginal mucosa. The use of localized vaginal estrogen will induce an increase in thickening of vulvar and vaginal epithelium over a 6–8-week period. Studies suggest that the use of localized vaginal estrogen in small amounts (ie, micronized estradiol, Vagifem, or the estradiol ring, Estring), as recommended by the U.S. Food and Drug Administration (FDA), will not appreciably increase systemic estrogen levels but will provide a suitable local vaginal epithelial effect. Many of the commonly used vaginal estrogen preparations provide detectable systemic estrogen levels even in patients with long durations of use.

Nonmodifiable and potentially modifiable risk factors for osteoporosis are summarized in Appendix C. The bisphosphonate, alendronate, is an effective agent for prevention of osteoporosis. However, the bone density changes from the DXA scan show mild osteopenia at the spine and hip sites (defined as a T-score of greater than -1 and less than -2.5). The National Osteoporosis Foundation has recommended medical therapy for prevention and treatment of osteoporosis for individuals without risk factors when the T-score is less than -2 or less than -1.5 in individuals who have associated risk factors. The use of alendronate would not address this patient's immediate symptoms.

The patient is currently taking a daily multivitamin containing 1,500 mg of calcium and 800 IU of vitamin D. Such daily administration can be effective in reducing bone loss in patients who are in the mid to late menopause.

Oral estrogen therapy is a less viable option in this patient. Recent findings from the Women's Health Initiative trial suggest that estrogen and progestin use may be associated with slightly increased incidences of cardiovascular events and breast cancer. Currently, the FDA and the American College of Obstetricians and Gynecologists recommend that oral estrogen therapy be limited to use for vasomotor symptoms and as an alternative medication for osteoporosis prevention and treatment. In this patient, who is asymptomatic with regard to vasomotor symptoms, her genital atrophy would respond to systemic estrogen but local estrogen therapy would provide similar efficacy. The risk–benefit ratio would need to be discussed carefully and documented before considering oral estrogen therapy.

Raloxifene hydrochloride (Evista) is a selective estrogen receptor modulator (SERM) that is approved by the FDA at a dose of 60 mg per day for prevention and treatment of osteoporosis. Selective estrogen receptor modulators are unique compounds that have the ability to compete with estradiol for binding at estrogen receptor sites. The class of compounds include raloxifene, tamoxifen citrate (Nolvadex), and clomiphene citrate (Clomid, Serophene).

In the presence of high estradiol levels, SERMs function as antiestrogens by competing with estrogen for estrogen receptor binding sites. At lower estrogen levels, such as during menopause, SERMs bind to estrogen receptor sites. However, the raloxifene-bound estrogen receptor results in a slightly altered receptor conformation. Thus, in tissues such as bone and liver, raloxifene-bound estrogen receptors can effectively bind estrogen response elements and induce estrogenlike changes. The estrogenlike properties of raloxifene include antiresorptive effects on bone turnover, an increased risk of venous thrombotic disorders, and a modest 6–11% decrease in total and LDL cholesterol levels.

In other tissues (eg, breast, endometrium, and hypothalamus), raloxifene induces antiestrogenic effects. Such effects include a potential antiproliferative effect on breast tissue, an absence of endometrial growth, and a potential increase in hot flushes in patients taking raloxifene.

Clinical trials in patients with advanced osteoporosis and vertebral fractures, such as the Multiple Outcomes of Raloxifene Evaluation Trial (MORE), show that raloxifene is effective at reducing the overall incidence of vertebral fractures. On the basis of the MORE trial, raloxifene was approved for prevention and treatment of osteoporosis. This study failed to demonstrate a reduced incidence of hip fractures in the treatment group; however, the study was not adequately powered to examine this endpoint. Other findings suggest that raloxifene may be effective in reducing the risk of breast cancer, but the study lacked sufficient power to draw this conclusion. An ongoing clinical trial, the Study of Tamoxifen and Raloxifene trial, will assess the efficacy of tamoxifen versus raloxifene in reducing breast cancer risk in women at high risk for breast cancer. Another ongoing clinical trial, the Raloxifene Use for the Heart study, will assess the efficacy of raloxifene versus placebo in reducing the risk of coronary disease events. The use of raloxifene would not be helpful at this time for management of the patient under discussion.

Cummings SR, Eckert S, Krueger KA, Grady D, Powles TJ, Cauley JA, et al. The effect of raloxifene on risk of breast cancer in postmenopausal women: results from the MORE randomized trial. Multiple Outcomes of Raloxifene Evaluation. JAMA 1999;281:2189–97.

Delmas PD, Bjarnason NH, Mitlak BH, Ravoux AC, Shah AS, Huster WJ, et al. Effects of raloxifene on bone mineral density, serum cholesterol concentrations, and uterine endometrium in postmenopausal women. Multiple Outcomes of Raloxifene Evaluation Investigators. N Engl J Med 1997;337:1641–7.

Ettinger B, Black DM, Mitlak BH, Knickerbocker RK, Nickelsen T, Genant HK, et al. Reduction of vertebral fracture risk in postmenopausal women with osteoporosis treated with raloxifene: results from a 3-year randomized clinical trial. JAMA 1999;282:637–45.

Fisher B, Constantino JP, Wickerham DL, Redmond CK, Kavanah M, Cronin WM, et al. Tamoxifen for prevention of breast cancer: report of the National Surgical Adjuvant Breast and Bowel Project P-1 Study. J Natl Cancer Inst 1998;90:1371–88.

Rossouw JE, Anderson GL, Prentice RL, LaCroix AZ, Kooperberg C, Stefanick ML, et al. Risks and benefits of estrogen plus progestin in healthy postmenopausal women: principal results from the Women's Health Initiative randomized controlled trial. Writing Group for the Women's Health Initiative Investigators. JAMA 2002;288:321–33.

28
Late-onset adrenal hyperplasia and nonclassic congenital adrenal hyperplasia

A 19-year-old Hispanic woman with a history of hepatitis comes in for management of hirsutism present since puberty that has become more severe despite therapy with oral contraceptives. She has dark facial hair on the sides of her face, upper lip, and chin. She has neither acanthosis nigricans nor clitoromegaly. Her dehydroepiandrosterone sulfate (DHEAS), serum testosterone, and androstenedione levels are at the upper limits of normal. Thyroid-stimulating hormone and prolactin concentrations are normal. Her basal 17α-hydroxyprogesterone level is 230 ng/dL. Following administration of corticotropin, her 17α-hydroxyprogesterone level increases to 510 ng/dL. The next best step in management is to continue OCs and prescribe

      (A) flutamide
*   (B) spironolactone
      (C) finasteride
      (D) gonadotropin-releasing hormone (GnRH) agonist

Polycystic ovary syndrome (PCOS) is the most common cause for androgen excess. Hirsutism occurs in approximately 70–80% of women with androgen excess but may not be apparent in women of Asian extraction. The steps that should be taken to establish the etiology of hirsutism start with examination of the patient to confirm the presence of coarse, terminal hairs in a malelike pattern. Thereafter, an evaluation of the patient's hormonal status should provide information regarding etiology. In most women with PCOS, circulating androgen (DHEAS, testosterone, and androstenedione) concentrations are within the normal range or at the upper limit of normal as seen in this patient.

In the evaluation of women with hirsutism, various disorders should be excluded, including thyroid dysfunction, hyperprolactinemia, nonclassic congenital adrenal hyperplasia (CAH), the hyperandrogenic insulin-resistant acanthosis nigricans syndrome, and adrenal tumor. In the latter case, serum testosterone levels usually are in the normal male range and commonly exceed 200 ng/dL. Nonclassic CAH can be eliminated by determination of the basal concentration of 17α-hydroxyprogesterone during the follicular phase of the ovarian cycle. If the basal 17α-hydroxyprogesterone level is higher than 200 ng/dL, the patient should undergo an acute adrenal stimulation test to identify nonclassic CAH. This can be accomplished by the intravenous administration of 0.25 mg of adrenocorticotropin hormone-(1-24) (Cortrosyn) followed by determination of serum concentration of 17α-hydroxyprogesterone. If the concentration of 17α-hydroxyprogesterone 30–60 minutes following administration of Cortrosyn exceeds 1,000 ng/dL (and commonly 1,500 ng/dL), a diagnosis of nonclassic CAH can be made.

Because this patient has a basal concentration of 17α-hydroxyprogesterone of 230 ng/dL, an adrenal stimulation test is warranted. Her response to Cortrosyn administration demonstrates an increase in 17α-hydroxyprogesterone concentration to 510 ng/dL that effectively eliminates nonclassic CAH as a diagnosis. Because her serum testosterone, DHEAS, and androstenedione levels are normal, adrenal tumor also can be eliminated. This patient has had hirsutism since puberty. It appears that she has PCOS.

The appropriate management of hirsutism should include androgen suppression, blockade of peripheral androgen action, and mechanical amelioration or destruction of unwanted hair. Androgen suppression and peripheral androgen blockade should proceed simultaneously and once androgen levels are under good control, elimination of the unwanted hair can proceed.

Treatment with OCs should be the initial step in the management of hirsutism for most women unless there is a contraindication to their use. Oral contraceptives suppress circulating luteinizing hormone and follicle-stimulating hormone concentrations and lead to diminished ovarian androgen production. They also are associated with decreased adrenal androgen production observed as decreased DHEAS concentrations. The progestin in OCs may antagonize 5α-reductase and compete for androgen receptors. In addition, estrogen in the OCs increases sex hormone-binding globulin levels and, therefore, decreases free testosterone levels. Oral contraceptives provide a cost-effective initial step for the treatment of this patient.

When OCs alone have failed to improve hirsutism, additional therapy is warranted. Further suppression of androgen production or androgen receptor blockade may be accomplished by the additional administration of other medications. Flutamide (Eulexin) is an androgen receptor blocker approved by the U.S. Food and Drug Administration (FDA) as adjuvant treatment for prostate cancer. It is effective for the management of women with hirsutism at doses of 500 mg daily, although a single dose of 250 mg per day may be effective in some patients. Side effects include excessive dryness of skin or scalp hair, the appearance of greenish urine, liver enzyme abnormalities, and, rarely, fatal hepatotoxicity. Because of its potential for serious side effects, flutamide would not be the best choice for this patient who has a history of hepatitis.

Spironolactone is an aldosterone antagonist and a mild diuretic. It competes with androgens for the androgen receptor, 5α-reductase, and sex hormone-binding globulin, and inhibits 5α-reductase directly. Spironolactone is an effective agent for reducing hirsutism. Although daily doses of 100 mg per day usually are effective for the management of hirsutism, higher doses (200–300 mg per day) may be used. Patients should start at a dose of 100 mg twice daily. If the dose is slowly increased by 25 mg per day in a progressive fashion over 3 weeks, side effects are minimal. The most common side effects include dyspepsia, nausea, polyuria, nocturia, fatigue, headache, ovulatory changes, breast tenderness, decreased libido, hypersensitivity to the sun, and atopic reactions. Patients with hypertension who are already taking a potassium-saving diuretic have been reported rarely to develop hyperkalemia. Spironolactone is inexpensive, has few side effects, and is very effective when used in combination with OCs. Because spironolactone theoretically might cause feminization of male infants, it should not be administered to women of reproductive age without OCs. It would be the next best step in the management of this patient.

Finasteride is a 5α-reductase inhibitor approved by the FDA for the treatment of benign prostatic hyperplasia. It is useful for the management of hirsutism in women at doses of 5 mg per day, although it may be less effective than the androgen receptor blockers. It has the least side effects of the drugs used for hirsutism. Finasteride also has the potential to cause feminization of male infants. However, there is much less clinical experience with the use of finasteride than with spironolactone. Thus, for a woman of childbearing age, such as this patient, finasteride would not be the best choice.

Long-acting GnRH agonists have been found to be useful in ameliorating hirsutism and may be required to suppress the hypothalamic–pituitary–ovarian axis in severely androgenized patients. Treatment for 2–3 months may be required before the full suppressive effect is observed. Treatment with a GnRH agonist should be combined with estrogen–progestin therapy or an OC and an androgen blocker. Because of the expense involved in treatment with a GnRH agonist, this should be used only when other more cost-effective treatments have been tried and proved unsuccessful.

Azziz R. The evaluation and management of hirsutism. Obstet Gynecol 2003;101:995–1007.

Rittmaster RS. Clinical review 73: Medical treatment of androgen-dependent hirsutism. J Clin Endocrinol Metab 1995;80:2559–63.

Waggoner W, Boots LR, Azziz R. Total testosterone and DHEAS levels as predictors of androgen-secreting neoplasms: a populational study. Gynecol Endocrinol 1999;13:394–400.

29

Management of ruptured endometrioma

A 32-year-old nulligravid woman seeks consultation because of a 1-year history of progressively worsening pelvic pain. She refuses therapy with a gonadotropin-releasing hormone agonist. Pelvic examination reveals fullness in the right adnexa, a retroverted uterus, and cul-de-sac tenderness, particularly when palpating the uterosacral ligaments. An ultrasound examination is done and the findings are shown in Fig. 29-1 (see color plate). The best treatment for this patient is

    (A) oophorectomy
    (B) irrigation of the cyst cavity
    (C) evacuation and cautery of the cyst
*   (D) excision of the endometrioma

Endometriomas have a very characteristic appearance on ultrasound. A hypoechoic area has been described in 82% of surgically proven endometriomas. Although this finding is not pathognomonic, the surgeon should have a high suspicion for an endometrioma in this case and be prepared to deal with it at surgery.

In a young patient who desires future fertility, ovarian preservation is preferable to oophorectomy. Even when relatively large cysts are present, there is normal ovarian cortex with abundant oocytes present in the ovarian tissue adjacent to the cyst wall. Thus, oophorectomy would not be the first choice in this case.

Removal of the endometrioma by cystectomy consists of peeling the cyst wall from the affected ovary. This necessitates familiarity with operative laparoscopic technique. The cyst wall may peel free from the ovary easier if it can be loosened from the normal ovarian cortex by filling the cyst cavity with irrigant (saline), then evacuating the irrigant and repeating this several times. The cyst wall is then grasped with one instrument, the normal appearing ovarian cortex with another, and the cyst wall is twisted and peeled off the ovary. Bleeding can occur and should be managed with prudent use of bipolar cautery. This technique appears preferable to drainage of the chocolate appearing fluid and bipolar coagulation of the cyst wall. In a randomized study of 64 patients with 1 of these 2 treatments, patients with excision had significantly lower rates of dysmenorrhea, deep dyspareunia, nonmenstrual pain, and a higher rate of pregnancy than patients with drainage and coagulation.

For surgeons who are inexperienced with ovarian cystectomy, copious irrigation of the base of the endometrioma and cautery of the base and postsurgical treatment is recommended. Drainage of the endometrioma followed by ovarian suppression has proved effective. If drainage of an endometrioma is carried out without ovarian suppression, this can lead to quick recurrence of the cyst and may promote the formation of pelvic adhesions.

Beretta P, Franchi M, Ghezzi F, Busacca M, Zupi E, Bolis P. Randomized clinical trial of two laparoscopic treatments of endometriomas: cystectomy versus drainage and coagulation. Fertil Steril 1998;70:1176–80.

Donnez J, Nisolle M, Gillerot S, Anaf V, Clerckx-Braun F, Casanas-Roux F. Ovarian endometrial cysts: the role of gonadotropin-releasing hormone agonist and/or drainage. Fertil Steril 1994;62:63–6.

Kupfer MC, Schwimer SR, Lebovic J. Transvaginal sonographic appearance of endometriomata: spectrum of findings. J Ultrasound Med 1992;11:129–33.

Muzii L, Marana R, Caruana P, Catalano GF, Mancuso S. Laparoscopic findings after transvaginal ultrasound-guided aspiration of ovarian endometriomas. Hum Reprod 1995;10:2902–3.

30
Diagnosis of ectopic pregnancy

A 25-year-old woman, gravida 3, para 0, with history of 2 previous miscarriages and unexplained secondary infertility, conceives after her second cycle of clomiphene citrate (Clomid, Serophene) with intrauterine insemination. The patient had an initial normal increase in her serum β-hCG levels and then a plateau at 2,500 mIU/mL at 6 weeks of gestation. She reports pelvic cramping and vaginal spotting. Which of the following ultrasound scans would be most consistent with this clinical scenario?

(A) 12-Week intrauterine pregnancy
* (B) Pseudogestational sac with an adnexal mass
(C) Molar pregnancy
(D) Sonohysterogram demonstrating an endometrial polyp

Ectopic pregnancy continues to be a leading cause of maternal mortality in the first trimester of pregnancy. Current advanced diagnostic technology that uses serum β-hCG along with transvaginal ultrasonography has made early detection possible. This technology can facilitate medical therapy with tubal preservation and, thus, avoid surgical intervention except in more advanced cases. A delay in diagnosis of ectopic pregnancy, however, can lead to complications, such as acute tubal rupture with severe anemia, that can be life threatening. Accurate diagnosis of ectopic pregnancies is essential for proper timely management.

The increase in serum β-hCG levels often is correlated with the appearance of a gestational sac within the uterine cavity. This essentially rules out the possibility of an ectopic gestation. There is always a risk of heterotopic pregnancy where 2 developing gestations co-exist. In the general population, the risk of intrauterine pregnancy with a concurrent ectopic gestation is 1 in 40,000 pregnancies. With the use of fertility treatments, this risk increases to 1–3%.

However, the presence of a pseudogestational sac can confuse the clinician and delay diagnosis. This term was first introduced by Mueller in 1979 when he described a decidual reaction within the uterus that was misinterpreted as a normal gestational sac. In actuality, this finding was caused by a hyperplastic endometrium or decidual cast with an anechoic central blood collection. Studies have shown its incidence ranges from 2% to 20% of ectopic pregnancies.

A pseudogestational sac associated with an ectopic pregnancy differs from the normal intrauterine pregnancy in the following ways:

• Pseudogestational sac is an endometrial decidual reaction in response to the ectopic pregnancy
• The sac is located centrally and has a symmetrical appearance
• An anechoic central blood collection without fetal pole or cardiac activity is seen

The normal gestational sac, on the other hand, has a sonolucent center surrounded by an echogenic "double ring" and may exhibit an eccentrically placed gestational sac with an asymmetrical pattern.

The plateauing hCG levels in this clinical scenario concern an early pregnancy complication. The most appropriate choice of the ultrasounds listed is that of the pseudogestational sac accompanied by an adnexal mass (choice C). Rather than a normal gestational sac with chorionic villi, there is an anechoic blood collection inside a decidual cast, which raises the suspicion of an ectopic pregnancy. Notice there is no echogenic ring noted or presence of a fetal pole. A normal gestational sac should be visualized by most transvaginal ultrasonograms with a β-hCG level higher than 2,000 mIU/mL. To confirm an ectopic pregnancy in this patient, a dilation and curettage should be considered.

Although the absence of an intrauterine gestational sac in the presence of a positive pregnancy test is suggestive of an ectopic pregnancy, other conditions, such as an early intrauterine gestation, must be considered. Awareness of risk factors and close evaluation of early pregnancy will allow the clinician to identify these complicated pregnancies in a timely manner. Demonstrating a structure that appears to be a gestational sac is not enough to exclude an ectopic pregnancy. The only sign confirming this is a fetal heart beat. Providers should maintain their current skills in transvaginal ultrasonography and consult a radiologist if there are suspicious findings that cannot be interpreted clearly.

Abramovici H, Auslender R, Lewin A, Faktor J. Gestational-pseudogestational sac: a new ultrasonic criterion for differential diagnosis. Am J Obstet Gynecol 1983;145:377–9.

Heard MJ, Buster JE. Ectopic pregnancy. In: Danforth's obstetrics and gynecology. 9th ed. New York (NY): Lippincott; 2003. p. 89–103.

O'Neil AG, Hammond IG, Reid SE. Problems in the diagnosis of ectopic pregnancy: the pseudogestational sac. Aust N Z J Obstet Gynaecol 1982;22:94–5.

Wexler S, Yedwab G, Golan A, David MP. Pseudogestational sac in ectopic pregnancy. Acta Obstet Gynecol Scand 1984;63: 63–5.

31
Ancillary surgery for pelvic pain

A 29-year-old woman with a 4-year history of pelvic pain and severe dysmenorrhea is taken to the operating room for a laparoscopic procedure. At the time of the laparoscopy, lesions consistent with endometriosis are observed. Your assistant is a resident in training, and you discuss treatment options. The surgical procedure that will result in the greatest likelihood of pain relief in this patient is

- (A) presacral neurectomy
- (B) uterosacral nerve ablation
- * (C) simple destruction of lesions
- (D) uterosacral nerve ablation and destruction of lesions

Many gynecologic surgeons choose to perform an ancillary surgical procedure in addition to destruction or removal of endometriosis lesions in an attempt to increase the likelihood of pain relief following surgery. Presacral neurectomy and uterosacral nerve interruption are procedures that can both be performed laparoscopically. A number of practitioners believe that these procedures can increase the rates of success with laparoscopic treatment of endometriosis-related pelvic pain.

Presacral neurectomy is based on the fact that the superior hypogastric plexus is the primary pathway for nociceptive (painful) stimuli that originate in the uterus and adjacent structures. Theoretically, destruction of the plexus would be expected to interrupt the nociceptive pathway and eliminate or ameliorate pain sensations that arise from inflammation, irritation, or dysfunction of the uterus. One of the problems in the performance of this procedure is the difficulty in identification and isolation of the nerve bundles so that they can be ligated completely. Significant bleeding secondary to the injury to the middle sacral artery or the venous plexus must be recognized. The concept behind uterosacral nerve ablation is similar to that for presacral neurectomy. The sensory parasympathetic nerve fibers from the cervix and the sensory sympathetic fibers from the corpus of the uterus traverse the cervical division of the Lee-Frankenhaeuser plexus that lies in, under, and around the uterosacral ligaments. In theory, transection of the nociceptive fibers anywhere along their pathway should ameliorate pain sensation.

Transection of the uterosacral nerves involves ligation or desiccation of the nerves in the paracervical region. The nerve bundles are not identified per se but the uterosacral ligaments are transected and ligated or desiccated at the time of laparotomy. The procedure has been used for relief of pelvic pain, especially pain described as midline.

Uncontrolled studies support the use of laparoscopic uterine nerve ablation for both primary and secondary dysmenorrhea with either complete relief or substantial reduction in menstrual pain in most subjects. Presacral neurectomy, by virtue of the surgical location, is believed to interrupt a greater number of nerve pathways than laparoscopic uterine nerve ablation. Presacral neurectomy, for these same reasons, is a more complex procedure than laparoscopic uterine nerve ablation and entails more operative risk. Despite these potential drawbacks, however, uncontrolled studies of presacral neurectomy are indicative of effectiveness similar to that for laparoscopic uterine nerve ablation for women with primary and secondary dysmenorrhea.

Both laparoscopic uterine nerve ablation and presacral neurectomy have limitations as treatment for dysmenorrhea or centralized pelvic pain. It has been shown that the success rates with laparoscopic uterine nerve ablation decreased rapidly over time from 72% in the first year to 39% in the fourth year. Anatomic distortion, such as subsequent uterine prolapse and bladder dysfunction, has been reported following laparoscopic uterine nerve ablation. Both procedures only partially interrupt some of the cervical sensory nerve fibers in the pelvic area; therefore, women with dysmenorrhea associated with additional pelvic pathology may not always benefit from this type of surgery. For this reason, these techniques often are combined with additional management (eg, ablation of endometriosis implants).

The laparoscopic uterine nerve ablation technique has been shown to be effective for primary dysmenorrhea in one small controlled study, but the results indicate a decrease in the effectiveness of pain relief over time. Another study of women with primary dysmenorrhea reported a dramatic decrease in the pain relief afforded by laparoscopic uterine nerve ablation where pain relief was compared 3 and 12 months following surgery. Therefore, although laparoscopic uterine nerve ablation may be effective for pain relief in the short term, the long-term results are uncertain.

A meta-analysis demonstrated that laparoscopic uterine nerve ablation and presacral neurectomy were not significantly different in effectiveness for the management of primary dysmenorrhea in the short term, but presacral neurectomy is significantly more effective in reducing pain in the long-term. One drawback of presacral neurectomy is the significantly higher level of adverse effects, such as constipation and urinary urgency. Symptoms of constipation are easily manageable and seem to improve over time.

In evaluating the effectiveness of laparoscopic uterine nerve ablation for the management of secondary dysmenorrhea associated with endometriosis, 2 authors reported no significant difference between the treatment and control groups when an interim analysis was performed after 6 months and after 9 months of follow-up. Thus, laparoscopic uterine nerve ablation combined with surgical treatment of endometriosis is no more effective than surgical treatment of the endometriosis alone for treatment of secondary dysmenorrhea.

Based on available scientific evidence, either laparoscopic uterine nerve ablation or presacral neurectomy may be somewhat effective for the relief of primary dysmenorrhea, but long-term results remain uncertain. Neither procedure appears to add benefit in terms of pain relief to laparoscopically directed removal or destruction of endometriosis lesions. Surgeons should consider the potential complications associated with performance of either ancillary procedure and weigh the risks against the somewhat dubious benefits when causes of pelvic pain are identified. The simple destruction of endometriotic lesions alone offers the highest likelihood of pain relief with the lowest incidence of complications.

Candiani GB, Fedele L, Vercellini P, Bianchi S, Di Nola G. Presacral neurectomy for the treatment of pelvic pain associated with endometriosis: a controlled study. Am J Obstet Gynecol 1992; 167:100–3.

Chen FP, Chang SD, Chu KK, Soong YK. Comparison of laparoscopic presacral neurectomy and laparoscopic uterine nerve ablation for primary dysmenorrhea. J Reprod Med 1996;41:463–6.

Nezhat CH, Seidman DS, Nezhat FR, Nezhat CR. Long-term outcome of laparoscopic presacral neurectomy for the treatment of central pelvic pain attributed to endometriosis. Obstet Gynecol 1998;91:701–4.

Papasakelariou C. Long-term results of laparoscopic uterosacral nerve ablation. Gynaecol Endosc 1996;5:177–9.

Proctor ML, Farquhar CM, Sinclair OJ, Johnson NP. Surgical interruption of pelvic nerve pathways for primary and secondary dysmenorrhoea (Cochrane Review). In: The Cochrane Library, Issue 2, 2004. Chichester, UK: John Wiley & Sons, Ltd.

32

Therapy for hyperprolactinemia

A 36-year-old woman, gravida 2, para 2, presents with amenorrhea for the past 6 years. Her medical history is significant for a diagnosis of paranoid schizophrenia, which is well controlled with medication. Her current medications include haloperidol decanoate (Haldol), benztropine mesylate (Cogentin), and lorazepam (Ativan). Her physical examination is unremarkable except for galactorrhea from the left breast. Laboratory studies are normal except for an elevated serum prolactin level of 142 ng/mL. A magnetic resonance imaging (MRI) scan of her pituitary shows no evidence of tumor. The most appropriate next step in her management is

    (A) visual field
    (B) reduce antipsychotic medications
    (C) mammography
*   (D) dual-energy X-ray absorptiometry (DXA) scan

The development of hyperprolactinemia in patients taking long-term antipsychotic medication is a problem that is underappreciated by clinicians. A variety of psychiatric illnesses, such as schizophrenia, psychotic depression, bipolar disorder, and anxiety disorders, require long-term treatment with antipsychotic drugs that are predominantly dopamine receptor antagonists. These drugs have been postulated to exert antidopaminergic action within the mesolimbic system. The potency of the compounds in terms of antipsychotic efficacy appears proportional to their dopamine receptor binding affinity. The antagonist action also carries over to the dopamine D_2 receptors localized to pituitary lactotropes, which causes a persistent and long-term elevation in prolactin levels. In most of these patients, prolactin levels usually are less than 100 ng/mL.

The endocrine-related disorders that arise from persistent hyperprolactinemia in this patient population include galactorrhea, amenorrhea, oligomenorrhea, sexual dysfunction, infertility, hirsutism, acne, and vaginal atrophy. The long-term estrogen deficiency caused by the hypogonadal state may have other consequences, such as changes in cognition and development of osteoporosis. Because hyperprolactinemia also could be caused by a common underlying prolactin-secreting microadenoma, an MRI of the pituitary sella should be performed to exclude an occult lesion. In the presence of a normal MRI, visual field evaluation is not indicated. An assessment of bone mineral density (BMD) would be appropriate for patients who remain hypoestrogenic, such as this patient. Although prolactin does not have a direct effect on BMD, in the long term hyperprolactinemia may result in osteoporosis and, therefore, BMD should be assessed by DXA scan.

Patients with documented long-term drug-induced hyperprolactinemia may benefit from estrogen therapy to reduce vaginal atrophy and prevent bone loss. Simultaneous use of an antipsychotic drug along with bromocriptine mesylate (Parlodel) to correct hyperprolactinemia may exacerbate psychotic symptoms and, thus, would not be appropriate for this patient. Reducing the dose of antipsychotic medications also may result in return of psychotic symptoms without correcting the hyperprolactinemia. Alternatively, one management option open to psychiatrists is the use of the newer anti-psychotics that have little or no effect on prolactin secretion, such as olanzapine (Zyprexa), clozapine (Clozaril), and quetiapine (Seroquel). Clinicians should caution patients who switch to these compounds that they may resume ovulation and be at risk for pregnancy.

Oral contraceptives may be appropriate in patients who have long-term amenorrhea and osteopenia or osteoporosis on bone density scanning. Mammography is not currently indicated for this patient because she is younger than 40 years.

Ataya K, Mercado A, Kartaginer J, Abbasi A, Moghissi KS. Bone density and reproductive hormones in patients with neuroleptic-induced hyperprolactinemia. Fertil Steril 1988;50:876–81.

Miller KK, Klibanski A. Clinical review 106: Amenorrheic bone loss. J Clin Endocrinol Metab 1999;84:1775–83.

Perovich RM, Lieberman JA, Fleischhacker WW, Alvir J. The behavioral toxicity of bromocriptine in patients with psychiatric illness. J Clin Psychopharmacol 1989;9:417–22.

Smith S, Wheeler M, Murray R, O'Keane V. The effects of antipsychotic induced hyperprolactinaemia on the hypothalamic-pituitary-gonadal axis. J Clin Psychopharmacol 2002;27:109–14.

33

Diagnosis and management of delayed puberty

A 13-year-old adolescent comes in for evaluation of "lack of sexual development." The patient's medical history and family history are unremarkable. Vital signs are normal. Physical examination reveals a height of 142 cm (56 in.), Tanner stage I breast and pubic hair development (see Appendix D), webbed neck, high-arched palate, broad chest, small uterus, normal cervix, and nonpalpable ovaries. Bone age is 11.2 years. Laboratory analysis reveals a follicle-stimulating hormone level of 41 mIU/mL, a luteinizing hormone level of 24 mIU/mL, estradiol level of less than 10 pg/mL, and karyotype of 45,X. Appropriate initial management for this patient is

    (A) thyroxine
    (B) calcium
*   (C) recombinant human growth hormone
    (D) medroxyprogesterone acetate

This patient presents with delayed puberty, specifically hypergonadotropic hypogonadism. She has multiple signs of gonadal dysgenesis (Turner's syndrome), which the karyotype confirms. Individuals with these conditions may present in infancy with lymphedema. Later, they may present with the findings seen in this patient.

The following studies should be done in women when a karyotype confirms the diagnosis of Turner's syndrome:

- Intravenous pyelogram or ultrasonographic examination to exclude a renal anomaly
- Echocardiography or magnetic resonance imaging study to assess cardiovascular function and to rule out coarctation of the aorta and bicuspid aortic valves
- Hearing examination, if multiple prior inner ear infections
- Evaluation of thyroid function and thyroid antibodies
- Fasting plasma glucose test (Table 33-1)

Particular emphasis should be placed on long-term monitoring for cardiovascular disease (including hypertension, aortic dilatation, and the risk of aortic dissection), regular screening for thyroid dysfunction, recognition of hearing impairment that worsens in adult life, monitoring for scoliosis and bone density in late adolescence and adulthood for evidence of osteopenia, and being prepared to discuss any request for assisted conception.

The prevalence of cardiovascular abnormalities varies from 20% to 50%. Coarctation of the aorta is found in 10% of patients. The prevalence of bicuspid aortic valves in patients with Turner's syndrome determined by echocardiograph ranges from 9% to 34%. Bicuspid aortic valves carry an increased risk for subacute bacterial endocarditis and may evolve with age into stenotic or insufficient aortic valves. These cardiac abnormalities also are risk factors for developing aortic dilatation, dissection, and rupture.

TABLE 33-1. Assessments That Should Be Completed for Females When the Diagnosis of Gonadal Dysgenesis (45,X; Turner's syndrome) Is Made and Then at Regular Specified Intervals

Baseline	Yearly	3–5-Year Intervals
Karyotype	Physical examination	Echocardiogram
Thyroid function tests	Thyroid function tests	Bone mineral density
Thyroid autoantibodies	Fasting blood glucose	Audiogram
Fasting blood glucose	Fasting lipid panel	
Fasting lipid panel	Renal function tests	
Gonadotropins	Liver function tests	
Echocardiogram		
Renal ultrasound or intravenous pyelogram		
Audiogram		

Data from Elsheikh M, Dunger DB, Conway GS, Wass JA. Turner's syndrome in adulthood. Endocr Rev 2002;23:120–40.

Malformation of the kidneys (eg, horseshoe kidney) and upper collecting system with an abnormal vascular supply are so common that intravenous pyelogram or renal ultrasonography should be obtained routinely at the time of diagnosis. Skeletal maturation is normal or slightly delayed in childhood and lags further in adolescence as a result of gonadal steroid deficiency. Patients not treated with estrogen often develop severe osteoporosis and may develop fractures.

The incidence of autoimmune disorders is increased; the most prevalent is autoimmune thyroiditis and Graves' disease, which occur in 15–30% of patients with gonadal dysgenesis. The prevalence of thyroid antibodies and hypothyroidism or hyperthyroidism increases during childhood and adolescence and may approach 50% in adulthood. Therapy, such as thyroxine for thyroid disorders, should not be initiated until a diagnosis is made.

Carbohydrate intolerance with mild insulin resistance is common, especially after age 16 years, and may become worse with obesity or during treatment with growth hormone. The risks of type 1 and type 2 diabetes mellitus are increased (relative risks, 2 and 4, respectively). Mean cholesterol levels may be elevated after age 11 years and are independent of age and body mass index.

Initial therapy should be directed toward augmentation of stature, correction of somatic anomalies, and counseling. Induction of secondary sexual characteristics should be initiated when the patient is psychologically ready and approximately at the expected age of puberty. Although calcium supplementation is an important consideration in patients with gonadal dysgenesis, the short stature in an adolescent must be addressed initially. The short stature in gonadal dysgenesis is not related to a deficiency of growth hormone, insulinlike growth factors, thyroid hormone, adrenal steroids, or gonadal steroids. However, administration of pharmacologic doses of biosynthetic growth hormone increases growth rate and augments final height by 5–10 cm. Growth hormone therapy is approved by the U.S. Food and Drug Administration for the treatment of patients with Turner's syndrome.

Studies in which growth hormone treatment was combined with early estrogen therapy (ie, in patients younger than 12 years) found a shorter final height than in patients who received early growth hormone treatment and later estrogen therapy. In all patients with gonadal dysgenesis whose height is more than 2 standard deviations below the mean value for age, especially those whose growth rate is less than 5 cm per year, the practitioner should discuss with the parents and patient growth hormone therapy, including its efficacy and side effects. Generally, the earlier growth hormone therapy is initiated, the more likely it is that greater final height will be achieved. Growth hormone therapy usually is continued until the growth rate decreases to less than 2 cm per year or the bone age exceeds 15 years. Growth may be further augmented by the addition of oxandrolone, an anabolic steroid, beginning after initiation of growth hormone.

In the past, the use of growth hormone and estrogen in combination with oxandrolone, an anabolic steroid, was recommended in selected cases. The initiation of low-dose, conjugated estrogen, synthetic estrogen therapy, or transdermal estradiol patch alone at approximately age 13 years (bone age greater than 11 years) elicits a brief growth spurt without inordinate advancement of skeletal maturation or reduction in final height. It is important to begin with low doses of estrogen therapy to achieve appropriate and optimal breast development (Fig. 33-1; see color plate). Likewise, estrogen therapy induces the development of secondary sexual characteristics at an age comparable to that of normal peers, thereby obviating the undesirable psychologic consequences and deficient bone mineralization of a prolonged delay in sexual maturation. To date, there are few data on the use of the transdermal estradiol patch in adolescent girls. Although the transdermal estradiol patch is more expensive, with this approach the natural estradiol reaches the systemic circulation directly without first undergoing metabolism by the intestine and liver.

The patient is maintained on the minimal dose of estrogen needed to maintain secondary sexual characteristics, permit withdrawal bleeding, and prevent osteopenia. Following 6 months of unopposed estrogen therapy, or when the patient has withdrawal bleeding, if this occurs first, a progestogen can be given for 12 days at periodic intervals to insure physiologic menses and to reduce the risks of endometrial cancer. After initial estrogen therapy, patients also may be treated with oral contraceptives to induce cyclic menses, but the estrogen in the oral contraceptives is far more than is needed by this patient.

Chernausek SD, Attie KM, Cara JF, Rosenfeld RG, Frane J. Growth hormone therapy of Turner syndrome: the impact of age of estrogen replacement on final height. Genentech, Inc., Collaborative Study Group. J Clin Endocrinol Metab 2000;85:2439–45.

Reiter EO, Blethen SL, Baptista J, Price L. Early initiation of growth hormone treatment allows age-appropriate estrogen use in Turner's syndrome. J Clin Endocrinol Metab 2001;86:1936–41.

Rosenfeld RG, Attie KM, Frane J, Brasel JA, Burstein S, Cara JF, et al. Growth hormone therapy of Turner's syndrome: beneficial effect on adult height. J Pediatr 1998;132:319–24.

Saenger P, Wikland KA, Conway GS, Davenport M, Gravholt CH, Hintz R, et al. Recommendations for the diagnosis and management of Turner syndrome. Fifth International Symposium on Turner Syndrome. J Clin Endocrinol Metab 2001;86:3061–9.

Sas TC, de Muinck Keizer-Schrama SM, Stijnen T, Jansen M, Otten BJ, Hoorweg-Nijman JJ, et al. Normalization of height in girls with Turner syndrome after long-term growth hormone treatment: results of a randomized dose-response trial. J Clin Endocrinol Metab 1999;84: 4607–12.

34

Diagnosis of amenorrhea

A 29-year-old nulligravid woman who recently immigrated from Asia to the United States undergoes a late luteal phase endometrial biopsy for infertility and amenorrhea. The biopsy results show lymphocytic infiltration, epithelioid tubercles, and several giant cells (Fig. 34-1). She has a history of oligomenorrhea, and her hysterosalpingogram is as shown (Fig. 34-2). The most frequent concurrent disease process in a patient with this presentation is

    (A) pleuritis
* (B) exudative salpingitis
    (C) caseating cervicitis
    (D) oophoritis
    (E) myometritis

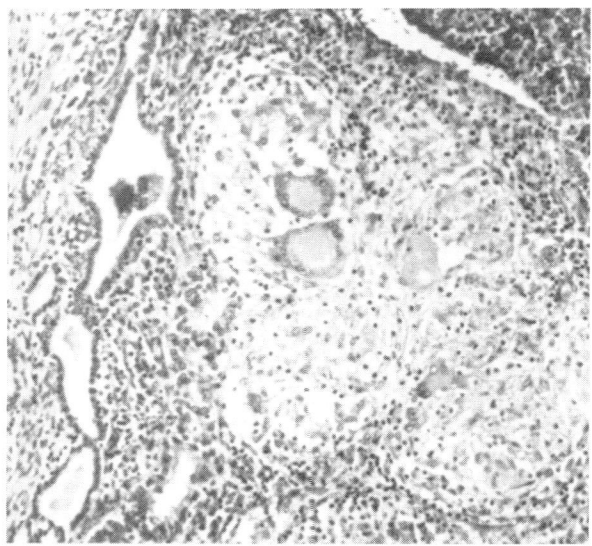

FIG. 34-1. Tuberculous encometritis with a nonnecrotizing granuloma containing Langerhans cells. (Kurman RJ, ed. Blaustein's pathology of the female genital tract. 5th ed. New York [NY]: Springer-Verlag; 2002. p. 429.)

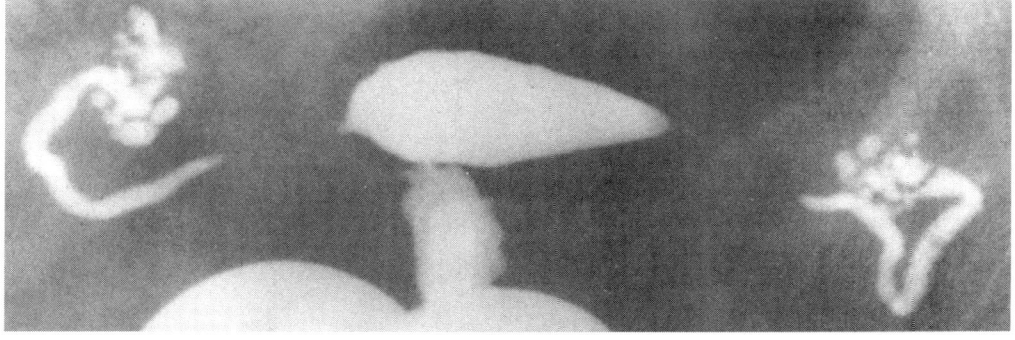

FIG. 34-2. Tubal tuberculosis with characteristic strictured "stiff" ampullary segments. (Reprinted from Wallach EE, Zacur HA. Reproductive medicine and surgery. 1st ed. St. Louis [MO]: Mosby; Copyright 1995, with permission from Elsevier.)

More than 30% of individuals worldwide harbor the tubercle bacillus. Although the prevalence of genital tuberculosis (TB) is increasing worldwide, the incidence of disease is difficult to determine because at least 11% of patients are asymptomatic. Genital TB usually is secondary to TB that originates from another organ system, usually the pulmonary system, with an eventual hematogenous mode of dissemination to the pelvis. A negative chest radiographic study does not preclude the diagnosis because most pulmonary lesions have resolved once the genital tract is involved. Most women with genital TB fail to mention prior or current respiratory problems, such as pleuritis or pneumonia.

The fallopian tube forms a favorable nidus for tubercle bacilli. Once infected, the fallopian tube enlarges and develops an exudative salpingitis but remains relatively free of adhesions. The fallopian tubes become saturated with a caseous material and release a purulent exudate. After initial involvement of the fallopian tubes, the TB infection spreads to the ovaries and uterus by direct extension. Extension to the uterus occurs along the endometrial surface and rarely extends into the depths of the myometrium. Similarly, perioophoritis, a superficial infection of the ovary, can sometimes be seen because spread of the TB infection from the fallopian tube often involves the ovarian epithelium.

A finding of TB endometritis generally indicates that TB salpingitis is present. The classic lesion of TB endometritis is the noncaseating granuloma, composed of epithelial cells, Langerhans giant cells, and lymphocytes. Cervical involvement in genital TB is less frequent and occurs in only 5–15% of cases. In fact, spread of TB occurs in decreasing magnitude from the fallopian tubes downward toward the cervix. Therefore, caseating cervicitis rarely occurs with genital TB. The peritoneal findings associated with genital TB often include pathognomonic study of peritoneal surfaces with granulomas.

A definitive diagnosis of genital TB requires isolation of the tubercle bacillus. The bacillus can be identified in a tissue specimen (eg, an endometrial biopsy) by the use of the acid-fast stain.

The most common initial symptom in genital tuberculosis is infertility, and the second most frequent symptom is lower abdominal or pelvic pain. Among women with genital TB, 75% have menstrual irregularities, 50% have tubal obstruction, and 15% have tuboovarian masses. It is important to realize that virtually all women with genital TB are sterile and that genital TB is a common cause of sterility worldwide. Endometrial destruction results in intrauterine synechiae, which even after hysteroscopic lysis portend a poor prognosis for pregnancy.

Bukulmez O, Yarali H, Gurgan T. Total corporal synechiae due to tuberculosis carry a very poor prognosis following hysteroscopic synechialysis. Hum Reprod 1960;14:1960–1.

Chow TW, Lim BK, Vallipuram S. The masquerades of female pelvic tuberculosis: case reports and review of literature on clinical presentations and diagnosis. J Obstet Gynaecol Res 2002;28:203–10.

Parikh FR, Nadkarni SG, Kamat SA, Naik N, Soonawala SB, Parik RM. Genital tuberculosis—a major pelvic factor causing infertility in Indian women. Fertil Steril 1997;67:497–500.

35
Premature ovarian failure

A 28-year-old nulliparous woman developed premature ovarian failure at age 22 years and, subsequently, 46,XX premature ovarian failure was diagnosed. Her older sister developed the same condition at age 31 years. At laparoscopy for pelvic pain, she was found to have very small round ovaries measuring 1 cm bilaterally. Before considering her youngest sister as an oocyte donor, the patient should be screened for which one of the following causes of familial ovarian failure?

   (A) Swyer syndrome
   (B) Galactosemia
 * (C) Fragile X premutation
   (D) Follicle-stimulating hormone (FSH) receptor gene mutation
   (E) 17α-Hydroxylase deficiency

Premature ovarian failure is the loss of germ cells from the ovary at an age 2.5 standard deviations before the mean. Age 40 years is the cutoff that meets this definition, given that the average age of menopause is 51 years.

A wide variety of both genetic and nongenetic causes of premature ovarian failure exist, many of which are relatively rare. One cause of premature ovarian failure that has gained recent attention is associated with the fragile X premutation. Mutations of the fragile X gene that lead to fragile X syndrome, the most common inherited cause of mental retardation, consist of an increased number of cytosine-guanine-guanine repeats. The *FMR1* gene usually has up to 60 such repeats. Expansion of this trinucleotide to greater than 200 repeats inactivates the gene and leads to fragile X syndrome in males. In addition to mild to severe mental retardation, these males have characteristic phenotypic features that include a long narrow face with increased head circumference, dysmorphic ears, prominent jaw and forehead, and macro-orchidism.

The premutation state, ie, 60–199 cytosine-guanine-guanine repeats, is unstable and prone to further expansion. It has been found that premature ovarian failure develops in approximately 21% of such premutation carriers. In addition, 2% of women with sporadic premature ovarian failure and 14% of women with familial premature ovarian failure have been found to harbor this unstable premutation state. Prior reports of nontwin sisters with premature ovarian failure have suggested an autosomal recessive disorder, and it is likely that a number of these sisters may have had the fragile X premutation instead. Because the fragile X mutation appears to occur so frequently, after obtaining a karyotype that demonstrates a 46,XX chromosomal compliment in a patient with premature ovarian failure, the next most important genetic test is analysis for the *FMR1* premutation state. Such an analysis is particularly important for individuals who are contemplating the use of their sister for oocyte donation. Not only may there be an insufficient ovarian response, but more importantly, should pregnancy occur in the face of an *FMR1* premutation, a son may be delivered with fragile X syndrome.

For women with 46,XY gonadal dysgenesis (ie, Swyer syndrome), or Turner's syndrome (ie, 45,X karyotype with or without mosaicism or other structurally abnormal X chromosomes), the insult leading to germ cell loss occurs largely in utero. All patients with Swyer syndrome and 85% of those with Turner's syndrome will have streak ovaries and will not spontaneously go through puberty. Although some women with 46,XX ovarian failure present similarly at puberty with streak ovaries and are given the diagnosis of gonadal dysgenesis, at least an equal number of these women will have a sufficient number of residual germ cells to allow both a normal pubertal progression and a menstrual life, however limited it might be. Their ovaries often are morphologically normal but very small rather than streak-like. Although most of these patients lack an identifiable etiology for germ cell loss, a number of rare disorders have been implicated, including iatrogenic, autoimmune, infectious, infiltrative, and genetic disorders such as galactosemia.

The most common iatrogenic etiology for premature ovarian failure is treatment for cancer, either as a child or adult. Historically, the treatment regimens most commonly associated with germ cell loss have included alkylating agents or radiation, with the resultant premature ovarian failure being both age- and dose-dependent. Although occurrence of premature ovarian failure is variable and potentially temporary at lower dosages, it is usual after high-dose chemotherapy, total body irradiation, or radiotherapy dosages higher than 6 Gy.

The presumption that autoimmune ovarian failure accounted for most patients with 46,XX premature ovarian failure has been based on 2 facts:

1. Premature ovarian failure is associated with other autoimmune endocrine disorders (ie, commonly Hashimoto thyroiditis and rarely hypoparathyroidism, adrenal insufficiency, pernicious anemia, and lupus erythematosus).
2. Because a large percentage of patients with premature ovarian failure do not have an identifiable etiology, it is not difficult to hypothesize that many have a relatively common condition, such as autoimmune disease.

Although some investigators have advocated the measurement of ovarian-specific autoantibodies, great variation has been reported in the ability to consistently make this diagnosis with such testing. A number of variables of the testing methodology and the patient populations studied exist which likely contribute to these inconsistent findings. It appears that multiple antigens within the ovary are targets for ovarian autoimmunity, and testing of individual antigens is insufficient to routinely identify ovarian autoimmune disease. Until standardized and proven testing is available, practitioners should keep in mind that patients with 46,XX premature ovarian failure are at risk for these associated autoimmune endocrinopathies (ie, Hashimoto thyroiditis, hypoparathyroidism, adrenal insufficiency, and pernicious anemia). Testing for adrenal antibodies with an indirect immunofluorescence assay that is commercially available will identify the 4% of women with premature ovarian failure who have steroidogenic cell autoimmunity and are at risk of adrenal insufficiency, a potentially fatal disorder. Although it has always been suggested that patients with premature ovarian failure be screened for lupus erythematosus, recent studies indicate that patients with lupus who develop premature ovarian failure are most likely to have been treated with cytotoxic agents.

Although infectious etiologies (eg, tuberculosis and viral agents) and infiltrative disorders (eg, mucopolysaccharidosis) usually are included among the causes for premature ovarian failure, such causal relationships have not been proved beyond isolated case reports. A more common association with premature ovarian failure, which has been shown with increasing regularity, is the presence of a genetic disorder. In addition to fragile X premutation as discussed previously, studies of patients with galactosemia, myotonic dystrophy, and ataxia telangiectasia have repeatedly reported premature ovarian failure as an association. The most recent additions to this list of genetic causes of premature ovarian failure are mutations in the *FOXL2* gene that cause blepharophimosis-ptosis-epicanthus inversus syndrome and the premutation for the fragile X (*FMR1*) gene. Different mutations of the *FOXL2* gene cause 2 forms of the disease, blepharophimosis-ptosis-epicanthus inversus syndrome type I and type II. Of these, blepharophimosis-ptosis-epicanthus inversus syndrome type I includes premature ovarian failure in the phenotype.

Patients with 46,XX hypergonadotropic hypogonadism also may have 2 other genetic syndromes. Resistant ovary syndrome, also called Savage syndrome, was classically reported in patients with a normal reserve of oocytes but elevated gonadotropin levels and a lack of an ovarian response. Gonadotropin resistance was suspected and mutations of the FSH receptor were subsequently identified. The syndrome in men causes variable degrees of reduced spermatogenesis. The second syndrome is 17α-hydroxylase deficiency. Women homozygous for mutations in this cytochrome *P450* gene also have a normal ovarian complement of oocytes. They are unable to produce steroids, either androgens or estrogens, in the ovaries and adrenal glands. Additionally, they are unable to produce glucocorticoids. They may have hypertension because of increased production of mineralocorticoids.

Aittomaki K, Lucena JL, Pakarinen P, Sistonen P, Tapanainen J, Gromoll B, et al. Mutation in the follicle-stimulating hormone receptor gene causes hereditary hypergonadotropic ovarian failure. Cell 1995; 82:959–68.

Bakalov VK, Vanderhoof VH, Bondy CA, Nelson LM. Adrenal antibodies detect asymptomatic auto-immune adrenal insufficiency in young women with spontaneous premature ovarian failure. Hum Reprod 2002;17:2096–100.

Blumenfeld Z. Preservation of fertility and ovarian function and minimalization of chemotherapy associated gonadotoxicity and premature ovarian failure: the role of inhibin-A and -B as markers. Mol Cell Endocrinol 2002;187:93–105.

Crisponi L, Deiana M, Loi A, Chiappe F, Uda M, Amati P, et al. The putative forkhead transcription factor FOXL2 is mutated in blepharophimosis/ptosis/epicanthus inversus syndrome. Nat Genet 2001; 27:159–66.

Luborsky J. Ovarian autoimmune disease and ovarian autoantibodies. J Womens Health Gend Based Med 2002;11:585–99.

Meirow D. Ovarian injury and modern options to preserve fertility in female cancer patients treated with high dose radio-chemotherapy for hemato-oncological neoplasias and other cancers. Leuk Lymphoma 1999;33:65–76.

Sherman SL. Premature ovarian failure in the fragile X syndrome. Am J Med Genet 2000;97:189–94.

Wheatcroft NJ, Salt C, Milford-Ward A, Cooke ID, Weetman AP. Identification of ovarian antibodies by immunofluorescence, enzyme-linked immunosorbent assay or immunoblotting in premature ovarian failure. Hum Reprod 1997;12:2617–22.

36
Ovarian cyst management during ovulation induction

A 28-year-old nulligravid woman with primary infertility has been treated with clomiphene citrate (Clomid, Serophene) for superovulation for the past 2 months. She presents on day 3 of her menstrual cycle with right lower quadrant pain and the ultrasonogram taken at that time is shown (Fig. 36-1). The most appropriate management is

    (A) continue the clomiphene citrate
    (B) combined oral contraceptives
    (C) ovarian cystectomy
* (D) expectant management
    (E) transvaginal cyst aspiration

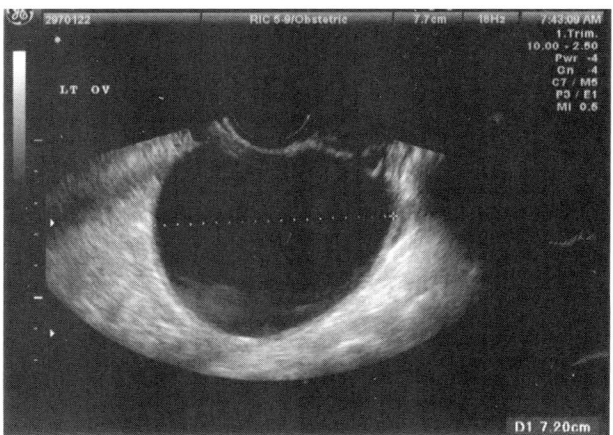

FIG. 36-1. Ultrasound of an ovarian cyst.

Ovarian cysts in reproductive-aged women usually are physiologic, either in the form of follicular or corpus luteum cysts. This is a frequent finding among patients who undergo ovulation induction and monitoring of follicular growth by ultrasonography. Ovarian stimulation should not be induced when symptomatic ovarian cysts are present. There is a small but real risk for rupture or torsion in any large cyst as shown.

Historically, some gynecologists have prescribed combined oral contraceptives for the resolution of functional ovarian cysts. Randomized controlled clinical trials in women who have undergone ovulation induction have suggested that functional ovarian cysts are not affected by oral contraceptives, although most studies to date have included not only functional cysts but also pathologic adnexal masses. In one study, 53 users of clomiphene citrate with functional ovarian cysts, identified by transvaginal ultrasonography within the first 5 days of a menstrual cycle, were randomized to expectant management or combined oral contraceptives for 1 cycle. If persistent, the patient was followed for another cycle without any treatment. Complete resolution of ovarian cysts was observed in 76% of oral contraceptive users compared with 72% in the observation group, which was not statistically significant. All of the persistent cysts disappeared after a second cycle without any treatment. This suggests that expectant management is as effective as combined oral contraceptives for the resolution of functional ovarian cysts induced by fertility drugs. The best next step in management for this patient would be to discontinue clomiphene citrate, observe, and repeat ultrasonography after her next menstrual period.

A high-rate of functional ovarian cysts are observed after ovulation induction. Therefore, a diagnostic laparoscopy or laparotomy with ovarian cystectomy would be inadvisable.

Although reports of its use during in vitro fertilization cycles have suggested a much quicker cyst resolution and initiation of ovulation induction, no studies to date have compared the efficacy of observation with transvaginal ovarian cyst aspiration. One study found a 27% overall recurrence rate after transvaginal cyst aspiration in the month after the procedure, which provides further support for an observational approach for the management of functional ovarian cysts.

MacKenna A, Fabres C, Alam V, Morrales V. Clinical management of functional ovarian cysts: a prospective and randomized study. Hum Reprod 2000;15:2567–9.

Steinkampf MP, Hammond KR, Blackwell RE. Hormonal treatment of functional ovarian cysts: a randomized, prospective study. Fertil Steril 1990;54:775–7.

Troiano RN, Taylor KJ. Sonographically guided therapeutic aspiration of benign-appearing ovarian cysts and endometriomas. AJR Am J Roentgenol 1998;171:1601–5.

37

Uterosacral ligament transection

A 33-year-old nulligravid woman undergoes a laparoscopic resection of deep endometriosis that primarily involves the right uterosacral ligament. The patient comes to the emergency department 4 days later with nausea, bloating, and inability to pass gas or have a bowel movement. Physical examination is unremarkable except for hypoactive bowel sounds. A flat plate and upright film of the abdomen and complete blood count are all normal. The next best diagnostic study is

* (A) computerized axial tomography (CAT) scan
* (B) upper gastrointestinal series with small bowel follow-through
* (C) pelvic and abdominal ultrasonography
* (D) repeat flat plate and upright film in 24 hours
* (E) blood urea nitrogen (BUN) and creatinine

Lateral and in close proximity to the uterosacral ligaments lie the ureters and uterine vasculature, with the potential for injury during pelvic surgery in this region. Wide resections in this area have the potential to lead to serious complications. Patients who present with nausea, bloating, and other gastrointestinal (GI) symptoms following pelvic operative procedures must be evaluated for pelvic hematoma or abscess or GI or urologic injury. As such, diagnostic procedures should have the potential to evaluate several types of pathology. Ureteral injury is hard to diagnose based on the patient's symptoms alone. The patient may present with unilateral or bilateral flank pain but also may present with mild ileus or can be completely asymptomatic. Bowel injury also can be difficult to diagnose based on the early symptoms of the patient. Early bowel injury may initially present as mild ileus, anorexia, and nausea before the later stages of actual bowel obstruction or sepsis. Electrosurgical bowel injuries, particularly with unipolar cautery, often are unrecognized at the time of surgery and can present several days after the procedure.

A CAT scan of the abdomen and pelvis with contrast has been shown to be just as reliable as intravenous pyelography for demonstrating injury. The CAT scan has the potential to identify ileus, bowel obstruction, hematoma, or abscess formation as well as urologic injury. This patient is at increased risk for ureteral injury because of the uterosacral ligament transsection. With her additional GI symptoms, the CAT scan has added value.

Upper GI series with small bowel follow-through is highly reliable in identifying small bowel obstruction but will miss ureteral injury, pelvic hematoma, or abscess. Thus, an upper GI series would not be the most appropriate diagnostic study for this patient.

Pelvic and abdominal ultrasonography will identify potential pelvic hematoma or abscess and hydronephrosis. However, it has limited utility in the diagnosis of small bowel obstruction and ureteral dilatation and would not be the diagnostic study of choice in this situation.

Repeat flat plate and upright films of the abdomen are valuable in noting the degree of bowel distension as well as air fluid levels but will not identify urinary tract injury nor fluid collections in the pelvis. Therefore, they would not be useful for this patient.

Serum creatinine and BUN levels will be significantly elevated in cases of bilateral ureteral obstruction. In cases in which there is only unilateral injury, the utility of these tests is extremely limited and, thus, would not be useful for this patient.

Harkki-Siren P, Sjoberg J, Kurki T. Major complications of laparoscopy: a follow-up Finnish study. Obstet Gynecol 1999;94: 94–8.

Lin P, Grow DR. Complications of laparoscopy. Strategies for prevention and cure. Obstet Gynecol Clin North Am 1999;26:23–38, v.

Maglinte DD, Reyes BL, Harmon BH, Kelvin FM, Turner WW Jr, Hage JE, et al. Reliability and role of plain film radiography and CT in the diagnosis of small-bowel obstruction. AJR Am J Roentgenol 1996;167: 1451–5.

McTavish JD, Jinzaki M, Zou KH, Nawfel RD, Silverman SG. Multidetector row CT urography: comparison of strategies for depicting the normal urinary collecting system. Radiology 2002;225:783–90.

38

Diagnosis of the menopausal transition

A 46-year-old woman presents with a 9-month history of irregular menstrual periods with unpredictable onset. She has noticed associated periodic hot flushes with profuse perspiration, which have caused her to awaken from sleep. Pelvic examination demonstrates a normal uterine size, without palpable adnexal masses. The most appropriate way to diagnose the menopausal transition in this patient is

(A) serum follicle-stimulating hormone (FSH)
(B) serum luteinizing hormone (LH)
(C) serum estradiol
* (D) menstrual history and symptoms
(E) basal body temperature chart

Menopausal transition, sometimes referred to as perimenopause, is defined as an interval of time that is before actual menopause and ends 12 months after the last menstrual period. Because the timing of the final menstrual period is established retrospectively, it is difficult to prospectively estimate when perimenopause ends. The hallmark of this period is the occurrence of intermittently irregular cycles, which leads to the clinical sign of irregular vaginal bleeding.

The World Health Organization defines the beginning of perimenopause as a break in a woman's regular menstrual cycles but not more than 3 months without a period. When a woman has 3–11 months of amenorrhea, she is considered to be in the late perimenopausal period. The Stages of Reproductive Aging Workshop has clarified terminology and established a staging system for reproductive aging. Because of the confusion concerning the use of the term "perimenopause," this consensus conference chose to use the term "menopausal transition" (Fig. 38-1). The early menopausal transition was defined to begin when a woman's regular menstrual cycles become greater than 7 days different from her normal cycle interval (eg, her regular cycles are now every 38 days instead of every 31 days). As cycles become more infrequent, the late menopausal transition is characterized by 2 or more skipped menstrual cycles and at least 1 interval of amenorrhea of 60 days or more. When 1 full year has elapsed from the final menstrual period, the menopausal transi-

Final Menstrual Period (FMP)

Stages:	-5	-4	-3	-2	-1	0	+1	+2
Terminology:	Reproductive			Menopausal transition			Postmenopause	
	Early	Peak	Late	Early	Late*		Early*	Late
				Perimenopause				
Duration of Stage:	variable			variable		(a) 1 yr	(b) 4 yrs	until demise
Menstrual Cycles:	variable to regular	regular		variable cycle length (>7 days different from normal)	≥2 skipped cycles and an interval of amenorrhea (≥60 days)	Amen x 12 mos	none	
Endocrine:	normal FSH	↑ FSH		↑ FSH			↑ FSH	

FIG. 38-1. The Stages of Reproductive Aging Workshop (STRAW) staging system. Abbreviations: ↑, elevated; FSH, follicle-stimulating hormone. (Reprinted from Fertility & Sterility, Vol 76, Soules MR, Sherman S, Parrott E, Rebar R, Santoro N, Utian W, et al. Executive summary: Stages of Reproductive Aging Workshop [STRAW], 875, Copyright 2001, with permission from Elsevier.)
*Stages most likely characterized by vasomotor symptoms.

tion is completed, and a woman is considered to be menopausal by definition. The duration of the menopausal transition is variable and can last 2–6 years, with an average of just more than 4 years. Because of the variability of this transition, it has been said that each woman goes through her own unique menopausal transition. The intermittent anovulation that may occur is similar to the pubertal period during which ovulatory cycles are interspersed among anovulatory periods.

Because of fluctuations in hormone levels, vasomotor symptoms and mood changes may be present. Unfortunately, laboratory studies are of little value in documenting the menopausal transition. In any single assessment, FSH and LH levels may not be elevated and relative hypoestrogenism or hyperestrogenism may be present. A single estradiol level is likely to be highly variable because of the intermittent nature of an ovulatory cycle present during menopausal transition. The charting of monophasic basal body temperatures can demonstrate the presence of an anovulatory cycle, but this method is more time-consuming and less convenient, and it will not add any additional information.

American College of Obstetricians and Gynecologists. Menopause. In: Precis: an update in obstetrics & gynecology. Reproductive endocrinology. 2nd ed. Washington, DC: ACOG; 2002. p.169–74.

Randolph JF Jr, Sowers M, Gold EB, Mohr BA, Luborsky J, Santoro N, et al. Reproductive hormones in the early menopausal transition: relationship to ethnicity, body size, and menopausal status. J Clin Endocrinol Metab 2003;88:1516–22.

Soules MR, Sherman S, Parrott E, Rebar R, Santoro N, Utian W, et al. Executive summary: Stages of Reproductive Aging Workshop (STRAW). Fertil Steril 2001;76:874–8.

39
Precocious thelarche

A 4-year-old child is referred for evaluation of precocious thelarche associated with a serum estradiol level of 382 pg/mL. The patient has Tanner stage III breast development and Tanner stage I pubic hair. Her longitudinal growth is in the 75th percentile, an increase from the 50th percentile of the previous years. The most appropriate next step in management is

(A) observation for 6 months
(B) gonadotropin-releasing hormone (GnRH) challenge test
* (C) pelvic ultrasound examination
(D) magnetic resonance imaging (MRI) of the head

Isolated precocious thelarche that represents a spontaneous temporary event related to the increase of gonadotropin levels during infancy usually occurs before age 2 years. It is not associated with other signs or symptoms of puberty, abdominal or pelvic pain, or central nervous system (CNS) problems. For such a presentation, observation often is all that is required. An evaluation is only necessary when there is evidence of true precocious thelarche with the appearance of additional pubertal landmarks (ie, adrenarche or vaginal bleeding), advanced skeletal growth, or both, or there are symptoms (ie, abdominal distention from ascites or pelvic abdominal pain) that would suggest an ovarian tumor or CNS lesion. In addition, isolated precocious thelarche is considered atypical if it appears after age 2 years because gonadotropin levels normally begin to decrease by this time, and the potential physiologic stimulus for estrogen production is gone. Isolated precocious thelarche is more likely to represent a pathologic entity when the initial signs of breast development occur after the second birthday.

This patient is atypical for the classical temporary form of isolated precocious thelarche. She is 4 years of age at presentation and has breast development beyond the initial breast bud associated with evidence of advanced bone growth. The referring clinician had obtained an estradiol level. Given the late age of presentation and the advancement of skeletal growth, this initial step was very appropriate. If the estradiol level had been normal, bone age radiographs would have been helpful to determine whether to begin the full investigation for true precocious puberty. Although bone age studies would likely be obtained at this initial referral visit, the high estradiol level is very suggestive of an ovarian tumor. The next important step, therefore, is to perform a pelvic ultrasound examination in this patient.

The most common ovarian neoplasms associated with sexual precocity in children are the granulosa cell tumor and rarely the feminizing Sertoli-Leydig cell tumor. Although it has been estimated that only 1% of sexual precocity in girls is caused by granulosa cell tumors, precocity is found in 70–80% of patients with these tumors. The mean age of diagnosis for such patients is 4 years. The most common symptoms are precocity and abdominal pain. Less frequently, these girls present with ascites or acute abdominal pain. The precocity usually is initiated with breast development but may progress to appearance of vaginal discharge and bleeding and less commonly the appearance of early pubic hair stages. Virilization is very rare. Accelerated bone and somatic growth also commonly occur. The sexual precocity has been reported to subside in most cases after removal of the tumors.

Estradiol levels rarely increase to more than 250 pg/mL in an adult spontaneous ovulatory menstrual cycle. Although a single value neither definitively rules in nor out primary ovarian pathology, the value presented here of 382 pg/mL raises the level of suspicion and warrants further investigation beginning with an ovarian ultrasound study. Other possible causes for an elevated estradiol value include isolated functional ovarian cysts and, less likely, gonadotropin independent precocity, such as McCune-Albright's syndrome. Recent evidence has determined that the granulosa cells of some of the isolated functional ovarian cysts that are identified at this age have the same activating somatic cell mutations of the Gs α-protein gene found in full-blown McCune-Albright's syndrome.

Other tumor markers have been used for identifying and following feminizing childhood ovarian tumors preoperatively and postoperatively. One such marker is inhibin. It has been found elevated in both granulosa cell and Sertoli-Leydig cell tumors and, when present, acts as an excellent indicator of cure and recurrence.

For this patient, if the estradiol value had been normal, further evaluation, beginning with bone age imaging, would have been appropriate. If more than 2 years discordant from chronologic age, further investigations would have been appropriate including an imaging study of the ovary and a GnRH challenge test to identify the predominant luteinizing hormone response associated with central true precocity. A head imaging study, such as an MRI, is an essential part of the evaluation for those patients identified with true precocity to rule out a pathologic central etiology.

Choong CS, Fuller PJ, Chu S, Jeske Y, Bowling F, Brown R, et al. Sertoli-Leydig cell tumor of the ovary, a rare cause of precocious puberty in a 12-month-old infant. J Clin Endocrinol Metab 2002;87: 49–56.

Cronje HS, Niemand I, Bam RH, Woodruff JD. Granulosa and theca cell tumors in children: a report of 17 cases and literature review. Obstet Gynecol Surv 1998;53:240–7.

Schumer ST, Cannistra SA. Granulosa cell tumor of the ovary. J Clin Oncol 2003;21:1180–9.

40

Metabolic syndrome

A 13-year-old adolescent comes in for evaluation and treatment of rapid weight gain and irregular menstrual cycles. She has a family history of obesity and diabetes mellitus in her father and endometriosis in her aunt. On physical examination, she is morbidly obese and has evidence of acanthosis nigricans. Her waist circumference is 90 cm, her fasting blood glucose level is 175 mg/dL, and her total cholesterol level is 300 mg/dL. The most common pathophysiologic basis for her disorder is

* (A) hyperlipidemia
* (B) hypothalamic dysfunction
* (C) hyperandrogenemia
* * (D) insulin resistance
* (E) leptin gene mutation

The metabolic syndrome (previously known as the insulin resistance syndrome or metabolic syndrome X) is a disorder associated with a number of risk factors (Box 40-1). The main underlying pathophysiology is acquired insulin resistance, where an associated postreceptor defect causes lack of response to insulin action leading to elevated levels of insulin and subsequent metabolic abnormalities. Along with co-existing medical disorders, insulin resistance has been closely linked to significant cardiovascular complications.

Metabolic syndrome is diagnosed when 3 or more of the following criteria are present: central obesity, elevated triglyceride level, low high-density lipoprotein (HDL) cholesterol level, elevated blood pressure level, and ele-

> **BOX 40-1**
>
> **Risk Factors for Metabolic Syndrome**
> - Abdominal obesity
> - Atherogenic dyslipidemia
>   - Elevated triglyceride level
>   - Small low-density lipoprotein particles
>   - Low high-density lipoprotein
> - Increased blood pressure levels
> - Insulin resistance
>   - With glucose intolerance
>   - Without glucose intolerance
> - Prothrombotic and proinflammatory states
>
> Data from Executive Summary of the Third Report of the National Cholesterol Education Program (NCEP) Expert Panel on Detection, Evaluation and Treatment of High Blood Cholesterol in Adults (Adult Treatment Panel III). JAMA 2001;285:2488.

TABLE 40-1. Guidelines for Clinical Identification of Metabolic Syndrome

Risk Factor	Defining Level
Waist circumference (abdominal obesity)	
Men	>102 cm (>40 in.)
Women	>88 cm (>35 in.)
High-density lipoprotein cholesterol level	
Men	<1 mmol/L (<40 mg/dL)
Women	<1.3 mmol/L (<50 mg/dL)
Triglyceride level	≥1.7 mmol/L (≥150 mg/dL)
Blood pressure level	≥130/85 mm Hg
Fasting plasma glucose level	≥6.6 mmol/L (≥110 mg/dL)

Modified from Executive Summary of the Third Report of the National Cholesterol Education Program (NCEP) Expert Panel on Detection, Evaluation and Treatment of High Blood Cholesterol in Adults (Adult Treatment Panel III). JAMA 2001;285:2493. Copyright © 2001, American Medical Association. All rights reserved.

vated fasting blood glucose level (Table 40-1). The measurement of waist circumference to estimate central obesity is more highly correlated with metabolic risk factors than is body mass index. Obesity leads to insulin resistance through several proposed mechanisms, the most common being an increased rate of nonesterified fatty acids, which can be associated with a postreceptor defect in insulin action.

The metabolic syndrome has been recognized as an important medical condition that should be diagnosed and treated aggressively. It is estimated to affect up to 22% of U.S. adults, a statistic that has continued to increase because of an increase in obesity in the United States. Individuals with sedentary lifestyles who exercise infrequently and who eat diets high in unsaturated fat are at highest risk. A genetic basis for the disease has been suggested, with individuals with a familial tendency for type 2 diabetes mellitus being at increased risk.

Metabolic syndrome often goes unrecognized and untreated by patients and providers and is associated with a high incidence of cardiovascular disease and premature death. Hyperinsulinemia represents a separate risk factor for the development of atherosclerotic plaques and is detrimental to the cardiovascular system. This combined with lifestyle factors that predispose to obesity, abnormal lipids, and diabetes mellitus can aggravate and worsen insulin sensitivity. Appropriate diet and exercise with weight reduction can help to decrease insulin resistance along with the related co-morbidities associated with this condition. Patients should be referred to providers who have experience with diet and exercise programs and who can follow patients on a long-term basis.

A realistic goal for weight reduction should be discussed with the patient. It has been shown that there is a 90% benefit to health status with only 5–7% reduction in body weight. The regimen to achieve this goal includes a low-calorie, low-cholesterol diet. Other modifications in lifestyle include smoking cessation, drinking alcohol in moderation, and engaging in regular exercise. Such improvements in lifestyle will likely decrease insulin resistance, low-density lipoprotein cholesterol levels, triglyceride levels, and blood pressure levels and elevate HDL cholesterol levels, thus improving the beneficial effects on cardiovascular function and decreasing coronary heart disease risk.

It often is difficult for patients with metabolic syndrome to remain dedicated to the recommended treatment. Treatment of severe obesity with medical therapy or bariatric surgery has proved to be successful for many patients in reducing significant long-term complications.

This patient presents with clinically recognizable metabolic syndrome. Even at a young age, she has a waist circumference greater than 88 cm and exhibits features of insulin resistance, signified by evidence of acanthosis nigricans and impaired glucose tolerance. A goal-directed health care plan for this patient is essential to prevent related gynecologic problems, maintain future fertility, and prevent cardiovascular complications along with an ultimate decrease in life expectancy.

Numerous endocrine manifestations are associated with insulin resistance and the development of the metabolic syndrome. Hyperlipidemia can lead to cardiovascular disease and complicate diabetes, but is not the cause of the underlying disorder. In addition, patients with polycystic ovary syndrome may exhibit features of the metabolic syndrome, but the presence of elevated androgen levels does not cause the disorder either. Finally, genetic mutations of the leptin gene have been the focus of obesity studies but to date have not been shown to play a significant role in the metabolic syndrome.

41
Glucocorticoid-induced osteoporosis

A 35-year-old African-American woman undergoes a dual-energy X-ray absorptiometry study. Her T-score at the hip is -2.8. She has eumenorrhea and a history of systemic lupus erythematosus. Her medications include daily prednisone (20 mg) for immunosuppression, a thiazide and ace inhibitor for hypertension, and Coumadin as prophylaxis. She also takes supplemental vitamin D and calcium. At this time, it would be most appropriate to

    (A) discontinue thiazide
* (B) add bisphosphonate
    (C) change Coumadin to heparin
    (D) add raloxifene
    (E) add calcitonin

Patients who receive prednisone doses greater than 2.5 mg per day for as short a time as 3 months are at increased risk for osteoporosis. Glucocorticoid-mediated effects responsible for reduction in bone mineral density (BMD) may include:

- Direct impairment of osteoblast and osteoclast function leading to reduced bone remodeling
- Enhanced effect of parathyroid hormone
- Antagonism of gonadal and adrenal function
- Increased renal elimination and reduced intestinal absorption of calcium, which might promote secondary hyperparathyroidism

Currently, risedronate and alendronate are the only bisphosphonates approved by the U.S. Food and Drug Administration (FDA) for the treatment of glucocorticoid-induced osteoporosis in men and women. Both drugs are potent inhibitors of bone resorption resulting in significant increases in BMD in the spine and hip. Increases in BMD at the spine and hip have resulted in significant decreases in the incidence of vertebral fractures in women with osteopenia and osteoporosis. Currently, a significant reduction in hip fractures in women with osteoporosis has only been observed with alendronate. Weekly rather than daily use of oral bisphosphonates has improved compliance and is associated with similar increases in BMD.

Thiazide, unlike loop diuretics, decreases renal calcium excretion. Hence, the use of a thiazide diuretic may reduce urinary calcium loss. In a randomized, double-blind crossover study that compared loop versus thiazide diuretics, urinary calcium levels decreased in a dose-dependent manner in response to thiazide treatment. Plasma calcium levels, as well as osteocalcin, a marker of bone formation, increased with the thiazide diuretic only.

Decreased BMD, secondary to heparin administration, was initially described in the mid-1960s. High doses and therapy for more than 6 months appear to be prerequisites. The exact mechanism responsible for heparin-induced osteoporosis is unknown. Heparin decreases lysosomal stability in bone cell homogenates, binds calcium ions because of its polyanionic nature, sensitizes bone to the resorptive activity of parathyroid hormone, and may cause resorption by partially replacing the normal mucopolysaccharide matrix of bone. Coumadin use has not been associated with osteoporosis.

Raloxifene, a selective estrogen receptor modulator, increases BMD to a lesser extent than bisphosphonates. Raloxifene is approved for treatment of osteoporosis in postmenopausal but not premenopausal women. Use of raloxifene in a premenopausal woman may be associated with ovarian cyst formation, vasomotor symptoms, menstrual irregularity, and an increased risk of thromboembolism. Calcitonin is FDA approved for the treatment of osteoporosis in postmenopausal women. Continuous use of calcitonin is associated with a persistent decrease in the rate of bone resorption. Calcitonin may have a beneficial short-term effect on pain in women who have sustained a vertebral fracture. Calcitonin use in postmenopausal osteoporosis often is limited because of its cost, relative inconvenience of intranasal administration, less improvement in BMD than other antiresorptive treatments, and the possible development of resistance to the drug. Neither calcitonin nor raloxifene have been shown to significantly reduce hip fractures.

Avioli LV. Heparin induced osteopenia: an appraisal. Adv Exp Med Biol 1975;52:375–87.

Doga M, Bonadonna S, Burattin A, Carpinteri R, Manelli F, Giustina A. Bisphosphonates in the treatment of glucocorticoid-induced osteoporosis. Front Horm Res 2002;30:150–64.

Patschan D, Loddenkemper K, Buttgereit F. Molecular mechanisms of glucocorticoid-induced osteoporosis. Bone 2001;29:498–505.

Rejnmark L, Vestergaard P, Pedersen AR, Heickendorff L, Andreasen F, Mosekilde L. Dose-effect relations of loop- and thiazide-diuretics on calcium homeostasis: a randomized, double-blinded Latin-square multiple cross-over study in postmenopausal osteopenic women. Eur J Clin Invest 2003;33:41–50.

Van Staa TP, Leufkens HG, Cooper C. The epidemiology of corticosteroid-induced osteoporosis: a meta-analysis. Osteoporos Int 2002;13:777–87.

42

Tubal anastomosis

A 24-year-old woman with a history of ectopic pregnancy and left total salpingectomy presents with findings consistent with a right tubal pregnancy. She underwent a tubal sterilization reversal 4 months ago. A laparoscopy is performed for worsening pain and anemia. A leaking ectopic pregnancy approximately 5 cm in size is visualized at the site of the tubal reversal in the isthmic portion of the fallopian tube, and she has distal peritubal adhesions. The remainder of the tube on either side of the ectopic pregnancy has a normal appearance. The most appropriate next step in the surgical management of this patient is

* (A) right salpingectomy
  (B) hysterectomy
  (C) salpingostomy with removal of ectopic pregnancy
  (D) partial salpingectomy to remove ectopic pregnancy
  (E) partial salpingectomy with immediate tubal anastomosis

Despite the fact that tubal sterilization is a permanent form of contraception, some women ultimately regret their decision and request a tubal ligation reversal. A change in marital status, desire for another child, or death of a child are common reasons why some women will request a reversal. Several studies have shown that 3–5% of women will ultimately regret their decision to have a voluntary tubal sterilization.

Pregnancy success rates following tubal sterilization reversal procedures are 50–70% in properly selected candidates. Along with surgical manipulation of the fallopian tubes comes the risk of ectopic pregnancy among women who conceive. Large studies reveal that the risk of ectopic pregnancy following tubal reversal is 2–8%.

Ectopic pregnancy is diagnosed by standard methods of serial monitoring of serum β-hCG levels combined with transvaginal ultrasonography. Contemporary methods of treatment include medical therapy using methotrexate and surgery. If diagnosed early, an ectopic pregnancy after tubal reversal may be treated with medical therapy. A salpingostomy with removal of the ectopic pregnancy may be performed if the tube is salvageable at the time of surgery and not destroyed by a large hematosalpinx or tubal rupture. In most cases, salpingectomy is the preferred treatment. A partial salpingectomy also may be performed if the possibility of tubal reanastomosis could be accomplished at a later time.

In this patient, the risk of ectopic pregnancy is even higher because of her previous history of ectopic pregnancy as well as tubal surgery. Salpingectomy with in vitro fertilization (IVF) may be considered a more appropriate option in this case. The other choices would not be considered the treatment of choice in the present patient's clinical situation. Expressing the ectopic pregnancy through the end of the fallopian tube via a tubal abortion or performing a salpingostomy with removal may result in residual trophoblastic tissue, which may require medical therapy with methotrexate or additional surgery.

Performing a partial salpingectomy and anastomosis on a tube that has already been altered through previous surgery and has an ectopic pregnancy would not be the best method of treatment in this patient. If anastomosis was ever considered after a partial salpingectomy, this type of surgery should be delayed to allow tubal healing to occur.

Risk factors for pregnancy complications are important when making decisions regarding treatment in a tubal reversal ectopic pregnancy. Postoperative follow-up care is important in the patient treated by laparoscopic salpingostomy. Monitoring of serum β-hCG levels is necessary to ensure that persistent trophoblastic disease is not present. Treatment with postoperative methotrexate or surgery is indicated if β-hCG levels persist or increase and do not decrease to undetectable levels.

Hysterosalpingography may be performed after treatment for an ectopic pregnancy to confirm tubal patency. If the fallopian tubes are occluded or the patient had a partial salpingectomy, the surgeon may consider a second anastomosis if the fallopian tubes are suitable for revision. Most practitioners recommend proceeding with IVF to avoid surgery and the future risk of complications.

Reversal of tubal sterilization using microsurgery poses a small but increased risk of ectopic pregnancy. Patients should be monitored closely after pregnancy confirmation to exclude the possibility of an ectopic pregnancy and treated with standard medical or surgical therapies if a diagnosis is made. Fortunately, most pregnancies following tubal ligation reversal are intrauterine and proceed normally.

Cantor B, Riggall FC. The choice of sterilizating procedure according to its potential reversibility with microsurgery. Fertil Steril 1979;31: 9–12.

Kim SH, Shin CJ, Kim JG, Moon SY, Lee JY, Chang YS. Microsurgical reversal of tubal sterilization: a report of 1,118 cases. Fertil Steril 1997;68:865–70.

Yadav R, Reddi R, Bupathy A. Fertility outcome after reversal of sterilization. J Obstet Gynaecol Res 1998;24:393–400.

43
Sheehan's syndrome

A 28-year-old woman, gravida 1, para 1, was admitted to labor and delivery with a retained placenta following a planned home delivery. The patient was managed with intravenous fluid therapy and manual removal of the placenta under anesthesia. Postoperatively, her hematocrit concentration was 19%. She was given 3 units of whole blood and her posttransfusion hematocrit concentration is now 32% and stable. She has experienced orthostatic symptoms and fatigue for the past 2 days but refuses further blood transfusions. She has no milk production and is concerned that her infant will become dehydrated. On examination, she appears tired and sleepy. In the supine position, her blood pressure level is 76/40 mm Hg and her pulse rate is 105 beats per minute. Her blood pressure level decreases to 60/30 mm Hg and pulse increases to 130 beats per minute 2 minutes after shifting into the sitting position. The most appropriate next step in her management is

    (A) blood transfusion
    (B) intravenous glucose
* (C) corticosteroid therapy
    (D) toxicology screen

Sheehan's syndrome, or postpartum pituitary necrosis, is an uncommon disorder associated with severe obstetric hemorrhage with hypotension, circulatory collapse, and shock. This condition, if not recognized, constitutes a medical emergency that can be life threatening.

The pathophysiology of Sheehan's syndrome is not entirely clear. During pregnancy, there is an increase in blood supply to many organs including the pituitary bed. The pituitary gland enlarges in part because of the increase in secretory activity of the prolactin-producing cells called lactotropes. Sheehan postulated that, during the period of obstetric hemorrhage and profound hypotension, there occurs vasospasm of the arteries that supply the pituitary gland and pituitary stalk. This in turn leads to venous stasis and thrombosis of the small pituitary portal vessels, which causes a variable degree of pituitary ischemia and pituitary cell death.

In the immediate postpartum period, many patients initially present with a failure to undergo breast engorgement and lactation because of the deficiency in pituitary prolactin secretion. Other anterior pituitary hormone deficiencies also can occur. In some patients, such as the one described, the absence of adrenocorticotropic hormone leads to inadequate cortisol secretion, causing hypotension, lethargy, nausea, and vomiting. Deficiency in thyroid-stimulating hormone (TSH) and thyroid hormone usually is noted later. Deficiencies in luteinizing hormone and follicle-stimulating hormone (FSH) would lead to amenorrhea and a hypogonadal state. The posterior pituitary usually is spared because this area is less dependent on the portal blood supply.

For the patient who presents with Sheehan's syndrome, hypotension, and lethargy, immediate intramuscular administration of corticosteroids is required. Once the patient has been stabilized, a maintenance dose of cortisone acetate or prednisone can be used. Under stressful conditions, such as infection or major surgery, the daily dose of corticosteroids should be doubled or tripled. The patient should be instructed to wear a medical alert bracelet.

The extent of pituitary gland deficiencies can be determined by provocative testing with a combined intravenous injection of the hypothalamic releasing factors gonadotropin-releasing hormone, corticotropin-releasing hormone, thyrotropin-releasing hormone, and growth hormone-releasing hormone. It is important to begin corticosteroid therapy before instituting thyroid hormone therapy because of the danger of circulatory collapse secondary to Addisonian crisis. For thyroid therapy, thyroxine (T_4) should be given gradually beginning at 25 µg per day and increased at 25 µg increments at 1-week intervals until a full dose of 0.1–0.2 mg per day is reached. In this case, the TSH levels may not be useful in guiding therapy, and free T_4 levels or clinical signs, such as basal pulse rate, can be used. Estrogen therapy will be needed in patients who remain amenorrheic. Gradual recovery of pituitary gland function has been reported in a few cases.

In this patient, her severe orthostatic hypotension, lethargy and fatigue is caused by hypocortisolism, a life-threatening condition that should be treated with corticosteroids. Additional blood transfusions will not correct her orthostatic hypotension. Intravenous fluid replacement or a fluid challenge will not improve her blood pressure level because she is no longer significantly intravascularly volume depleted. Because her lethargy is secondary to hypocortisolism and not hypoglycemia, intravenous glucose will not be effective. It is conceivable that her symptoms could be the result of recreational drug use. However, this is less likely given her clinical presentation.

Jackson IM, Whyte WG, Garrey MM. Pituitary function following uncomplicated pregnancy in Sheehan's syndrome. J Clin Endocrinol Metab 1969;29:315–8.

Sheehan HL, Davis JC. Pituitary necrosis. Br Med Bull 1968;24:59–70.

Sheldon WR Jr, DeBold CR, Evans WS, DeCherney SG, Jackson RV, Island DP, et al. Rapid sequential intravenous administration of four hypothalamic releasing hormones as a combined anterior pituitary function test in normal subjects. J Clin Endocrinol Metab 1985;60:623–30.

44

Evaluation of chronic pelvic pain

In a 25-year-old woman, gravida 2, para 2, with a 9-month history of dysmenorrhea and dyspareunia, the diagnosis that would most likely be confirmed by laparoscopy only is

* (A) endometriosis
(B) interstitial cystitis
(C) irritable bowel syndrome
(D) musculoskeletal disease

Abdominal and pelvic pain often occur together and may be secondary to a variety of gynecologic and nongynecologic disorders. Gynecologic causes of chronic pelvic pain commonly include leiomyomas, endometriosis, adenomyosis, pelvic adhesive disease, and chronic pelvic inflammatory disease. Nongynecologic causes include chronic interstitial cystitis, musculoskeletal disease, and irritable bowel syndrome.

A thorough history of the woman's symptoms, previous diagnoses, and previous treatments should be obtained. With chronic pelvic pain, symptoms tend to be vague and may have a psychologic component. A complete gynecologic examination should be conducted, including pelvic and abdominal examinations, with a focus on tenderness, nodularity, palpable masses, and referred pain. Laboratory and imaging studies should be considered to assist with developing an initial impression of the etiology of the chronic pelvic pain. These assessments should occur before consideration of any surgical intervention.

Endometriosis, characterized by the presence of functional endometrial glands and stroma outside the uterus, is the most likely cause of chronic pelvic pain that presents with dysmenorrhea and dyspareunia. The American

Society for Reproductive Medicine classifies endometriosis in a range from minimal (stage I) to severe (stage IV). Diagnosis can be confirmed by biopsy of suspicious lesions detected at the time of laparoscopy, a minimally invasive method for evaluating the pelvis for pathology.

Laparoscopy also allows management of the identified lesion at the time of diagnosis using numerous modalities, including carbon-dioxide, potassium titanyl phosphate, neodymium:yttrium-aluminum-garnet, and argon lasers; ultrasonic shears; and monopolar and bipolar electrical energy.

Chronic pelvic pain can be caused by endometriosis or interstitial cystitis or both; therefore, it is important to perform concurrent laparoscopic and cystoscopic examinations followed by hydrodistention in an initial evaluation, especially if the patient reports irritative bladder symptoms. Interstitial cystitis is diagnosed by the presence of glomerulations and terminal hematuria by National Institutes of Health criteria. Women also may be screened for interstitial cystitis using the Interstitial Cystitis Symptom Index and Problem Index (Box 44-1). In a study of 45 women scheduled to undergo laparoscopy and cystoscopy with hydrodistention and bladder biopsy for chronic pelvic pain, 17 (38%) met the diagnosis of interstitial cystitis, which included a combination of urgency, frequency or nocturia, and positive cystoscopic

---

BOX 44-1

Interstitial Cystitis Symptom and Problem Questionnaire for Identifying Interstitial Cystitis*

To help your physician determine if you have interstitial cystitis (IC), please put a check mark next to the most appropriate response to each of the questions shown below. Then add up the numbers to the left of the check marks and write the total below.

During the past month, how much has each of the following been a problem for you:

IC Symptom Index

Q1. How often have you felt the strong need to urinate with little or no warning?
   0. ___Not at all
   1. ___Less than 1 time in 5
   2. ___Less than half the time
   3. ___About half the time
   4. ___More than half the time
   5. ___Almost always

Q2. Have you had to urinate less than 2 hours after you finished urinating?
   0. ___Not at all
   1. ___Less than 1 time in 5
   2. ___Less than half the time
   3. ___About half the time
   4. ___More than half the time
   5. ___Almost always

Q3. How often did you most typically get up at night to urinate?
   0. ___Not at all
   2. ___A few times
   3. ___Almost always
   4. ___Fairly often
   5. ___Usually

Q4. Have you experienced pain or burning in your bladder?
   0. ___Not at all
   2. ___A few times
   3. ___Almost always
   4. ___Fairly often
   5. ___Usually

Add the numerical values of the checked entries.
Total score:

IC Problem Index

Q1. Frequent urination during the day?
   0. ___No problem
   1. ___Very small problem
   2. ___Small problem
   3. ___Medium problem
   4. ___Big problem

Q2. Getting up at night to urinate?
   0. ___No problem
   1. ___Very small problem
   2. ___Small problem
   3. ___Medium problem
   4. ___Big problem

Q3. Need to urinate with little warning?
   0. ___No problem
   1. ___Very small problem
   2. ___Small problem
   3. ___Medium problem
   4. ___Big problem

Q4. Burning, pain, discomfort, or pressure in your bladder?
   0. ___No problem
   1. ___Very small problem
   2. ___Small problem
   3. ___Medium problem
   4. ___Big problem

Total score:

---

*Indices are not meant as screening tools. They can be used as an aid in the diagnosis and management of IC. Summary scores range from 0 to 24 for both indices. Almost no patients with IC score less than 6 on either index.

Reprinted from O'Leary MP, Sant GR, Fowler FJ Jr, Whitmore KE, Spolarich-Kroll J. The interstitial cystitis symptom index and problem index. Urology 1997;49(suppl):62. Copyright 1997 with permission from Elsevier.

findings. Based on their responses before surgery, independent risk factors for a diagnosis of interstitial cystitis were an elevated symptom index score and an elevated dyspareunia pain score.

Interstitial cystitis should be included in the differential diagnosis of chronic pelvic pain. Patients with interstitial cystitis have a history of being treated for urinary tract or vaginal infections, and the condition can be exacerbated by menses, coitus, and stress. In 1988, the National Institute of Diabetes and Digestive and Kidney Diseases published criteria for diagnosing interstitial cystitis for research purposes, but the criteria may be too rigid to manage patients in an active clinical setting. Besides urinary tract symptoms, the hallmark of this diagnosis is its chronicity, with a pattern of intermittent flaring interspersed with periods of remission. Urinary frequency is a key historical symptom, but often patients are not aware of the number of times they void per day. Any patient who voids more than 15 times per day should be strongly suspected of having interstitial cystitis. The pathogenesis is thought to be related to the activation of the bladder sensory nerves related to urothelium dysfunction. Tests include a potassium sensitivity test using a dilute solution of intravesical potassium solution. Patients with interstitial cystitis experience urgency, pain, or both in response to this potassium challenge. More than 80% of patients with interstitial cystitis will have positive test results, whereas only 2% of controls will experience discomfort. Experts are divided on the diagnostic usefulness of cytoscopy to observe the characteristic bladder ulcerations.

A retrospective study of women referred to a tertiary care center with interstitial cystitis and exacerbation of symptoms during the menstrual cycle found 15 had undergone laparoscopy followed immediately by cystoscopy and bladder hydrodistention and treatment with gonadotropin-releasing hormone agonist or oral contraceptive pills. Ten of the patients (67%) also had peritoneal endometriosis. In this first report of hormonal treatment for chronic, cyclic irritative bladder symptoms, improvement occurred even when endometriosis was not identified by laparoscopy.

Pain secondary to irritable bowel syndrome is easily confused with endometriosis-associated chronic pelvic pain. However, one of the most common distinctions is the relief of pain following bowel movements.

Finally, a woman who presents with pain that occurs with walking and radiates around her flank region and leg most likely is experiencing the result of lumbar spinal disease. This includes arthritis, spondylolosis, disk rupture, or spinal stenosis.

Clemons JL, Arya LA, Myers DL. Diagnosing interstitial cystitis in women with chronic pelvic pain. Obstet Gynecol 2002;100:337–41.

Chung MK, Chung RR, Gordon D, Jennings C. The evil twins of chronic pelvic pain syndrome: endometriosis and interstitial cystitis. JSLS 2002;6:311–4.

Guarnaccia MM, Olive DL. Diagnosis and management of endometriosis. In: Carr BR, Blackwell RE, eds. Reproductive medicine. 2nd ed. Stamford (CT): Appleton and Lange; 1998. p. 641–63.

Lentz GM, Bavendam T, Stenchever MA, Miller JL, Smalldridge J. Hormonal manipulation in women with chronic, cyclic irritable bladder symptoms and pelvic pain. Am J Obstet Gynecol 2002;186:1268–71; discussion 1271–3.

Winkel CA. Evaluation and management of women with endometriosis. Obstet Gynecol 2003;102:397–408.

45

Ovarian androgen-secreting tumors

A 57-year-old woman (Fig. 45-1; see color plate), 6 years postmenopausal, presents with new onset hirsutism and increased sensitivity and size of the clitoris. Physical examination shows normal blood pressure level and increased muscle mass but is negative for hypertension, acanthosis nigricans, adnexal mass, or striae. Pelvic ultrasonography reveals normal appearing ovaries, and computed tomography (CT) scan shows normal adrenal glands. Her serum testosterone level is 300 ng/dL. The most likely diagnosis is

    (A) adult onset congenital adrenal hyperplasia
    (B) adrenal tumor
* (C) hilus cell tumor
    (D) Cushing's syndrome
    (E) hyperinsulinemia and hyperthecosis

Given the clinical description of this patient, it is probable that she has an androgen-producing tumor. Although such tumors are extremely rare, they have a dramatic presentation and evoke substantial clinical interest. The rapid onset of virilization is the first clue to reaching this diagnosis. Serum testosterone levels greater than 200 ng/dL in the premenopausal woman or greater than 100 ng/dL in the postmenopausal woman are associated with ovarian tumor. Generally, there is a palpable adnexal mass or ultrasonographic evidence of ovarian enlargement. Nearly any ovarian tumor is capable of producing testosterone, and, thus, narrowing down the histologic diagnosis preoperatively is difficult.

Hilus cell tumors of the ovary often are very small and can secrete testosterone. They are typically 1 cm or less, usually unilateral but can be bilateral, and may present in the postmenopausal years. They may go undetected by bimanual pelvic examination or by ultrasonography. Bilateral oophorectomy would be appropriate for this patient. Selective venography may be possible to lateralize the tumor and potentially allow preservation of a normal ovary.

When there is no ovarian mass by ultrasonography, the diagnosis is more elusive, and imaging studies are appropriate. Vaginal ultrasonography is better than magnetic resonance imaging (MRI) or CT scan for imaging the ovary. When screening for an adrenal tumor, imaging by CT scan is most appropriate and provides better resolution for the adrenal gland than both ultrasonography and MRI. A CT scan of the adrenal gland is sensitive for small tumors that produce Cushing's syndrome, as well as for virilizing adrenal adenomas. Cushing's syndrome can feature virilization, but not before initial presentation with hirsutism, and often is associated with hypertension and striae.

Postmenopausal hyperthecosis of the ovaries is rare. It can occur, though, when high circulating insulin stimulates the ovarian theca. Acanthosis nigricans is a common clinical finding. Testosterone levels are not known to exceed 200 ng/dL, and the progress from hirsutism to masculinization is gradual. An ultrasonogram reveals bilateral ovarian enlargement. Hyperthecosis is responsive to suppression with a gonadotropin-releasing hormone agonist.

Late onset congenital adrenal hyperplasia does not present with virilization, and baseline 17-hydroxycorticosteroids progesterone levels usually are greater than 200 ng/dL. Initial presentation of congenital adrenal hyperplasia would be unlikely in the sixth decade of life. Heterozygotes for 21-hydroxylase deficiency often do not have clinically relevant hirsutism.

Duun S. Bilateral virilizing hilus (Leydig) cell tumors of the ovary. Acta Obstet Gynecol Scand 1994;73:76–7.

Hayes FJ, Sheahan K, Rajendiran S, McKenna TJ. Virilization in a postmenopausal woman as a result of hilus cell hyperplasia associated with a simple ovarian cyst. Am J Obstet Gynecol 1997;176:719–20.

Knochenhauer ES, Cortet-Rudelli C, Cunnigham RD, Conway-Myers BA, Dewailly D, Azziz R. Carriers of 21-hydroxylase deficiency are not at increased risk for hyperandrogenism. J Clin Endocrinol Metab 1997; 82:479–85.

Krug E, Berga SL. Postmenopausal hyperthecosis: functional dysregulation of androgenesis in climacteric ovary. Obstet Gynecol 2002;99(5 Pt 2):893–7.

White FE, White ME, Drury PL, Fry IK, Besser GM. Value of computed tomography of the abdomen and chest in investigation of Cushing's syndrome. Br Med J (Clin Res Ed) 1982;284:771–4.

46

Chromosomal abnormalities in couples with recurrent abortion

Five couples come in for further evaluation for recurrent pregnancy loss. Of the following pregnancy histories, the couple most likely to have a parental balanced chromosome translocation as the cause for their loss(es) has

(A) 6 spontaneous abortions
(B) 2 spontaneous abortions
(C) 3 spontaneous abortions, each separated by a healthy term infant
* (D) 1 spontaneous abortion, 2 term infants (1 with unbalanced translocation)
(E) 1 term infant followed by 3 spontaneous abortions

The most common method of ascertainment that will identify individuals who harbor balanced chromosome abnormalities is the history of multiple spontaneous abortions. Although both the definition of recurrent abortion and a number of the purported etiologies have been long questioned, the fact that specific structural alterations of the chromosomes may lead to aneuploidy is well documented and understood. What often is overlooked, in regard to identifying these findings, however, is the setting in which such parental chromosome abnormalities may or may not exist. The number of abortions is not as important compared with reproductive history (eg, for the patient in scenario D).

The reported incidence of a parental chromosome abnormality that is etiologic for spontaneous abortions has varied from 0.2% to more than 20%. This wide variation reflects the differences in the patient populations studied and argues against several long-held misconceptions: that the couples with the highest risk for such abnormalities have a large number of spontaneous abortions and that they either do not have a history of liveborn normal children or, if they do, the abortions are consecutive.

The most common chromosome abnormality in this patient population is the chromosome translocation. Balanced reciprocal translocations often are more common than the Robertsonian translocation; however, both may be identified in the recurrent abortion population. In addition, some series identify translocations more commonly in female partners than in males because some of the translocations interfere with normal spermatogenesis and cause male subfertility or sterility.

Most chromosome translocations are familial and are inherited intact from a normal parent who usually has had a mixture of pregnancy outcomes (ie, scenarios C, D, and E). Although the history of a mixed pregnancy outcome that includes a newborn infant with anomalies (ie, scenario D) has the greatest likelihood of being caused by a chromosome translocation, it is a misconception that birth of a normal child rules out the presence of a parental chromosome translocation. The chromosome pairs involved in a chromosome translocation may segregate into gametes in any number of ways that can result in a variety of outcomes. Fig. 46-1 (see color plate) illustrates the segregation possibilities for a translocation involving chromosomes 14 and 21, probably the most common Robertsonian translocation. This example demonstrates that both normal and abnormal gametes (and pregnancy outcomes) can be expected to result from the meiotic process. Although it would appear that the 4 segregation possibilities would each occur equally and one third of liveborn children resulting from the $t(14q\ 21q)$ translocation heterozygote would have Down syndrome, this only occurs for 10% of female carriers and 2% of male carriers. Such a sex difference in segregation outcomes has not been reported for other translocations, which may reflect the relative rarity of the other translocations.

Parents who harbor chromosome translocations may have phenotypically normal children with either completely normal chromosomes or the balanced translocation carrier state. Although most of the unbalanced outcomes of these translocations result in spontaneous abortion, liveborn children with anomalies, developmental delays, or mental retardation also may be found. Because most translocations may result in either normal or abnormal gametes, it is rare for them to be found in only couples with a history of multiple abortions and no liveborn children as suggested previously (ie, scenario A). A number of series have demonstrated that the incidence of parental chromosome abnormalities is not different in couples with only 2 abortions compared with couples with 3 or more abortions (ie, scenario B). In fact, studies that limit the patient population to a pure history of abortions only or to 4 or more abortions have found the lowest incidence of parental translocations. Studies that include the history of either normal or abnormal children in addition to 2 or more abortions report higher incidences of chromosome translocations. If only those couples with abortions and defective children (with or without normal siblings) were separated out, the incidence of this finding would be even higher.

The previous insistence on counting the number of abortions that a couple has to define recurrent abortion has prevented more appropriate focus on the reproductive setting in which the abortions have occurred. If an individual has a translocation, the first pregnancy could be a liveborn child with mental retardation and anomalies, a normal child, or a spontaneous abortion. Therefore, this risk may be ascertained during a preconceptional counseling discussion by disclosure of a family history with multiple spontaneous abortions and children with anomalies or mental retardation. For such an individual, obtaining a karyotype may be appropriate before becoming pregnant. Couples who have a child with anomalies, developmental delays, or obvious mental retardation should be considered for chromosome analysis, as should couples with normal children and 2 or more spontaneous abortions.

Other chromosome abnormalities that lead to unbalanced gametes include large paracentric or pericentric inversions, ring chromosomes, and mosaicism. The most common of these chromosome abnormalities is X chromosome mosaicism. Low-level mosaicism may represent in vitro cultural artifact. However, it also may be the etiology for single cell line X chromosome aneuploidy (eg, 45,X), which usually is lethal and can result in spontaneous abortion.

Phung Thi Tho, Bryd JR, McDonough PG. Etiologies and subsequent performance of 100 couples with recurrent abortion. Fertil Steril 1979; 32:389–95.

Sachs ES, Jahoda MG, Van Hemel JO, Hoogeboom AJ, Sandkuyl LA. Chromosomes studies of 500 couples with two or more abortions. Obstet Gynecol 1985;65:375–8.

Schwartz S, Palmer CG. Chromosomal findings in 164 couples with repeated spontaneous abortions: with special consideration to prior reproductive history. Hum Genet 1983:63:28–34.

Simpson JL, Meyers CM, Martin AO, Elias S, Ober C. Translocations are infrequent among couples having repeated spontaneous abortions but no other abnormal pregnancies. Fertil Steril 1989;51:811–4.

47

Vascular injury with laparoscopy

A 26-year-old woman, weighing 92 kg (205 lb), has a 6 cm × 7 cm persistent complex left adnexal mass. She is scheduled to have a laparoscopy and left ovarian cystectomy. After placing the laparoscope, you unsuccessfully attempt to transilluminate the deep inferior epigastric vessels before insertion of the accessory trocars. The best strategy to avoid damage to the deep inferior epigastric vessels during placement of secondary trocars is to

    (A) place the trocars 2 cm lateral to and 2 cm above the iliac crest
* (B) identify the umbilical ligaments
    (C) use only a single suprapubic midline trocar
    (D) insert the trocars 5 cm medial to the iliac crest

Operative laparoscopy allows the gynecologic surgeon to evaluate and manage a wide variety of pelvic pathology on an outpatient basis. The ability to remove adnexal pathology safely via the laparoscope is dependent on the operator's ability to place multiple trocars to allow for visualization and manipulation of the pelvic pathology. This usually requires the placement of at least 2 additional 5-mm or 10-mm trocars in the right and left lower quadrants in addition to the infraumbilical trocar. Other locations can be used, such as the suprapubic or left upper quadrant sites. Regardless of which accessory trocar site is used, the surgeon must be aware of the relevant anatomy and potential complications related to the placement of these instruments.

Vascular injuries constitute some of the more common complications associated with operative laparoscopy. When placing trocars in the right and left lower quadrants, injury to the superficial and deep inferior epigastric vessels are the most frequent. The deep inferior epigastric vessels originate from the external iliac, while the superficial epigastric vessels are a branch of the femoral. Several alternative techniques can be used by the operator to avoid these types of injuries. A commonly accepted method for avoiding injury to the superficial epigastric vessels is through transillumination, where the operator shines the intraabdominal laparoscope light under the skin of the patient in an attempt to identify those arteries and veins. However, this method is limited when the patient is overweight, as in the case of patient described. In addition, the technique is not consistently effective in identifying the deep epigastric vessels. Therefore, knowledge of the course of the vessels is extremely important.

A strategy used to limit the possibility of damaging the deep inferior epigastric vessels includes placement of lateral secondary trocars 4–5 cm above the symphysis pubis at the lateral border of the rectus muscle, which usually is 3–4 cm medial to the iliac crest (Fig. 47-1). This will allow placement of the secondary trocars 2–3 cm lateral to the deep inferior epigastric vessels. However, in cases of obesity, these landmarks become less reliable because of the potential distortion of the anatomy.

The deep inferior epigastric vessels run lateral to the umbilical ligaments. The ligaments can be seen intraperitoneally. The vessels pass the round ligament, proceed to the anterior abdominal wall, and usually can be seen just above the peritoneum. Injury to these vessels can be avoided by inserting the secondary trocars lateral or medial to the umbilical ligaments (Fig. 47-2). Although aberrant vessels can be present, this technique for avoiding the deep inferior epigastric vessels will provide the greatest consistency and is the optimum choice in this patient.

The use of a single midline suprapubic trocar will allow the surgeon to accomplish some operative laparoscopic procedures. When complex anatomic dissections or suturing is anticipated, the surgeon usually will require several port sites and must be prepared to place these in a safe manner. Therefore, use of a single suprapubic trocar is not an option in this patient. Because the deep epigastric vessels will run approximately 4–5 cm medial to the iliac crest, the operator should avoid placement of trocars in this area.

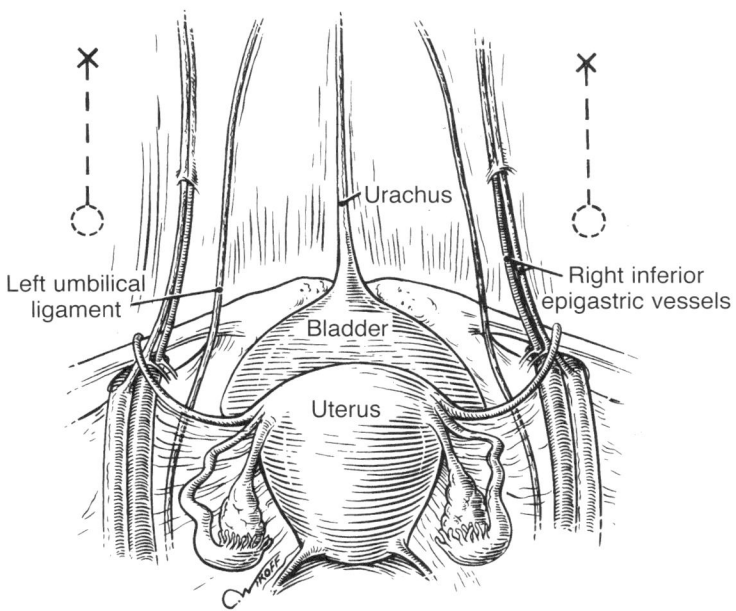

FIG. 47-1. Deep inferior epigastric vessels run lateral to the umbilical ligaments. (Nezhat CR, Nezhat FR, Luciano AA, Siegler AM, Metzger DA, Nezhat C. Operative gynecologic laparoscopy, principles and techniques. New York [NY]: McGraw-Hill; 1995. p. 88. Reproduced with permission of The McGraw-Hill Companies.)

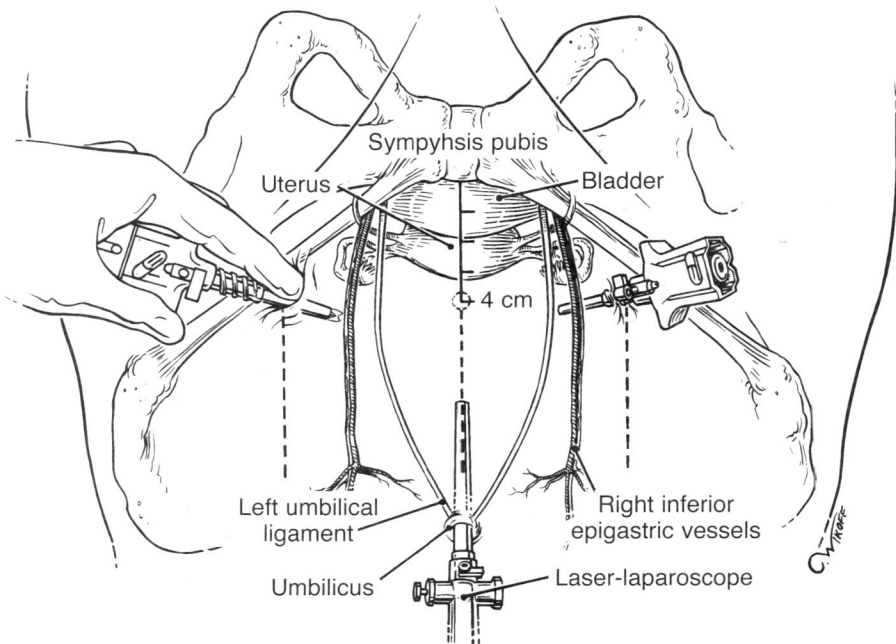

FIG. 47-2. Accessory trocars are placed under direct vision to avoid injury to the inferior epigastric vessels and any organs that may be adherent to the pelvic side wall or the anterior abdominal wall. The trocar is inserted lateral to the left umbilical ligament, avoiding inferior epigastric vessels that are invariably lateral to the umbilical ligaments. (Nezhat CR, Nezhat FR, Luciano AA, Siegler AM, Metzger DA, Nezhat C. Operative gynecologic laparoscopy, principles and techniques. New York [NY]: McGraw-Hill; 1995. p. 88. Reproduced with permission of The McGraw-Hill Companies.)

Jansen FW, Kapiteyn K, Trimbos-Kemper T, Hermans J, Trimbos JB. Complications of laparoscopy: a prospective multicentre observational study. Br J Obstet Gynaecol 1997;104:595–600.

Lin P, Grow DR. Complications of laparoscopy. Strategies for prevention and cure. Obstet Gynecol Clin North Am 1999;26:23–38, v.

Munro MG. Laparoscopic access: complications, technologies, and techniques. Curr Opin Obstet Gynecol 2002;14:365–74.

Quint EH, Wang FL, Hurd WW. Laparoscopic transillumination for the location of anterior abdominal wall blood vessels. J Laparoendosc Surg 1996;6:167–9.

48

Hereditary cancer syndromes

A 45-year-old woman, gravida 1, para 1, presents with abnormal uterine bleeding and is given a diagnosis of endometrial cancer. She tells you that colorectal cancer was diagnosed in her brother, her only sibling, at age 45 years, and her mother developed ovarian cancer at age 62 years. The mutation that is most likely to test positive in this woman is

    (A) *BRCA1*
* (B) *MSH2*
    (C) *APC*
    (D) *TP53*
    (E) *MEN1*

Although hereditary cancer syndromes have been recognized for many years, only recently have the molecular mutations of several been identified. In most cases, the increased risk of cancer is transmitted in an autosomal dominant fashion (Table 48-1). An important implication of autosomal dominant inheritance is that one half of all women with a hereditary risk of cancer of the breast, ovary, or endometrium inherit that risk from their father rather than from their mother because men carry and transmit these mutations just as often as women. Thus, the family history must include an assessment of both paternal and maternal disorders. Mutations in any of 3 major types of genes—tumor suppressor, DNA repair enzyme, and proto-oncogenes—can cause hereditary cancer syndromes. Because there are so many familial syndromes, it is not unreasonable to have a genetic counselor take a detailed history from patients with a strong family history of cancer.

This patient has a family history of colorectal, ovarian, and endometrial cancer. Consultation with a genetic counselor in this case would be appropriate. The presence of a colorectal cancer in that history should lead to a consideration of hereditary nonpolyposis colorectal cancer or Lynch II syndrome. This syndrome is characterized by markedly increased susceptibility to cancers of the large bowel, but, as is true for this patient's family history, ovarian and endometrial cancer can occur frequently as well. The most likely mutation is *MSH2*. The increased risk of cancer in these families has been shown to be caused by defects in DNA repair enzyme genes, which are responsible for the repair of nucleotide mismatches during DNA replication and prevent propagation of potentially harmful mutations. Mutations in the genes *MSH2*, located on chromosome 2p, and *MLH1*, found on chromosome 3p, account for 70% of hereditary nonpolyposis colorectal cancer cases, and mutations in *PMS1*, *PMS2*, and *MSH3* account for most of the remaining hereditary nonpolyposis colorectal cancer cases. Mutations in either *MLH1* or *MSH2* increase the risk of colorectal cancer to as much as 82% by age 70 years, compared with a risk of 2% in the population at large. Women who inherit either of these mutations also have an increased risk of endometrial cancer of approximately 60% by age 70 years. Of particular note, the risk of cancer before age 50 years is 20% for endometrial cancer and 25% for colorectal cancer, compared with a risk of 0.2% for each in the general population. The risk of ovarian cancer associated with this syndrome is 12% by age 70 years, a 10-fold increase over that seen in the general population. Mutations in *MSH2* and *MLH1* also increase the risk of other cancers, especially cancers of the stomach and urinary and biliary tracts but are not associated with any significant increase in the risk of breast cancer. Individuals with hereditary nonpolyposis colorectal cancer who survive the first cancer have a significantly increased risk of a second malignancy. The American Gastroenterological Association has recommended that genetic testing be considered for individuals with colorectal or endometrial cancer who have a first-degree relative with an hereditary nonpolyposis colorectal cancer-related cancer diagnosed before age 50 years and for individuals with 2 hereditary nonpolyposis colorectal cancer-associated cancers.

It is now well known that mutations in *BRCA1*, a tumor surveillance gene which may play a role in genetic recombination and DNA repair and which is found at chromosome 17q21, are associated with increased risks for breast and ovarian cancer. There is no increased risk of colorectal or endometrial cancer associated with mutations in *BRCA1*. Germ-line *BRCA1* mutations also are responsible for fallopian tube and primary peritoneal carcinomas.

Mutations in the tumor suppressor gene *APC*, localized to chromosome 5q21, can result in familial adenomatous polyposis syndrome. Individuals with this disorder characteristically develop as many as thousands of adenomatous polyps throughout the colon and rectum during adolescence. The polyps are more common on the left side of the colon and in the rectum. Approximately 15%

TABLE 48-1. Genes Associated With Autosomal Dominant Hereditary Cancer Syndromes

Type of Gene	Gene	Syndrome	Tumors
DNA repair	BRCA1	Breast and ovarian	Breast carcinoma, ovarian carcinoma
DNA repair	BRCA2	—	Female and male breast carcinoma, prostate cancer
DNA repair	MSH2	Hereditary nonpolyposis colorectal cancer	Colorectal and endometrial adenocarcinoma
DNA repair	MSH6	—	—
DNA repair	MLH1	—	—
DNA repair	PMS1	—	—
DNA repair	PMS2	—	—
Proto-oncogene	CDKN2A	Familial melanoma	Cutaneous malignant melanoma, pancreatic cancer
Proto-oncogene	CDK4	—	—
Proto-oncogene	MET	Hereditary papillary renal cell carcinoma	Papillary renal cell carcinoma
Tumor suppressor	PRKAR1A	Carney complex	Pituitary adenoma, testicular neoplasms, thyroid adenoma carcinoma, breast ductal adenoma
Tumor suppressor	PTEN(MMAC1/TEP1)	Cowden	Breast carcinoma, thyroid (follicular adenoma, follicular carcinoma and papillary carcinoma), endometrial carcinoma
Tumor suppressor	APC	Familial adenomatous polyposis	Adenomatous polyps of the colorectum, increased gastrointestinal cancer risk, papillary thyroid carcinoma
Tumor suppressor	SDHD, SDHC, SDHB	Hereditary paraganglioma and phaeochromocytoma	Paraganglioma, pheochromocytoma
Tumor suppressor	SMAD4(DPC4), BMPR1A	Juvenile polyposis coli	Multiple juvenile polyps in the gastrointestinal malignancy
Tumor suppressor	TP53, hCHK2	Li-Fraumeni	Breast cancer, soft tissue sarcoma, brain tumors, adrenocortical tumors, leukemia
Tumor suppressor	MEN1	Multiple endocrine neoplasia type 1	Primary hyperparathyroidism, pancreatic islet cell tumors, anterior pituitary tumors
Tumor suppressor	PTC	Nevoid basal cell carcinoma	Basal cell carcinoma
Tumor suppressor	NF1	Neurofibromatosis type 1	Neurofibrosarcoma, astrocytoma, pheochromocytoma, melanoma, rhabdomyosarcoma, and chronic myeloid leukemia
Tumor suppressor	NF2	Neurofibromatosis type 2	Bilateral vestibular schwannomas, meningiomas, spinal tumors, skin tumors

Reprinted from Cancer Letters, Vol 181, Marsh DJ, Zori RT, Genetic insights into familial cancers—update and recent discoveries, 127–8, Copyright 2002, with permission from Elsevier.

of patients develop polyps by age 10 years and 90% by age 30 years. Malignancies on average are detected by age 35 years in these individuals. Individuals with familial adenomatous polyposis syndrome also are at risk of extracolonic malignancies, including papillary thyroid carcinoma, pancreatic adenocarcinoma, and premalignant duodenal polyps. Endometrial and ovarian carcinoma generally are not associated with mutations in the APC gene.

Mutations in the tumor suppressor gene TP53 can result in the Li-Fraumeni syndrome. The TP53 gene also is frequently mutated in sporadic human cancers. Malignancies in the Li-Fraumeni syndrome often occur by age 30 years and include breast, adrenocortical, and brain cancer; soft tissue and osteogenic sarcomas; and leukemia. Colorectal, ovarian, and endometrial cancer are not part of this syndrome. Although this disorder is autosomal dominant, one mutant allele in the germ-line does not result in cancer. However, when a second somatic cell mutation occurs in a particular tissue (such as the breast), both alleles are inactivated, permitting malignancy.

Mutations in the proto-oncogene MEN1, located at chromosome 11q13, can result in the autosomal dominant multiple endocrine neoplasia type I. The proto-oncogene MEN1 involves 1 or more types of tumors of parathyroid, anterior pituitary, or pancreatic islet origin. If there is a family history, only 1 type of neoplasm is needed for diagnosis. In an isolated case, malignancies in 2 organ systems are needed. Affected individuals also may have carcinoid, adrenocortical, or lipoid tumors. These individuals do not have the tumors present in the case history. Signs and symptoms usually occur in the fourth decade, and nearly 50% of *MEN1* patients succumb to their disease.

Detailed mutation summaries for all of these genes are available. See the Human Gene Mutation Database at http://archive.uwcm.ac.uk/uwcm/mg/hgm0.html.

Coukos G, Rubin SC. Prophylactic oophorectomy. Best Pract Res Clin Obstet Gynecol 2002;16:597–609.

Frank TS, Critchfield GC. Hereditary risk of women's cancers. Best Pract Res Clin Obstet Gynaecol 2002;16:703–13.

Lynch HT, Coronel SM, Okimoto R, Hampel H, Sweet K, Lynch JF, et al. A founder mutation of the MSH2 gene and hereditary nonpolyposis colorectal cancer in the United States. JAMA 2004;291:718–24.

Marsh DJ, Zori RT. Genetic insights into familial cancers—update and recent discoveries. Cancer Lett 2002;181:125–64.

Pharoah PDP, Ponder BA. The genetics of ovarian cancer. Best Pract Res Clin Obstet Gynaecol 2002;16:449–68.

Wooster R, Weber BL. Breast and ovarian cancer. N Engl J Med 2003;348:2339–47.

49

Levonorgestrel intrauterine system

A 40-year-old woman, gravida 3, para 3, requests contraception. Her past medical history is significant for chronic hypertension, which is currently controlled with a diuretic and a β-blocker. Which of the following methods of contraception would be the most cost-effective for this patient?

    (A) Combined oral contraceptive
    (B) Transdermal patch
    (C) Progestin-only pill
* (D) Intrauterine device (IUD)
    (E) Laparoscopic bilateral tubal ligation

A compelling argument can be made for recommending an IUD for this patient and many other reproductive-aged women who seek contraception. The IUD is a highly effective method of contraception that is underused in the United States. It is the most common method of reversible contraception in most other countries. Although concerns about the safety of this method contribute to its lack of universal use, several published reviews dispel some of the myths associated with the IUD. One study determined the clinical and economic impact associated with 15 contraceptive methods. The main outcome measures were the 1- and 5-year costs and number of pregnancies avoided compared with use of no contraceptive method. The investigators found that all 15 contraceptive methods were more effective and less costly than no method. Over 5 years, the copper-T IUD, vasectomy, the contraceptive implant, and the injectable contraceptive were the most cost-effective methods, saving $14,122, $13,899, $13,813, and $13,373, respectively, and preventing approximately the same number of pregnancies (4.2) per individual. Because of their high failure rates, barrier methods, spermicides, withdrawal, and periodic abstinence were costly but still saved from $8,933 to $12,239 over 5 years. Oral contraceptives fell between these groups, saving $12,879, and preventing 4.1 pregnancies. All IUDs are safe to use in patients who have hypertension.

Transdermal contraceptive patches deliver a constant rate of ethinyl estradiol and norelgestromin over 7 days, with contraceptive success rates comparable to combined oral contraceptives. With perfect use, the failure rate is 0.7 pregnancies per 100 women per year. In women who weigh more than 90 kg (198.4 lb), there is a lower effectiveness. The side effects and contraindications are similar to combined oral contraceptives, and there are no long-term data on the use of contraceptive transdermal patches and chronic hypertension.

Especially for women in whom estrogen is contraindicated, progestin-only pills offer an excellent method of contraception in women older than 40 years because of the reduced fecundity associated with this age. However, patients who use this method may experience irregular menstrual periods and spotting that, for some women, may prove a major drawback. The typical pregnancy rate for the progestin-only pill during the first year of use is 3%, which is the highest among the choices given, and, therefore, would not be the most effective method of contraception for this patient.

Laparoscopic bilateral tubal ligation would be another option for this individual. Studies have shown that the pregnancy rate in women who are undergoing interval tubal sterilization is significantly higher than previously thought. The 10-year risk of pregnancy is 7.5–36.5 per 1,000 procedures, which is significantly higher than other methods of contraception. The U.S. Collaborative Review of Sterilization found a failure rate of 12.3 per 1,000 procedures in the first year of use after tubal sterilization among women aged 34–44 years. Although it could be argued that tubal sterilization would be a good choice in this patient, the surgical risk, complications, and cost associated with this method of contraception must be considered.

Arias RD. Compelling reasons for recommending IUDs to any woman of reproductive age. Int J Fertil Womens Med 2002;47:87–95.

Burkman RT. The transdermal contraceptive patch: a new approach to hormonal contraception. Int J Fertil Womens Med 2002;47:69–76.

French RS, Cowan FM, Mansour D, Higgins JP, Robinson A, Procter T, et al. Levonorgestrel-releasing (20 microgram/day) intrauterine systems (Mirena) compared with other methods of reversible contraceptives. BJOG 2000;107:1218–25.

Trussell J, Leveque JA, Koenig JD, London R, Borden S, Henneberry J, et al. The economic value of contraception: a comparison of 15 methods. Am J Public Health 1995;85:494–503.

50
Craniopharyngioma

A 23-year-old woman comes to the emergency department following a minor motor vehicle accident. A skull film (Fig. 50-1) demonstrates a large lesion in the intrasellar and suprasellar spaces, with scattered areas of calcification throughout. On further questioning, the patient states that although she initiated pubertal development, she has never had a menstrual period. On physical examination, she has Tanner stage I breast development, confused by a very chubby chest, and Tanner stage IV pubic hair. Laboratory evaluation reveals a follicle-stimulating hormone level of less than 2 mIU/mL, luteinizing hormone level of less than 2 mIU/mL, serum prolactin level of 800 ng/mL, and thyroid-stimulating hormone level of 0.1 µU/ml. The most appropriate next step in treatment is

    (A) observation
*   (B) transfrontal surgical removal
    (C) dopamine agonist therapy followed by transsphenoidal resection
    (D) transsphenoidal resection
    (E) dopamine agonist therapy alone

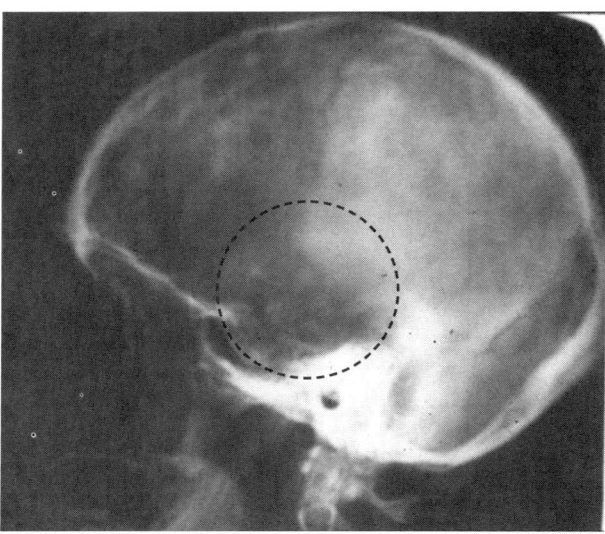

FIG. 50-1. Skull film of a patient with craniopharyngioma.

The 2 most common tumors associated with primary amenorrhea are prolactinoma and craniopharyngioma. Previously, the craniopharyngioma was considered to be the most common tumor for this age group. However, the prolactinoma now outnumbers the craniopharyngioma as a cause of pubertal delay and primary amenorrhea in girls. These tumors have both differences and similarities.

Craniopharyngiomas, such as the one described, have a bimodal distribution in occurrence in the late childhood and early to mid-adolescent years and, similar to dermoid tumors of the ovary, later in life, at approximately age 50–60 years. Craniopharyngioma is dysembryogenetic in origin, and it arises from squamous rest cells of the remnants of Rathke's pouch and, in 90% of cases, from a suprasellar location. It occurs in both intrasellar and suprasellar regions concomitantly in less than 20% of patients and only rarely within the pituitary alone. Although benign, these tumors can aggressively invade surrounding areas. Although some of craniopharyngiomas may develop silently, as in the patient presented here, most are associated with neurologic symptoms or endocrine deficits. Headache and visual problems are the most common neurologic symptoms, and seizures occur less frequently. The most common endocrine disturbances are pubertal abnormalities and stunted growth from deficiencies of gonadotropins and growth hormone. Pituitary stalk compression causes hyperprolactinemia in 20% of patients; the prolactin levels in these patients increase to occasionally very high levels as seen here. Because these tumors often develop in the late childhood years, they often delay the onset of breast development rather than occur after puberty has begun. Diabetes insipidus is rare. These tumors consist of 3 components with solid, cystic, and calcified areas. The most common features of the pediatric craniopharyngiomas are cystic changes and calcification. All of these features are very characteristic on magnetic resonance imaging and computed tomography, which makes them relatively easy to diagnose.

Prolactinoma usually occurs after puberty has been initiated, with estrogen being the apparent stimulus for increasing messenger RNA production for prolactin synthesis. It is almost always intrasellar in location with only rare suprasellar extension. These tumors are very slow growing, rarely interfere with other endocrine functions, and are much less likely to produce neurologic symptoms than craniopharyngiomas.

Because the tumor diagnosed in this patient is large and calcified, associated with a high prolactin level, and present in a patient who likely has never had breast development, these facts are highly suggestive that it is a craniopharyngioma. Observation would not be appropriate. The primary treatment is surgical resection with adjunctive radiotherapy reserved for those with incomplete resection or recurrence. Although the transsphenoidal approach can be used for some of these tumors, many require craniotomy and a transfrontal approach when large, as in this patient. Postoperative morbidity is high because partial or total hypopituitarism occurs in most patients. Appetite disorders, hypothalamic obesity, and neuropsychologic sequelae also have been observed. Although survival rates following surgery for these patients now approach 100% at 15 years, survival is sometimes as low as 85%.

In contrast to craniopharyngiomas, treatment of prolactinoma is virtually always accomplished with medical therapy alone. Shrinkage of tumors occurs in the vast majority of such tumors. Compliance has improved with newer dopamine agonists. Surgery is only rarely required for special circumstances because these tumors are very slow growing and recurrence after surgery is high with a risk for pituitary failure, especially for the macroadenomas. Gamma knife radiation also has been used in special circumstances.

Kalapurakal JA, Goldman S, Hsieh YC, Tomita T, Marymont MH. Clinical outcome in children with craniopharyngioma treated with primary surgery and radiotherapy deferred until relapse. Med Pediatr Oncol 2003;40:214–8.

Reindollar RH, Byrd JR, McDonough PG. Delayed sexual development: a study of 252 patients. Am J Obstet Gynecol 1981;140:371–80.

Sklar CA. Craniopharyngioma: endocrine abnormalities at presentation. Pediatr Neurosurg 1994;21(suppl 1):18–20.

Van Effenterre R, Boch AL. Craniopharyngioma in adults and children: a study of 122 surgical cases. J Neurosurg 2002;97:3–11.

Zhang YQ, Wang CC, Ma ZY. Pediatric craniopharyngiomas: clinicomorphological study of 189 cases. Pediatr Neurosurg 2002;36:80–4.

51
Environmental toxicity and sperm counts

A tobacco farmer is concerned that his occupation may be contributing to his documented oligoasthenospermia (ie, reduced sperm count with low motility). He admits to occasional use of marijuana. The factor that is most likely to be responsible for his increased risk of asthenospermia is

* (A) polychlorinated biphenyl hydrocarbons (PCBs)
* (B) lead
* (C) tetrahydrocannabinol
* (D) ionizing radiation
* (E) nicotine

There is a perception worldwide that semen quality has decreased. This may be the result of work-related activities that frequently expose men to toxic chemicals. Polychlorinated biphenyl hydrocarbons are halogenated, lipophilic, aromatic hydrocarbons with known estrogenic effects that have been detected as potential hazards in almost every global ecosystem. They are components of a number of insecticides and, thus, may be encountered by farmers. Because of the ubiquitous nature of these environmental contaminants, it has proved difficult to detect their adverse effect on semen parameters. Although absent in fertile control males, PCBs have been detected in the semen of infertile men who have sperm counts less than 25–30% of normal counts. It has been demonstrated that the total motile sperm counts in infertile men are inversely proportional to concentrations of estrogenlike substances found in the environment (ie, xenoestrogens) and may be responsible for poor semen quality in infertile men without an obvious etiology. Little is known about the effects of xenoestrogens on reproduction.

As in the case presented, chronic occupational exposure to PCB in farmers is associated with damage to the spermatogenic process. The reasons why PCBs adversely effect sperm parameters are unclear but are hypothesized to be the result of the following factors:

- Direct antiandrogen activity in the testes
- Modulatory effects on enzymes that control receptor metabolism
- Direct inhibition of enzymes involved in testosterone steroidogenesis
- Loosening of intercellular contacts between germ cells and Sertoli cells
- Possible direct influence of PCBs on the thyroid, pituitary, and adrenal glands

Long-term exposure to toxic substances can lead to decreases in total sperm count, sperm motility, and the proportion of morphologically normal spermatozoa. Reserve cells of spermatogonia, because of their decreased mitotic rate, appear to be less susceptible to toxic hydrocarbons. Hence, many estrogenic compounds may not affect testicular sperm production, but epididymal sperm transit or storage may be specifically affected. This is reflected in compromised parameters measuring sperm motility and fertilizing ability. Increased viscosity of ejaculates and decreased capacity for liquefaction suggest that toxic substances may affect seminal plasma.

Tetrahydrocannabinol, a component of marijuana, may adversely affect sperm parameters, but would not be specific to an agricultural-specific occupation. Tetrahydro-cannabinol inhibits morphologic alterations in the acro-somal cap, which may significantly impair sperm binding to the zona pellucida.

Heavy metals and certain physical agents may affect male reproductive function. Painters, plumbers, and printers, but generally not farmers, are exposed to lead at work. High levels of lead also are seen in individuals who smoke, drink alcohol, or fail to exercise. High levels of lead in semen have been associated with low fertilization rates in in vitro fertilization.

Spermatogonia are extremely sensitive to radiation. Doses as low as 600 cGy cause irreversible sterility. A farmer is no more likely to be exposed to ionizing radiation than individuals in other occupations.

Smoking studies have demonstrated a dose-response reduction in sperm density, motility, and possibly morphology. These reductions, compared with nonsmokers, often are still within normal parameters for the standard semen analysis. The effect of smoking on male fecundity is more difficult to discern. In vitro studies, such as the zona-free hamster egg penetration assay, a predictor of fertilization capability of sperm, is decreased in smokers. Unless the farmer grows and handles large quantities of tobacco without the use of gloves, he would not be exposed to nicotine on the job. Even in that event, the impact on sperm count should not be great.

Benoff S, Centola GM, Millan C, Napolitano B, Marmar JL, Hurley IR. Increased seminal plasma lead levels adversely affect the fertility potential of sperm in IVF. Hum Reprod 2003;18:374–83.

De Celis R, Feria-Velasco A, Gonzalez-Unzaga M, Torres-Calleja J, Pedron-Nuevo N. Semen quality of workers occupationally exposed to hydrocarbons. Fertil Steril 2000;73:221–8.

Pflieger-Bruss S, Hanf V, Behnisch P, Hagenmaier H, Rune GM. Effects of single polychlorinated biphenyls on the morphology of cultured rat tubuli seminiferi. Andrologia 1999;31:77–82.

Robins TG, Bornman MS, Ehrlich RI, Cantrell AC, Pienaar E, Vallabh J, et al. Semen quality and fertility of men employed in a South African lead acid battery plant. Am J Ind Med 1997;32:369–76.

Rozati R, Reddy PP, Reddanna P, Mujtaba R. Role of environmental estrogens in the deterioration of male factor fertility. Fertil Steril 2002;78:1187–94.

Schuel H, Burkman LJ, Lippes J, Crickard K, Mahony MC, Giuffrida A, et al. Evidence that anandamide-signaling regulates human sperm functions required for fertilization. Mol Reprod Dev 2002;63:376–87.

Sofikitis N, Miyagawa I, Dimitriadis D, Zavos P, Sikka S, Hellstrom W. Effects of smoking on testicular function, semen quality and sperm fertilizing capacity. J Urol 1995;154:1030–4.

52

Males with oligospermia and assisted reproductive technologies

A 36-year-old nulligravid woman and her husband come in for consultation regarding the best method for them to achieve a pregnancy. The husband has undergone 2 semen analyses, which have documented sperm concentrations of 1–2 million sperm per mL, sperm motilities of 10–15%, and normal sperm morphologies of 10–15%. His urologist has documented a small nonpalpable varicocele on ultrasonography. The woman has an ovulatory menstrual history and no history suspicious for pelvic adhesions. The most cost-effective means of achieving a pregnancy in this couple not concerned about paternity is

    (A) varicocele repair for the husband
    (B) clomiphene citrate (Clomid, Serophene) for the husband
    (C) in vitro fertilization with intracytoplasmic sperm injection (ICSI)
*   (D) donor insemination
    (E) intrauterine inseminations with the husband's sperm

Male infertility accounts for approximately 40% of all causes of infertility in couples who wish to achieve pregnancy and is the sole cause in 20% of couples. Semen parameters typically associated with normal probabilities of conception if the female has no confounding factors include sperm concentrations greater than 20 million per mL, sperm motility greater that 50%, and normal sperm morphology of least 30% by World Health Organization standards (see Appendix E).

Varicocele is the presence of dilated veins in the testicle. The condition is present in 15% of the normal male population and in approximately 40% of men with infertility. It is presumed that these veins increase the scrotal temperature, promote venous efflux, and, thus, affect a wide variety of semen parameters and potentially induce some degree of subfertility or infertility. Varicoceles are classified as clinically palpable versus subclinical (ie, nonpalpable, noted on scrotal ultrasonography only). A variety of surgical and nonsurgical approaches are available for the treatment of varicocele. However, the absolute affect of varicocele on male fertility remains controversial. Recently, there has been a consensus regarding the lack of impact of subclinical varicocele on male fertility. Varicocele repair may improve motility but is unlikely to increase sperm count appreciably in the husband in the present scenario.

Several medical therapies have been proposed to treat men with significant abnormalities of their semen parameters. Clomiphene citrate (Clomid, Serophene) historically has been promoted because of its known ability to increase follicle-stimulating hormone and luteinizing hormone levels and potentially to improve sperm quality. However, the ability of this medication to lead to significant and consistent improvements in semen parameters with resultant pregnancy has been disappointing. Although clomiphene citrate is a relatively inexpensive medication, its utility is extremely questionable in this situation because of the woman's age and potentially decreasing egg quality. During the interval of time that the couple would be waiting for possible improvements in the husband's semen parameters, her egg quality may be decreasing.

The use of donor sperm is a well-established means of achieving pregnancy in cases of male infertility and subfertility. The donor pool is intensively screened for sexually transmitted diseases as well as for common inherited disorders (eg, cystic fibrosis). Cost in many programs that offer donor insemination averages several hundred dollars per insemination. The cumulative pregnancy and delivery rates in cases where there is no female factor approach 30–40% after 6 months of therapy. Because paternity is not an issue for this couple, the use of donor sperm is the most cost-effective means of achieving a pregnancy.

In vitro fertilization (IVF), with the ability to inject individual sperm into oocytes (ie, intracytoplasmic sperm injection or ICSI), has allowed men with markedly abnormal semen parameters to father children. The average cost of IVF with ICSI can range from several thousand dollars to more than $10,000 per attempt, with reported delivery rates of 30% per cycle. The female partner must undergo ovulation induction in conjunction with ultrasonographic monitoring and ultimately transvaginal ultrasound-guided egg retrieval under anesthesia. Although IVF is a very reasonable means for this couple to have a biologic child from both partners, it is not the most cost effective means of achieving a pregnancy if paternity is not an issue.

Intrauterine insemination is commonly used to treat couples with unexplained infertility or in cases of minimal abnormalities in the semen parameters. Recent studies have demonstrated the extremely poor prognosis when the total motile numbers of sperm after sperm processing is less than 10 million. In this case, where the sperm concentration is already less than 10 million and the motility between 10% and 15%, the prognosis for achieving this minimum standard with sperm washing is extremely poor and should not be offered to this couple.

A double-blind trial of clomiphene citrate for the treatment of idiopathic male infertility. World Health Organization. Int J Androl 1992;15: 299–307.

Schlegel PN. Is assisted reproduction the optimal treatment for varicocele-associated infertility? A cost-effectiveness analysis. Urology 1997; 49:83–90.

Sharlip ID, Jarow JP, Belker AM, Lipshultz LI, Sigman M, Thomas AJ, et al. Best practice policies for male infertility. Fertil Steril 2002;77: 873–82.

Shenfield F, Doyle P, Valentine A, Steele SJ, Tan SL. Effects of age, gravidity, and male infertility status on cumulative conception rates following artificial insemination with cryopreserved donor semen: analysis of 2998 cycles of treatment in one centre over 10 years. Hum Reprod 1993;8:60–4.

Van Voorhis BJ, Barnett M, Sparks AE, Syrop CH, Rosenthal G, Dawson J. Effect of the total motile sperm count on the efficacy and cost-effectiveness of intrauterine insemination and in vitro fertilization. Fertil Steril 2001;75:661–8.

53
Hysteroscopic endometrial ablation

A 43-year-old multiparous woman presents with unpredictably heavy menstrual bleeding for the past 2 years. Her medical history and review of systems are unremarkable, and she is using no medications. The physical examination is unremarkable, and the uterus is felt to be of normal size. No adnexal masses are palpated. The Pap test and endometrial biopsy results are normal. Ultrasonography is done (Fig. 53-1). She refuses all forms of medical therapy as well as hysterectomy. Her best option for therapy will be

    (A) balloon ablation
    (B) radiofrequency ablation
    (C) hot circulating saline ablation
    (D) hysteroscopic ablation
*   (E) hysteroscopic resection

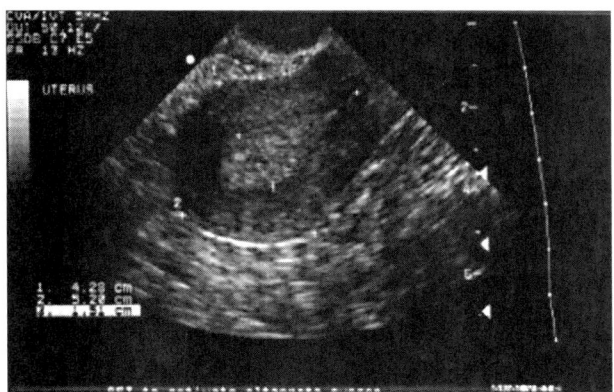

FIG. 53-1. Ultrasonogram showing pelvic mass.

In the United States, hysterectomy is the second most common gynecologic surgical procedure after cesarean delivery. There has been a growing interest in technologies to reduce the number of hysterectomies in patients with or without identifiable pathology.

One of the relative contraindications to nonhysteroscopic and hysteroscopic endometrial ablation is the presence of undiagnosed intrauterine pathology (eg, submucous myomas, intrauterine polyps, atypical hyperplasia, and endometrial cancer). Because this patient has ultrasound evidence of intrauterine pathology, this pathology must be evaluated before performing any of the nonhysteroscopic and hysteroscopic ablation techniques. The best means of performing this evaluation will be the use of directed hysteroscopic visualization and resection.

Endometrial ablation was first performed in the United States using a hysteroscope and a neodymium:yttrium-aluminum-garnet laser in the late 1980s. Since that time, operative hysteroscopy in conjunction with electrosurgical techniques (endometrial ablation, endomyometrial resection) have dominated the picture. Hysteroscopic surgery offered the opportunity to visualize the entire uterine cavity and directly treat intrauterine pathology or ablate the endometrium. Endometrial ablation techniques have typically required the use of liquid distension media, electrosurgical loops or balls, and an operative hysteroscope. Hysteroscopic techniques require significant skills in endoscopic surgery and have the potential complications of fluid overload leading to pulmonary edema, hyponatremia, and seizures, leading to possible death. In the late 1990s, techniques for endometrial ablation were developed that do not require operative hysteroscopy. These techniques include the use of thermal balloons, hot circulating saline, radiofrequency waves, and cryoprobes.

Amenorrhea rates following hysteroscopic techniques and each of the alternative techniques range from 20% to 36% with little difference between the various technologies. Overall, patient satisfaction with each of these techniques approaches 70–85%, with most women noting hypomenorrhea or acceptable menses. Although hysteroscopic techniques generally are viewed as the criterion standard, thermal balloon ablation technology has very similar success rates in terms of amenorrhea and overall patient satisfaction.

Lethaby A, Hickey M. Endometrial destruction techniques for heavy menstrual bleeding: a Cochrane review. Hum Reprod 2002;17: 2795–806.

Loffer FD, Grainger D. Five-year follow-up of patients participating in a randomized trial of uterine balloon therapy versus rollerball ablation for treatment of menorrhagia. J Am Assoc Gynecol Laparosc 2002;9: 429–35.

Onyeka BA, Arthur ID, Wilcox FL. Exclusion of abnormal endometrial histology before balloon endometrial ablation: lessons to be learnt. J Obstet Gynaecol 2002;22:453–4.

Roy KH, Mattox JH. Advances in endometrial ablation. Obstet Gynecol Surv 2002;57:789–802.

54
Prolactin-secreting pituitary microadenoma

A 27-year-old woman presents with a history of irregular menstrual cycles for the past 8 months. Menses are unpredictable and occur at 27–60-day intervals punctuated by vaginal spotting or full flow. She has gained approximately 7.3 kg (16 lb) during the past year. Menarche occurred at age 11 years, and she had regular cycles of 26–29 days' duration until age 19 years. She was started on oral contraceptives and remained on them until age 26 years when she discontinued them to attempt pregnancy. She denies having headaches, hot flushes, or visual disturbances and is not taking any medications. There have been no changes in her diet or exercise pattern. On examination, her thyroid gland is not enlarged, and her breasts have no masses or discharge. Her thyroid-stimulating hormone (TSH), total thyroxine, and follicle-stimulating hormone levels are normal. Two basal serum prolactin values are elevated at 57 ng/mL and 65 ng/mL. A magnetic resonance imaging (MRI) scan with contrast of the pituitary region shows an isolated nodule 2.5 mm in diameter in the left lateral anterior pituitary. The most appropriate next step in her management is

(A) observation
(B) exogenous gonadotropins
* (C) dopamine receptor agonist
(D) clomiphene citrate (Clomid, Serophene)

Prolactin-producing tumors are the most common tumors that involve the pituitary gland. These benign tumors usually occur during the reproductive years but can be seen in children, postmenopausal women, and men. The pituitary lactotropes are distributed mostly in the lateral wings of the anterior pituitary. They increase in size and number during pregnancy, accounting for an almost doubling in anterior pituitary volume.

Prolactin secretion is primarily regulated by the inhibitory factor dopamine with lactotropes having an abundance of dopamine type II receptors. Any central nervous system (CNS) tumors that compress the pituitary stalk or prevent the delivery of dopamine to the pituitary gland will result in increased prolactin secretion. Prolactin release also can be stimulated by thyroid-releasing hormone because thyroid-releasing hormone receptors also are present on the lactotropes. Because patients with primary hypothyroidism can present with hyperprolactinemia as well as TSH elevations, a TSH level should be obtained in all patients with elevations in prolactin.

It has been postulated that prolactinomas initially arise because of inadequate delivery of dopamine to a localized area within the pituitary and that they result in hyperplasia of small nests of lactotropes. These lactotropes eventually increase in size and number until they form a radiologically defined microadenoma (size 10 mm or less). These lesions can be readily imaged on computed tomography or MRI. In most cases, the optic chiasm is clearly seen on imaging and additional visual field testing is not necessary. Generally, prolactinomas are slow-growing functional tumors that can on occasion achieve sizes in the macroadenoma range (greater than 10 mm).

Normal serum prolactin levels range from 5 ng/mL to 20 ng/mL. Prolactin levels can increase in a physiologic fashion with a noon meal, during sleep onset, and with increased stress. Thus, any elevation in serum prolactin level should be confirmed by a second measurement. Ideally, prolactin should be drawn fasting in the morning. If the second prolactin level is elevated above 25 ng/mL and TSH level is normal, the patient should undergo further radiologic imaging studies, such as an MRI with contrast enhancement.

A common clinical presentation for prolactinomas in reproductive-aged women is the presence of amenorrhea with or without galactorrhea. It is thought that prolactin elevations lead to an increase in hypothalamic dopamine and β-endorphin activity, which in turn reduces pulsatile gonadotropin-releasing hormone secretion, resulting in a disruption of the menstrual cycle. In the patient described, prolactin elevations have begun to disrupt the normal cycle interval without amenorrhea. Galactorrhea alone in the presence of a normal menstrual cycle is not a reliable marker for hyperprolactinemia and often other risk factors for galactorrhea, such as breast stimulation, could cause the hyperprolactinemia.

The primary approach to treatment of prolactinomas is medical. Two dopamine D_2 receptor agonists, bromocriptine mesylate (Parlodel) and cabergoline (Dostinex), are available for the treatment of hyperprolactinemia. Bromocriptine is administered at a starting dose of 2.5 mg at bedtime for 1 week, followed by an increase to 2.5 mg twice per day. The half-life of bromocriptine is approximately 10–12 hours. Prolactin levels decrease quickly to a nadir within 6 hours of bromocriptine administration.

Cabergoline is a longer-acting dopamine analog and is given at a dose of 0.25 mg twice weekly. Prolactin levels can be re-evaluated 3–4 weeks after initiating medical therapy. Side effects of both medications include nausea, mild postural hypotension, and nasal congestion. These side effects usually diminish with long-term use. If side effects, such as nausea, become significant, vaginal administration of bromocriptine can be an option.

If prolactinomas enlarge, they do so slowly. They can decrease in size during treatment with dopamine agonists. Treatment usually is successful at suppressing prolactin levels, which allows return of normal menstrual cycles. Prolactin levels obtained at 6-month intervals usually will confirm response and compliance to treatment. Routine repeat radiologic imaging may not be necessary unless prolactin levels become elevated or CNS symptoms reappear. Although medical treatment usually is not curative for prolactinomas, it is not unreasonable to stop medical treatment after 1–2 years of suppression to determine if prolactin levels will rebound. For individuals that have prolactin level elevations associated with a microadenoma without menstrual disturbances, observation or expectant management can be an option. The use of birth control pills is not contraindicated in patients with prolactin-secreting pituitary microadenomas.

Surgical excision of prolactinomas should be limited to macroadenomas that cause space-occupying and compression symptoms. Generally, success with surgical resection is limited and is directly proportional to tumor size. Presurgical treatment with dopamine agonists to shrink macroadenomas may increase resection success rates. In this patient, the use of gonadotropins or clomiphene citrate to induce ovulation and regular menstrual cycles is not indicated because suppression of prolactin levels into the normal range with dopamine agonists usually will result in return of regular menstrual cycles.

Kletzky OA, Vermesh M. Effectiveness of vaginal bromocriptine in treating women with hyperprolactinemia. Fertil Steril 1989;51:269–72.

Molitch ME. Pathologic hyperprolactinemia. Endocrinol Metab Clin North Am 1992;21:877–901.

Molitch ME, Elton RL, Blackwell RE, Caldwell B, Chang RJ, Jaffe R, et al. Bromocriptine as primary therapy for prolactin-secreting macroadenomas: results of a prospective multicenter study. J Clin Endocrinol Metab 1985;60:698–705.

Serri O, Rasio E, Beauregard H, Hardy J, Somma M. Recurrence of hyperprolactinemia after selective transsphenoidal adenomectomy in women with prolactinoma. N Engl J Med 1983;309:280–3.

55

Chemotherapy, irradiation, and premature ovarian failure

A 25-year-old single woman in whom stage III Hodgkin's disease was recently diagnosed is scheduled to begin systemic chemotherapy and pelvic irradiation. She is referred to you to discuss how to preserve her ovarian function and future fertility. On the basis of available data, the most effective proven treatment is

    (A) gonadotropin-releasing hormone (GnRH) agonist during therapy
    (B) combination oral contraceptive during therapy
    (C) collection of oocytes for cryopreservation
*   (D) laparoscopic transposition of the ovaries
    (E) removal and cryopreservation of ovarian tissue strips

As treatment and survival for several malignancies common to young women have improved, increasing emphasis has been placed on improving the quality of life for these patients. Abundant data have documented that systemic chemotherapy, particularly with alkylating agents, and pelvic irradiation frequently result in ovarian failure. The risk is proportional to the patient's age, with older women running a higher risk of permanent ovarian failure. It appears that a dose of 800 rads (800 cGy) is sufficient to induce ovarian failure in all women. Chemotherapy is more likely to induce ovarian failure when administered as part of a regimen including irradiation. Thus, the patient in this case is likely at high risk of experiencing ovarian failure and consequent infertility.

A number of older studies documented that transposition of the ovaries by laparotomy before radiotherapy can reduce the dose administered to the ovaries by approximately 90% and reduce the incidence of ovarian failure. More recent studies indicate that laparoscopic transposition of the ovaries is equally effective and will preserve ovarian function in almost 90% of women who are undergoing pelvic irradiation. Thus, laparoscopic transposition of the ovaries should be offered to the woman in this case. It has been suggested that the ovaries should be transposed at least to the level of the pelvic brim. In most cases, this can be accomplished simply by dividing the ovarian ligament and mesovarium to facilitate mobilization of the ovary and then by suturing the ovary laterally to the pelvic peritoneum (Fig. 55-1; see color plate). Because this patient will be receiving pelvic irradiation including the uterus, it may be necessary to offer her in vitro fertilization with the use of a surrogate host for the pregnancy, but there are no published data to support this approach. Even without pelvic irradiation, chances for pregnancy might be increased with in vitro fertilization.

Few clinical studies have evaluated the effects of GnRH agonists in preventing chemotherapy-induced ovarian failure. What studies exist have produced conflicting results. Yet, the use of prior and concomitant GnRH agonists with chemotherapy has been promising in preventing ovarian failure in animals. Although further controlled trials involving GnRH analogs are needed, this approach has not been proved at this time. Similarly, data do no support the usefulness of administration of combination oral contraceptives during therapy to protect ovarian function. Even though these approaches are unproved, they can be considered and are unlikely to cause significant harm.

Oocyte cryopreservation is a potential realistic technique for preservation of fertility in women who must undergo chemotherapy or irradiation. However, at this time, success rates are sufficiently low, both with regard to oocyte survival and with regard to subsequent pregnancy, that the procedure must be considered experimental, should only be conducted under the auspices of an Institutional Review Board, and should only be offered together with transposition of the ovaries. Term pregnancies have resulted from less than 2% of frozen oocytes.

Oocytes, which are arrested in the meiotic process, appear particularly sensitive to the freezing process. In an effort to prevent freezing injury, the traditional slow cooling rates of 1–2° C per minute are being replaced by vitrification (ie, ultrarapid freezing), so that ice does not have a chance to form within the egg. More research, however, is still needed to prove the effectiveness of this approach.

Cryopreservation of ovarian cortical strips rich in primordial and primary follicles is another alternative approach. A high proportion of viable oocytes survive in human tissue after freeze-thawing. Animal studies have indicated the possible efficacy of this approach, but this approach remains experimental.

Transposition of the ovaries is currently the most appropriate and effective measure for young women who desire to preserve their potential fertility before treatment. However, clinicians should keep abreast of this advancing field to offer appropriate choices to their cancer patients.

Bisharah M, Tulandi T. Laparoscopic preservation of ovarian function: an underused procedure. Am J Obstet Gynecol 2003;188:367–70.

Blumenfeld Z. Preservation of fertility and ovarian function and minimalization of chemotherapy associated gonadotoxicity and premature ovarian failure: the role of inhibin-A and -B as markers. Molec Cell Endocrinol 2002;187:93–105.

Blumenfeld Z, Dann E, Avivi I, Epelbaum R, Rowe JM. Fertility after treatment for Hodgkin's disease. Ann Oncol 2002;13 (Suppl 1):138–47.

Revel A, Laufer N. Protecting female fertility from cancer therapy. Molec Cell Endocrinol 2002;187:83–91.

Tulandi T, Al-Took S. Laparoscopic ovarian suspension before irradiation. Fertil Steril 1998;70:381–3.

56
Hormone therapy and risk of breast cancer

A 52-year-old woman comes to your office to discuss her options regarding her hormone therapy (HT) regimen in view of the results of the Women's Health Initiative trial. The patient had her last menstrual period approximately 5 years ago and has been taking combination HT for the past 2 years for treatment of vasomotor symptoms. The patient believes this regimen has helped control her hot flushes and insomnia. She is concerned that remaining on HT may increase her risk for breast cancer, although she has no family history of this disease. You counsel her that

(A) combination HT does not increase her risk of breast cancer
(B) the progestin protects her from developing cancer
(C) only medroxyprogesterone acetate is associated with an increased risk of breast cancer
(D) only conjugated estrogen is associated with an increased risk of breast cancer
* (E) there appears to be some increased risk of breast cancer with any combination HT

Breast cancer is the most common invasive cancer in U.S. women. Results of a number of randomized controlled trials and observational studies have found an increased risk of breast cancer with both current and recent HT use.

One of the largest studies of breast cancer to date, the Million Women Study, investigated the effects of specific types of HT not only on incidence of but mortality from the disease in a cohort study of British women aged 50–64 years. One half of the women were found to have used HT. After an average of 2.6 years of follow-up, 9,364 invasive breast cancers were registered and, after 4.1 years, 637 breast cancer deaths. Current HT users at study recruitment were found to be more likely than never users to develop breast cancer (adjusted relative risk [RR] = 1.66) and to die from this disease (RR = 1.22). Past use did not convey an increased risk of breast cancer (RR = 1.01) or fatal disease (RR = 1.05).

When specific HT regimens were examined, the estrogen-progestin combination conferred a substantially greater risk (RR = 2) than estrogen alone (RR = 1.3) or tibolone (Livial) (RR = 1.45), a drug not currently approved for use in the United States. These results were similar regardless of specific estrogen or progestin doses or whether the regimen was administered sequentially or continuously. Relative risks also were increased for oral (RR = 1.32), transdermal (RR = 1.24), and implanted (RR = 1.65) estrogen-only formulations. Breast cancer risk increased with duration of use, so 10 years of HT use was estimated to result in 5 additional breast cancers per 1,000 users of estrogen-only formulations and 19 per 1,000 users of estrogen-progestin combinations.

In a follow-up analysis, the Women's Health Initiative trial found that estrogen plus progestin increased total and invasive breast cancers. The invasive breast cancers tended to be similar in histology and grade but displayed larger tumor size and more advanced stage than cancers diagnosed in the placebo group. In addition, after 1 year, more women in the HT group had abnormal mammograms, which could hinder a diagnosis of breast cancer.

For this patient, a switch to an estrogen-only regimen would not be an appropriate option, partly because of similar breast cancer risks but also because administration of unopposed estrogen in a woman with an intact uterus may result in endometrial hyperplasia. The results of the Million Women Study indicated that use of a different progestin formulation also would not reduce risk of breast cancer. Remaining on a combination HT regimen would convey the highest RR of invasive breast cancer, although the patient's 2-year use of this regimen places her at less risk (RR = 1.74) than if her duration of therapy had been 5–9 years (RR = 2.17) or 10 years or more (RR = 2.31).

The estrogen-only trial of the Women's Health Initiative trial reported that use of estrogen alone reduced the risk of breast cancer, although not significantly so. Because these results are not consistent with those from other randomized trials, further assessment is warranted.

This patient is counseled that there appears to be some increased risk of breast cancer with any combination HT. Therefore, the best option for the patient, given her concerns, would be to taper off HT. Although there are no published methods for the best way to proceed with tapering, many clinicians recommend a 1–3-month time frame. The patient should be seen in 3 months to assess her vasomotor symptoms. Her risks of cardiovascular disease and osteoporosis also should be assessed to determine if other interventions (eg, diet and lifestyle modifications or medical therapy) may be indicated.

Anderson GL, Limacher M, Assaf AR, Bassford T, Beresford SA, Black H, et al. Effects of conjugated equine estrogen in postmenopausal women with hysterectomy: the Women's Health Initiative randomized controlled trial. JAMA 2004;291:1701–12; discussion 1769–71.

Beral V. Breast cancer and hormone-replacement therapy in the Million Women Study. Million Women Study Collaborators. Lancet 2003;362: 419–27.

Beral V, Banks E, Reeves G. Evidence from randomised trial on the long-term effects of hormone replacement therapy. Lancet 2002;360: 942–4.

Breast cancer and hormone replacement therapy: collaborative reanalysis of data from 51 epidemiological studies of 52,705 women with breast cancer and 108,411 women without breast cancer. Collaborative Group on Hormonal Factors in Breast Cancer. Lancet 1997;350: 1047–59.

Chlebowski RT, Hendrix SL, Langer RD, Stefanick ML, Gass M, Lane D, et al. Influence of estrogen plus progestin on breast cancer and mammography in healthy postmenopausal women: The Women's Health Initiative Randomized Trial. JAMA 2003;289:3243–53.

Ettinger B, Grady D, Tosteson AN, Pressman A, Macer JL. Effect of the Women's Health Initiative on women's decisions to discontinue postmenopausal hormone therapy. Obstet Gynecol 2003;102:1225–32.

Grady D, Ettinger B, Tosteson ANA, Pressman A, Macer JL. Predictors of difficulty when discontinuing postmenopausal hormone therapy. Obstet Gynecol 2003;102:1233–9.

Rossouw JE, Anderson GL, Prentice RL, LaCroix AZ, Kooperberg C, Stefanick ML, et al. Risks and benefits of estrogen plus progestin in healthy postmenopausal women: principal results from the Women's Health Initiative randomized controlled trial. Writing Group for the Women's Health Initiative Investigators. JAMA 2002;288:321–33.

57
Depot medroxyprogesterone acetate and appetite

A 24-year-old woman, gravida 2, presents for contraceptive management. She has been using depot medroxyprogesterone acetate for contraception for the past 3 years and reports that her weight has increased by more than 22.7 kg (50 lb). She reports no menstrual bleeding over the past 18 months. Physical examination reveals a blood pressure level of 136/87 mm Hg, a plump facies, a small fat pad in the posterior neck, and scattered white stretch marks near the hips and buttocks. Laboratory evaluations show normal levels of thyroid-stimulating hormone (TSH), human chorionic gonadotropin, serum prolactin, and follicle-stimulating hormone. Her serum cortisol level is less than 5 µg/dL after an overnight dexamethasone suppression test. The factor that has most likely contributed to her current weight gain is

    (A) Cushing's syndrome
*   (B) depot medroxyprogesterone acetate
    (C) polycystic ovary syndrome
    (D) acromegaly

Obesity has emerged as a major health problem in the United States, and it now affects more than 50% of the U.S. population. Although diet and lifestyle variables are major factors in the obesity epidemic, an association also has been observed between the use of steroid contraception, in particular depot medroxyprogesterone acetate, and excessive weight gain. Although depot medroxyprogesterone acetate is a highly effective contraceptive method, the discontinuation rates are primarily because of weight gain and irregular vaginal bleeding. Retrospective clinical studies suggest that in adolescents who take depot medroxyprogesterone acetate for more than 1 year, the average weight gain ranges from 2.2–5.5 kg (4.8–12.2 lb). In one study that compared intrauterine device (IUD) users versus depot medroxyprogesterone acetate users over 5 years, depot medroxyprogesterone acetate users gained 4.3 kg (9.5 lb) versus 1.8 kg (4 lb) among the IUD users. When studies have stratified the subjects by race, African-American adolescents appear to gain more weight than white adolescents. Adolescents who are initially overweight tend to gain more weight than those who are not overweight, although these findings are not consistently seen in all studies.

The mechanism(s) for weight gain in depot medroxyprogesterone acetate users is not known. A possible mechanism is the weak glucocorticoid activity of depot medroxyprogesterone acetate. Alternatively, depot medroxyprogesterone acetate might alter the hormones that affect fat metabolism or appetite.

Recently, 2 major hormones have been linked to obesity and appetite: 1) leptin and 2) ghrelin. Leptin is a hormone product of the adipocyte. Leptin has demonstrated effects on key organs that regulate energy homeostasis, including the brain, muscle, fat, liver, and pancreas. Patients with a mutation in the leptin gene and a complete deficiency of leptin are morbidly obese from infancy and also have hypogonadotropic hypogonadism and insulin resistance. Replacement with recombinant leptin in such a patient resulted in substantial weight loss and improvement in hormonal abnormalities. These findings have led investigators to study the effects of leptin on obesity.

Low levels of leptin are seen in anorexia and signal starvation. Leptin appears to direct the body to adapt to this condition by reducing energy expenditure with increased conversion of total triiodothyronine (T_3) to reverse T_3. By contrast, higher levels of leptin would be expected to increase energy expenditure or reduce food intake. Subjects who are obese have higher levels of endogenous leptin, which suggests that these individuals are leptin-resistant.

Ghrelin is an appetite-stimulating hormone that is secreted primarily by the stomach and duodenum. In humans, ghrelin levels increase before meals and decrease after meals, which may indicate that this hormone may play a major role in appetite stimulation. In rodents, constant ghrelin administration induces weight gain, decreases metabolic rate, and decreases fat catabolism while blocking ghrelin in the brain leads to reductions in food intake. In humans, diet-induced weight loss leads to significant elevations in the pattern of ghrelin release, which suggests that increased ghrelin secretion may play a role in the adaptive response to constrain weight loss. As more information becomes available regarding the possible links between the appetite-stimulating effects of ghrelin and obesity, new approaches to understanding energy homeostasis and fat metabolism are certain to emerge.

In this patient, a normal TSH level excludes hypothyroidism whereas the normal overnight dexamethasone suppression test excludes Cushing's syndrome. Although the patient is anovulatory by history, there are no clear stigmata for polycystic ovary syndrome or androgen excess, such as facial hirsutism or acne. The patient also fails to demonstrate signs of acromegaly, such as an increase in hat or foot size, frontal bossing, or an elevated prolactin level.

Bahamondes L, Del Castillo S, Tabares G, Arce XE, Perrotti M, Petta C. Comparison of weight increase in users of depot medroxyprogesterone acetate and copper IUD up to 5 years. Contraception 2001; 64:223–5.

Cummings DE, Weigle DS, Frayo RS, Breen PA, Ma MK, Dellinger EP, et al. Plasma ghrelin levels after diet-induced weight loss or gastric bypass surgery. N Engl J Med 2002;346:1623–30.

Mangan SA, Larsen PG, Hudson S. Overweight teens at increased risk for weight gain while using depot medroxyprogesterone acetate. J Pediatr Adolesc Gynecol 2002;15:79–82.

Nakazato M, Murakami N, Date Y, Kojima M, Matsuo H, Kangawa K, et al. A role for ghrelin in the central regulation of feeding. Nature 2001;409:194–8.

Risser WL, Gefter LR, Barrattt MS, Risser JM. Weight change in adolescents who used hormonal contraception. J Adolesc Health 1999; 24:433–6.

Taneepanichskul S, Reinprayoon D, Khaosaad P. Comparative study of weight change between long-term DMPA and IUD acceptors. Contraception 1998;58:149–51.

58

Chronic labial agglutination

A 7-year-old girl presents with findings of chronic labial agglutination. Her mother reports that the labia are adherent periodically, but there is no redness or problems with urinating. Her symptoms recur despite repeated application of estrogen cream. On physical examination, the child exhibits Tanner stage I breast development and Tanner stage I pubic hair (see Appendix D). The labia are adherent in the midline with minimal erythema without bleeding or discharge. The urethra is patent and unobstructed. The most appropriate next step in management is

(A) surgery for failed medical therapy
(B) vulvar biopsy to determine the etiology of the chronic symptoms
* (C) reassurance and discontinuation of use of estrogen therapy
(D) corticosteroid cream
(E) office adhesiolysis under local anesthesia

Although some labial adhesions remain asymptomatic and untreated, complications such as frequent urinary tract infections with dysuria as well as vulvar pain with movement may lead to chronic symptoms with worsening adhesions or a chronic urinary disorder. Labial agglutination is a common condition and involves the fusion of the labial minora in the midline. In the past, labial agglutination was treated with a short course of topical estrogen cream. Today, many centers prefer to observe patients and instruct on proper hygiene. Chronic recurrent cases often need careful evaluation and treatment.

Labial adhesions range in incidence from 0.6% to 3% and commonly affect girls from ages 2 months to 7 years, although they may persist through puberty. The most common etiologies include low estrogen levels in the prepubertal child or a chronic inflammatory process where thinning of surface epithelium causes the adherence of the labia.

The diagnosis may go unrecognized because of asymptomatic minor adhesions. Children who come in for evaluation have irritation or rash at the vaginal opening, dysuria, symptoms of a urinary tract infection, or discomfort with daily activity. Sometimes this condition may be confused with an imperforate hymen, vaginitis, or an intersex problem. A careful examination usually will easily differentiate these disorders.

Patients who remain asymptomatic without urinary problems or pain should be observed and treated conservatively. The standard treatment remains topical application of estrogen cream over a 2–4-week period. After labial separation, vitamin A and D ointment may be applied for 6–12 months to prevent recurrence. For patients who have failed medical therapy and remain symptomatic, in-office manual separation can be accomplished for selected patients using a topical anesthetic, such as EMLA cream (lidocaine 2.5% and prilocaine 2.5%). In patients who are not candidates for office treatment, a procedure in the operating room may be used to decrease pain and anxiety for the young child. The adherent labia should never be forcefully cut or separated, which can only induce emotional trauma and cause more adhesions to develop.

Prolonged use of estrogen cream for more than 2–3 months may cause hyperpigmentation, breast budding and tenderness, vulvar irritation, erythema, or the development of labial hair. In this case, the estrogen cream should be discontinued to allow symptoms to resolve.

The patient described presents with chronic and recurrent labial adhesions. Because she is asymptomatic without urinary or vaginal symptoms, a more conservative approach is warranted. The estrogen cream should be stopped to avoid side effects and surgery or manual separation should be avoided. Once pubertal development begins, her condition should resolve with time. Corticosteroid creams can thin the vulvar epithelium and should not be used in this case.

Appropriate education of parents and child care providers on proper hygiene is essential for long-term care of labial agglutination with repeated occurrence. Although most adhesions cause no problems, referral to a provider is necessary with the onset of new symptoms that involve the urinary tract or persistent vulvar pain.

Bacon JL. Prepubertal labial adhesions: evaluation of a referral population. Am J Obstet Gynecol 2002;187:327–31; discussion 332.

Leung AK, Robson WL. Labial fusion and urinary tract infection. Child Nephrol Urol 1992;12:62–4.

Muram D. Treatment of prepubertal girls with labial adhesions. J Pediatr Adolesc Gynecol 1999;12:67–70.

59
Precocious adrenarche

A 7-year-old white girl (Fig. 59-1; see color plate) presents with pubic hair growth, oily skin, and body odor. She has no signs of masculinization. Her blood pressure level is 90/60 mm Hg. Her longitudinal height and weight charts are shown in Fig. 59-2. The most likely pathophysiologic process responsible for these signs is

  (A) hyperprolactinemia
  (B) 11β-hydroxysteroid dehydrogenase deficiency
* (C) impaired insulin sensitivity
  (D) 5α-reductase deficiency
  (E) adrenal tumor

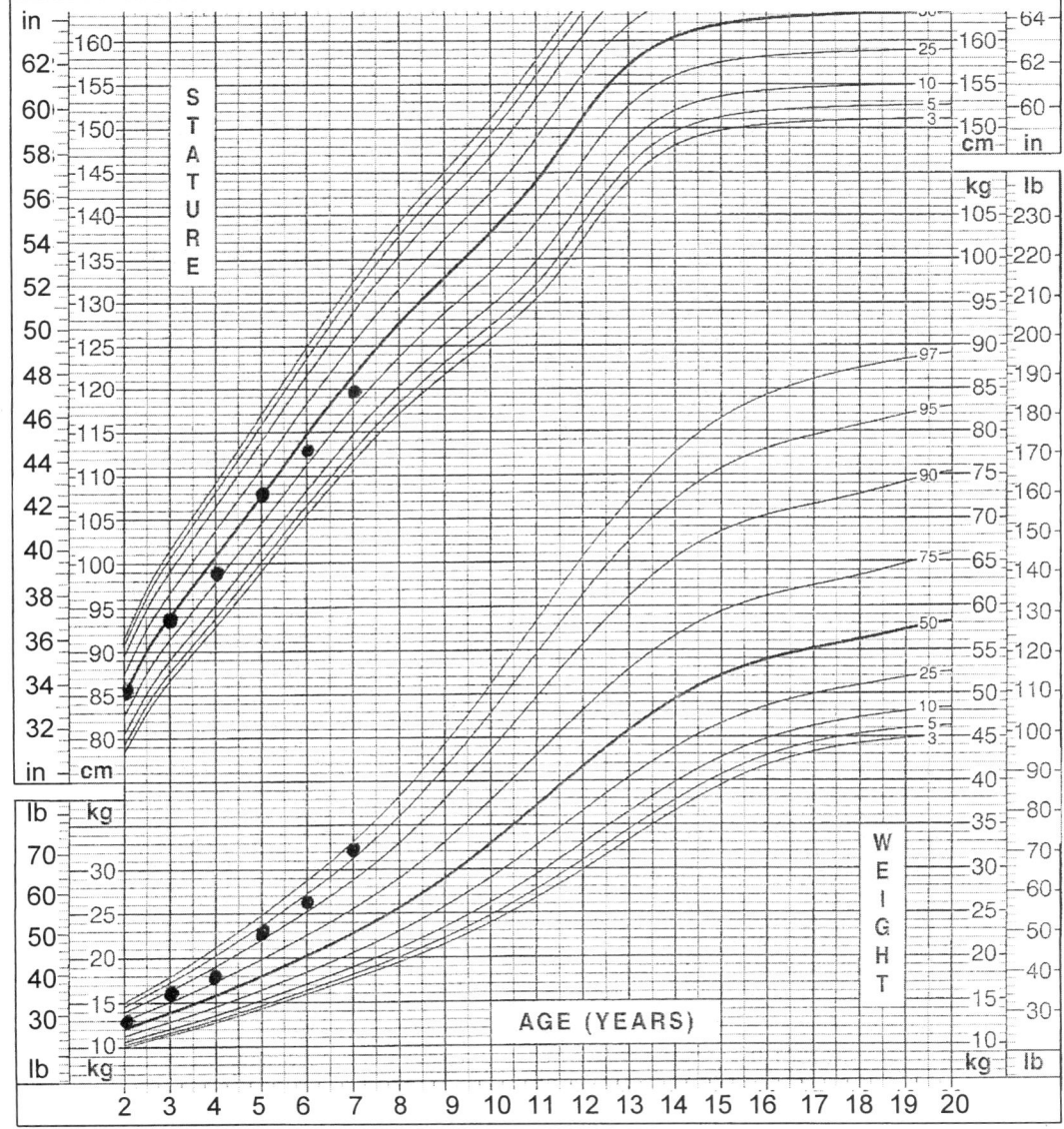

FIG. 59-2. Longitudinal growth chart showing height and weight of 7-year-old patient with complete pubic hair, oily skin, and body odor.

The classic definition of premature adrenarche, the appearance of pubic hair in girls younger than 8 years, originated from Marshall and Tanner's normative data of British white girls shortly after World War II. Recently, accumulating evidence has suggested that puberty may occur earlier, particularly in African-American girls. In a large cross-sectional study of 17,077 girls across the United States, nearly 30% of African-American girls had some evidence of puberty by age 7 years and one half of them by age 8 years. In contrast, only 15% of white girls had already initiated puberty by age 8 years. Adrenarche often precedes thelarche in African-American girls, with pubic hair present in nearly 20% of them by age 8 years. Although controversy exists about when to initiate the evaluation for precocious puberty, management of girls with premature adrenarche has largely consisted of observation after ruling out significant pathology. At a minimum, given the suspicion for insulin resistance in this patient, testing should include fasting glucose and insulin.

Although it is likely that many girls with isolated adrenarche before age 8 years have normal yet early puberty, a number of studies have demonstrated that some patients may have an identifiable cause. Recent studies have concentrated on insulin resistance and the metabolic syndrome and have shifted away from congenital adrenal hyperplasia (CAH). Insulin resistance and the metabolic syndrome now appear to be more commonly associated with premature adrenarche than is homozygous CAH. A high incidence of type 2 diabetes mellitus has been found in family members of these patients. Physical findings have consistently demonstrated high body mass index and signs of hyperandrogenism (eg, acne, increased body odor, and oily skin), both of which were observed in this patient. In addition, acanthosis nigricans has been identified in these young girls.

Laboratory findings of metabolic syndrome in patients with adult polycystic ovary syndrome (PCOS) include unfavorable lipid profiles, hyperandrogenism, and insulin resistance and are similarly found in young girls with premature adrenarche. Fasting glucose/insulin ratios less than 7 in these young patients have been consistently predictive of insulin resistance when correlated with results of intravenous glucose challenge tests with tolbutamide. This fasting glucose/insulin ratio is higher than in adults for prediction of insulin resistance (ie, a ratio less than 4.5). Additional evidence of this syndrome in girls with premature adrenarche are increased insulinlike growth factor (IGF)-1, IGF-1/IGF–binding protein 1 ratio, and leptin levels. Insulin resistance is more frequent in African-American and Caribbean Hispanic girls with premature adrenarche than in white girls. Other races have not been thoroughly studied. Although adult patients with PCOS have been found to have minimal hyperprolactinemia, this area has not been studied in prepubertal patients.

Preliminary longitudinal studies have demonstrated that premature adrenarche for many patients is likely a marker for the development of PCOS later in adolescence. No interventional studies have been reported for treatment of patients with these findings. However, lifestyle modifications, such as dietary restrictions and increased exercise programs, have been suggested for girls with premature adrenarche in whom insulin resistance is suspected or identified.

For many years, the focus of investigations for premature adrenarche has been to uncover nonclassical (ie, adult onset) CAH, notably 21-hydroxylase gene (*CYP21* gene) deficiency. Several recent studies, however, have identified the homozygous state of this disorder in less than 10% of children with premature adrenarche. Although earlier studies implicated other adrenal steroid enzyme blocks as etiologic for premature adrenarche, newer research has not replicated these findings and has excluded 3β-hydroxysteroid dehydrogenase, 11β-hydroxysteroid dehydrogenase, and 5α-reductase deficiencies.

Premature adrenarche is rarely associated with signs of virilization that usually are rapid in onset. The patients with premature adrenarche who have virilization are more likely to have significantly higher androgen levels produced from ovarian or adrenal tumors. Such neoplasms are occasionally malignant. The patient with premature adrenarche with virilization will probably require interventional management.

Cizza G, Dorn LD, Lotsikas A, Sereika S, Rotenstein D, Chrousos GP. Circulating plasma leptin and IGF-1 levels in girls with premature adrenarche: potential implications of a preliminary study. Horm Metab Res 2001;33:138–43.

Dacou-Voutetakis C, Dracopoulou M. High incidence of molecular defects of the CYP21 gene in patients with premature adrenarche. J Clin Endocrinol Metab 1999;84:1570–4.

DiMartino-Nardi J. Pre- and postpuberal findings in premature adrenarche. J Pediatr Endocrinol Metab 2000;13(suppl 5):1265–9.

Herman-Giddens ME, Slora EJ, Wasserman RC, Bourdony CJ, Bhapkar MV, Koch GG, et al. Secondary sexual characteristics and menses in young girls seen in office practice: a study from the Pediatric Research in Office Settings Network. Pediatrics 1997;99:505–12.

Vuguin P, Linder B, Rosenfeld RG, Saenger P, DiMartino-Nardi J. The roles of insulin sensitivity, insulin-like growth factor I (IGF-1), and IGF-binding protein-1 and –3 in the hyperandrogenism of African-American and Caribbean Hispanic girls with premature adrenarche. J Clin Endocrinol Metab 1999;84:2037–42.

60
Ovarian hyperstimulation syndrome

A 28-year-old nulligravid woman has polycystic ovary syndrome (PCOS). She undergoes controlled ovarian hyperstimulation using recombinant follicle-stimulating hormone for a cycle of intrauterine insemination with a peak estradiol level of 1,800 pg/mL on the day of human chorionic gonadotropin (hCG) stimulation. Four days after the insemination, she comes to the emergency department with abdominal distention, weight gain, generalized abdominal pain, and nausea. The most likely explanation for her symptoms is

  (A) ectopic pregnancy
  (B) acute appendicitis
  (C) ovarian cyst
* (D) ovarian hyperstimulation syndrome
  (E) ovarian torsion

Ovarian hyperstimulation syndrome is a recognized complication of assisted reproductive technology. This condition can be life threatening if left untreated. Anovulatory women with PCOS are at greatest risk for ovarian hyperstimulation syndrome. In mild cases, ovarian hyperstimulation syndrome consists of ovarian enlargement, abdominal distention, nausea, vomiting, and weight gain. In severe cases, there is a significant decrease in circulating volume, development of ascites or pleural effusion, and electrolyte imbalance that may lead to hypovolemia, hypotension, and oliguria. The ovaries are significantly enlarged with multiple cysts. Torsion of the adnexa is a potential complication, and patients should be warned to report any sudden increase of severe abdominal pain. Although mild forms of ovarian hyperstimulation syndrome occur frequently, moderate to severe forms appear in 1–2% of all in vitro fertilization cycles. Most of the cases resolve spontaneously usually within 7 days if the patient is not pregnant. When pregnancy occurs, endogenous hCG stimulation of the corpus luteum can extend the syndrome for up to 2–3 weeks.

Careful monitoring during a controlled ovarian stimulation cycle is a key component to the prevention of ovarian hyperstimulation syndrome. Withholding the hCG injection in patients with estradiol levels greater than 1,500 pg/mL or multiple (greater than 3) preovulatory ovarian follicles should be seriously considered to prevent ovarian hyperstimulation syndrome. The presence of many smaller follicles also increases the risk. The practice committee of the American Society for Reproductive Medicine has concluded that the weight of evidence does not provide direction for development of specific guidelines for the prevention of ovarian hyperstimulation syndrome.

Ectopic pregnancy is unlikely in the patient described because the insemination was done 4 days ago, and implantation has not yet occurred. Acute appendicitis also is part of the differential diagnosis of abdominal pain, but it is associated with right lower quadrant pain, fever, and gastrointestinal symptoms and would be unlikely in this case. During controlled ovarian hyperstimulation, an ovarian cyst and ovarian torsion should always be considered in any patient who presents with abdominal pain not associated with ascites and increased weight.

Al-Shawaf T, Zosmer A, Tozer A, Gillott C, Lower AM, Grudzinskas JG. Value of measuring serum FSH in addition to serum estradiol in a coasting programme to prevent severe OHSS. Hum Reprod 2002;17: 1217–21.

American Society for Reproductive Medicine. Multiple pregnancy associated with infertility therapy. ASRM Educational Bulletin. Birmingham (AL): ASRM; 2000.

Chen D, Burmeister L, Goldschlag D, Rosenwaks Z. Ovarian hyperstimulation syndrome: strategies for prevention. Reprod Biomed Online 2003;7:43–9.

Meldrum DR. Vascular endothelial growth factor, polycystic ovary syndrome, and ovarian hyperstimulation syndrome [editorial]. Fertil Steril 2002;78:1170–1.

61
Salpingitis isthmica nodosa

A patient with longstanding infertility undergoes hysterosalpingography, which shows bilateral proximal tubal occlusion (Fig. 61-1). In the proximal tube, there is a honeycomb pattern of contrast that seems to enter the tubal wall. Subsequent laparoscopy shows multiple 1–2 cm nodules in the isthmus of one fallopian tube. The most likely diagnosis is

    (A) chronic chlamydial salpingitis
    (B) tuberculous salpingitis
* (C) salpingitis isthmica nodosa
    (D) prenatal exposure to diethylstilbestrol
    (E) ectopic pregnancy

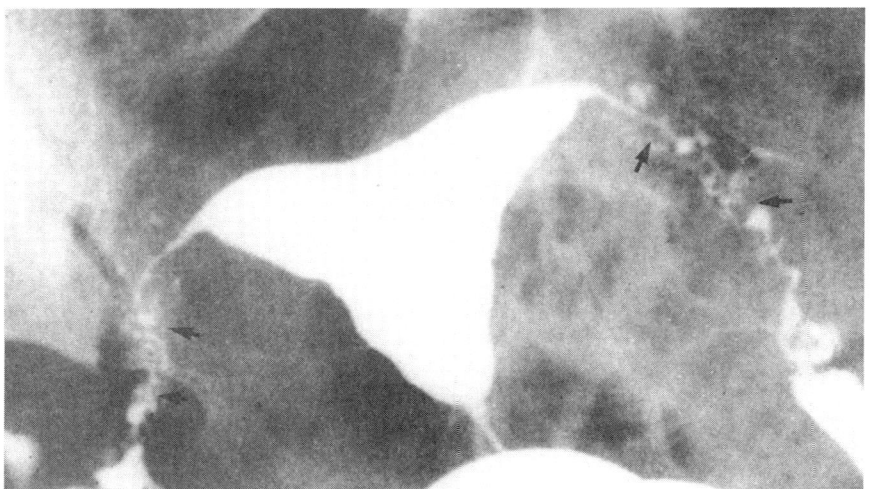

FIG. 61-1. Salpingitis isthmica nodosa. (Reprinted from Wallach EE, Zacur HA. Reproductive medicine and surgery. St. Louis [MO]: Mosby; 1995. p. 501. Copyright 1995, with permission from Elsevier.)

Salpingitis isthmica nodosa is a condition that consists of single or multiple outpouchings or diverticula of the fallopian tube. It often is bilateral and usually is accompanied by nodular hyperplasia of the surrounding muscularis. Some investigators believe that the origin of salpingitis isthmica nodosa is noninflammatory, much like uterine adenomyosis, whereas others believe it has an inflammatory origin. As in uterine adenomyosis, the presence of glands appears to stimulate muscular growth with subsequent mural thickening. The usual external gross appearance is 1 or more nodular swellings of up to 1–2 cm in diameter in the isthmic region. The prevalence of salpingitis isthmica nodosa in healthy, fertile women ranges from 0.6% to 11%, but it is significantly more common in infertile women or women with ectopic pregnancy.

Because salpingitis isthmica nodosa often is multifocal, surgical therapy is not uniformly successful. Segmental resection and anastomosis rarely result in successful pregnancy because of the progressive nature of salpingitis isthmica nodosa. Therefore, in vitro fertilization is the treatment of choice.

Postinflammatory salpingitis can have many appearances on hysterosalpingography. It can show evidence of proximal tubal occlusion, distal occlusion and hydrosalpinx, loculation of contrast about the end of the tube, or the examination may be normal.

Tuberculous salpingitis can cause nodular thickening of the fallopian tubes, mimicking salpingitis isthmica nodosa in its early stages, but progression often results in severe pelvic adhesive disease. Hysterosalpingography findings also may show extensive intrauterine adhesions.

Prenatal exposure to diethylstilbestrol shows a T-shape to the uterine cavity. The fallopian tubes often are patent, but there is a higher incidence of ectopic pregnancy and tubal malfunction.

Kurman RJ, ed. Blaustein's pathology of the female genital tract. Diseases of the fallopian tube. 3rd ed. New York (NY): Springer-Verlag; 1987. p. 414–23.

Jenkins CS, Williams SR, Schmidt GE. Salpingitis isthmica nodosa: a review of the literature, discussion of clinical significance, and consideration of patient management. Fertil Steril 1993;60:599–607.

Saracoglu FO, Mungan T, Tanzer F. Salpingitis isthmica nodosa in infertility and ectopic pregnancy. Gynecol Obstet Invest 1992;34: 202–5.

Thurmond AS, Burry KA, Novy MJ. Salpingitis isthmica nodosa: results of transcervical fluoroscopic catheter recanalization. Fertil Steril 1995;63:715–22.

62

Imperforate hymen versus transverse vaginal septum

A 14-year-old adolescent is referred from the local emergency department for recurrent severe pelvic–abdominal pain. A midline pelvic mass was palpated on rectal examination and a pelvic ultrasonogram suggests a hematocolpometra. Although less than optimal, a vaginal examination suggests that the upper vagina ends blindly. On repeat rectal examination, the bulging mass is found to extend cephalad from the top of the blind vagina. The next best step in management for this patient is

    (A) renal ultrasonography
    (B) bone malformation assessment
*   (C) imaging of the vagina, cervix, and uterus
    (D) examination under anesthesia
    (E) aspiration of the bulging mass

This patient demonstrates the classic presentation of an obstructed genital tract at puberty. Although these patients may present in the newborn period or during infancy with an abdominal mass and a mucocolpos, mucometra, or both, most do not become symptomatic until the obstructed genital tract fills with blood after concealed menarche and 1–2 years of subsequent obstructed menstrual cycles. These patients usually develop cyclic pain that corresponds to the time of concealed menses and eventually present with an acute episode of pain or difficulty with defecation or urination (ie, urinary retention). They are found to have a pelvic–abdominal mass, and an investigation is initiated. The observant clinician will identify the hematocolpos on rectal examination and begin to form a differential diagnosis that would include an imperforate hymen, transverse vaginal septum, or cervical atresia.

The most common of the disorders associated with this scenario is the imperforate hymen. Unlike the patient presented here, a bulging bluish colored mass is seen at the obstructed introitus for these patients. Valsalva maneuver often will make the bulging imperforate hymen even more prominent. The transverse vaginal septum occurs less frequently and is found in 1 in 30,000–80,000 females. Unlike the imperforate hymen, which usually is visible on inspection of the introitus, one half of the transverse vaginal septa are located in the upper vagina, as found in the present patient. Approximately 40% are located closer to the middle of the vagina and the remainder is found in the lower third of the vagina. For both of these disorders, microperforation is more common than is the imperforate state. The difference is that the microperforate hymen will resolve with estrogen production at puberty whereas the transverse vaginal septum will not. The imperforate hymen often is diagnosed during the childhood years while transverse vaginal septum is virtually always diagnosed after the normal time for menarche because of its high location. Cervical atresia is rare and may only be mistaken for the high transverse vaginal septum when a large and high midline mass is identified on rectal examination.

Unlike müllerian anomalies that are commonly associated with renal and skeletal abnormalities, the embryogenesis of the transverse vaginal septum and the imperforate hymen precludes such findings in all but the exceptional patient. For that reason, renal ultrasonography usually is not necessary, and a search for skeletal defects will be unrevealing. The most important part of the evaluation of the patient with a transverse vaginal septum is assessment of the location and width of the septum in preparation for surgery and to rule out cervical atresia. The very thin septum is easy to resect followed by an end-to-end anastomosis. However, a thick septum may require a Z-plasty for repair and in some situations a skin graft. Having this knowledge allows the surgeon to be prepared for any possible situation in the operating room.

A number of specialized imaging studies have been used to assist in the diagnosis (eg, MRI, transrectal ultrasonography, and sonocolpography). Sonocolpography involves placement of a distal vaginal balloon for contrast during abdominal ultrasonography. Most of the recent experience is with MRI. Aspiration of the hematocolpos at the time of the initial presentation to help with the diagnosis should be avoided because it may convert a hematocolpos into a pyocolpos. In the distant past, patients in this situation died from sepsis. In contrast with the transverse vaginal septum, the imperforate hymen needs little preoperative evaluation, and the surgery is easily accomplished with a cruciate incision or complete excision. In addition, repair of the imperforate hymen is best performed when it is diagnosed, including during the childhood years. The longer the time between repair and the psychosexual development of adolescence, the better it is for the individual.

Fedele L, Portuese A, Bianchi S, Zanconato G, Raffaelli R. Transrectal ultrasonography in the assessment of congenital vaginal canalization defects. Hum Reprod 1999;14:359–62.

Garcia RF. Z-plasty for correction of congenital transverse vaginal septum. Am J Obstet Gynecol 1967;99:1164–5.

Hugosson C, Jorulf H, Bakri Y. MRI in distal vaginal atresia. Pediatr Radiol 1991;21:281–3.

Reinhold C, Hricak H, Forstner R, Ascher SM, Bret PM, Meyer WR, et al. Primary amenorrhea: evaluation with MR imaging. Radiology 1997; 203:383–90.

Suidan FG, Azoury RS. The transverse vaginal septum: a clinicopathologic evaluation. Obstet Gynecol 1979;54:278–83.

Thabet SM, Thabet AS. Role of new sono-imaging technique "sonocolpography" in the diagnosis and treatment of the complete transverse vaginal septum and other allied conditions. J Obstet Gynecol Res 2002;28:80–5.

63

Donor oocyte in the older patient

A 43-year-old woman, gravida 4, para 1, comes in for infertility evaluation. She had a 5-year-old son who died in an accident, and she has a history of 3 early pregnancy losses since age 40 years. She and her husband have normal peripheral karyotypes. She has a normal pelvic ultrasonogram, hysterosalpingogram, glucose tolerance test result, serum thyroid-stimulating hormone level, lupus anticoagulant level, anticardiolipin antibody level, antinuclear antibody level, mammogram, and prenatal laboratory test result. A clomiphene citrate (Clomid, Serophene) challenge test shows a day 10 follicle-stimulating hormone level of 15 mIU/L. The therapy that will result in the greatest probability of a term pregnancy in this patient is

    (A) in vitro fertilization (IVF)
    (B) gestational surrogacy with the patient's eggs
*   (C) donor oocyte IVF
    (D) superovulation and intrauterine insemination
    (E) intravenous immunoglobulin

Age-related changes in the egg can hamper a woman's ability to reproduce. All oocytes enter into meiosis during fetal development but do not complete meiosis until after ovulation. Thus, an oocyte may be arrested in the first meiotic division from before birth until perhaps the fiftieth year of life. This prolonged period has led to speculation that there is an age-related effect on chromosomal nondisjunction. For proper chromosomal separation to occur during meiosis, the chromosomal pairs must properly align before being pulled to opposing ends of the cell during cell division. This chromosomal separation is performed with spindle fibers, which some investigators have noted may become tangled as a result of advancing maternal age. Spindle damage affects both meiosis I and II, leading to increased damage. Some species (eg, fruit fly and mouse) have tight control over meiosis with a very low frequency of chromosomal errors. An estimated 25% incidence in chromosomal error occurs in the oocyte of the 30-year-old human female. This incidence increases to 60–90% after age 40 years, compared with a rate of 1% or less in the human male.

Miscarriage frequency increases with advancing maternal age. Before age 35 years, the frequency of any clinically recognized pregnancy ending in a loss with a karyotypically proven trisomy is steady at a rate of less than 5%. However, this risk increases dramatically after age 35 years and exceeds 35% at age 42 years (Fig. 63-1). The reason for this is not entirely understood,

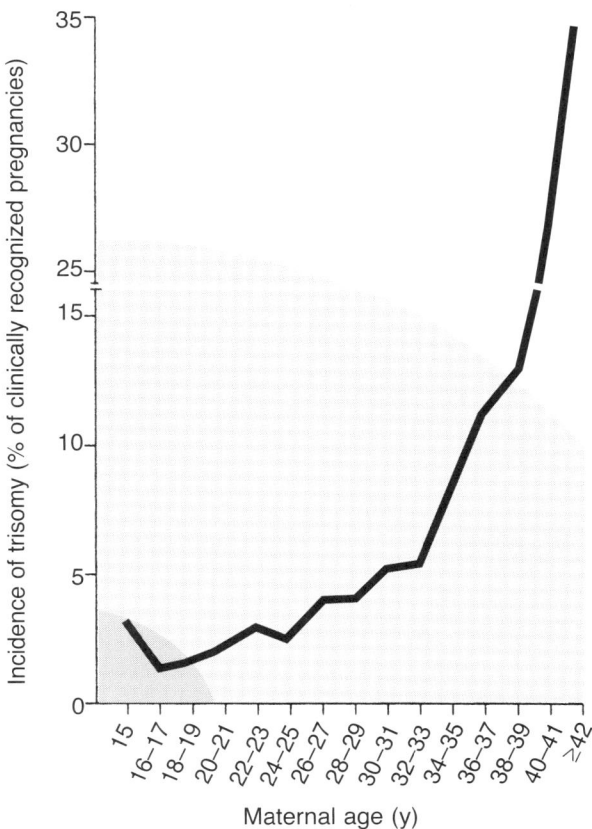

FIG. 63-1. The incidence of trisomy among clinically recognized pregnancies. (Reproduced with permission from Nature Reviews Genetics. Terry T, Hunt P. To err [meiotically] is human: the genesis of human aneuploidy. Nat Rev Genet 2001:2:288. Copyright 2001, Macmillan Magazines Ltd.)

but recent studies of human oocytes and chromosomal studies of human embryos may be helpful in explaining why the risk increases after age 35 years.

Preimplantation genetic diagnosis is now being performed selectively for couples with recurrent pregnancy loss and advanced maternal age. Fluorescent in situ hybridization confirms that there is a high rate of chromosomal error in embryos from women of advancing maternal age. One study using fluorescent in situ hybridization showed that women older than 38 years produce embryos that have a 60% chance of being chromosomally abnormal.

The success rate with donor oocyte IVF is independent of the recipient's age (Fig. 63-2; see color plate). There is a stark contrast in live birth rate between women older than 35 years who use their own eggs and women older than 35 years who use donor eggs. A uterus that is normal by hysterosalpingogram and ultrasonogram does not show an age-related decrease in fertility potential. Testing of the uterus is necessary because age-related increases exist in the incidence of fibroids and other uterine conditions. Therefore, gestational surrogacy with the patient's own eggs will not increase the likelihood of pregnancy. Moreover, superovulation will not improve the quality of an older woman's oocytes.

Testing of the oocyte recipient is dependent on her chronologic age and medical condition. A medical condition may be the reason that a woman's ovaries are failing. Women with previous radiation or chemotherapy deserve special attention. Older women have a higher chance of developing gestational diabetes mellitus and pregnancy-induced hypertension. Older women also should be screened for breast cancer. Medical clearance should be obtained if there is asthma, autoimmune disease, heart disease, diabetes, or hypertension. Women older than 40 years should have a mammogram. Women older than 45 years should have a thorough medical evaluation including cardiovascular testing and a high-risk obstetric consultation before undertaking IVF with donor oocytes. Intravenous immunoglobulin has no role in the treatment of this patient.

American Society for Reproductive Medicine. Guidelines for oocyte donation. Fertil Steril 2002;77(Suppl 5):S6–8.

American Society for Reproductive Medicine. Intravenous immunoglobulin (IVIG) and recurrent spontaneous pregnancy loss. ASRM Committee Opinion. Birmingham (AL): ASRM; 1998.

Battaglia DE, Goodwin P, Klein NA, Soules MR. Influence of maternal age on meiotic spindle assembly in oocytes from naturally cycling women. Hum Reprod 1996;11:2217–22.

Gianaroli L, Magli MC, Ferraretti AP, Munne S. Preimplantation diagnosis for aneuploidies in patients undergoing in vitro fertilization with a poor prognosis: identification of the categories for which it should be proposed. Fertil Steril 1999;72:837–44.

Hassold TJ, Jacobs PA. Trisomy in man. Annu Rev Genet 1984;18:69–97.

Hunt PA. The control of mammalian female meiosis: factors that influence chromosome segregation. J Assist Reprod Genet 1998;15:246–52.

Penzias AS. Oocyte donation 2002. Infert Reprod Med Clin N Am 2002;13:587–94.

64
Blastocysts and twinning

A 41-year-old woman and her husband have decided to try in vitro fertilization (IVF) in an attempt to conceive. The woman has had both fallopian tubes removed as treatment for ruptured ectopic pregnancies. The couple is concerned about the risks and complications associated with IVF techniques. They have heard about assisted reproductive technology (ART) that involves blastocyst culture and transfer. In counseling this couple, the most accurate statement based on current data is that blastocyst culture, compared with day 3 transfer, is associated with

* (A) reduced incidence of cycle cancellation
* (B) similar pregnancy rates
* (C) reduced incidence of twin pregnancy
* (D) higher pregnancy rates in women older than 40 years

According to the American Society for Reproductive Medicine and the Centers for Disease Control and Prevention's *2001 National Summary of Fertility Clinic Reports*, 39.7% of all births that occurred following conception through IVF and other ART were multiple births, of which 83.4% were twins and 16.6% were high-order multiple gestations. These rates are significantly elevated compared with an incidence of less than 3% for multiple births following spontaneous conception in the general population. Along with the high incidence of high-order multiple gestation following ART there occur increased incidences of multifetal reduction and pregnancy-related complications (eg, increased perinatal morbidity and mortality and maternal pregnancy complications) and increased economic problems.

To ensure success and increase the chance for ongoing pregnancy, most IVF centers transfer an average of 3 or more cleavage-stage embryos. Specific guidelines regarding the number of embryos transferred have been published by the Society for Assisted Reproductive Technology. Implantation rates have been sufficiently low enough that the success rate with transfer of a single cleavage-stage embryo was unacceptable. More recent studies have suggested improved success rates for select patients. Although the reasons for the low implantation rates are unknown, suggested possibilities are increased incidences of genetic abnormalities in IVF embryos, inadequacies in embryo culture techniques, and asynchrony between embryo stage and endometrium. The implantation rates following transfer of cleavage-stage embryos usually are reported at 10–20%.

By extending the culture period, it is possible to allow embryos to undergo further development to the blastocyst stage. Blastocysts are advanced-stage embryos with potential for higher implantation rates because of a number of factors (eg, natural selection of healthier embryos and greater synchronicity between embryo and endometrium). Although embryologists are able to culture embryos to the blastocyst stage, the percentage of embryos that survive until the blastocyst stage, to date, has been felt to be unacceptably low. Advances in culture techniques and the development of sequential culture media that support the changing nutritional requirements of the human embryo as it develops into the blastocyst has made blastocyst culture and transfer a viable option for introduction into clinical practice.

Current rates of blastocyst development have been reported to be as high as 50%. This might lead physicians to conclude that all patients should undergo this technique as part of IVF therapy. In patients who produce few embryos (eg, women who are poor responders to ovulation induction therapy and women of advanced age), cleavage-stage embryos may fail to develop to the blastocyst stage. These patients may have no embryos to transfer on day 5 following oocyte retrieval, the day when blastocyst transfer is commonly performed. When women older than 40 years are compared with women younger than 40 years, blastocyst development is found to be approximately 50% less in the older population (22.5% versus 40%, respectively). In addition, the age-related reduction in blastocyst development and implantation rates appears to mimic the data on IVF success in general for this population of women. Blastocyst transfer in women older than 40 years is associated with pregnancy rates per embryo transfer in the 10% range compared with rates in excess of 20% in younger women. Cancellation rates anticipating blastocyst transfer as high as 39% have been reported in older women compared with cancellation rates of 12% in younger women. Thus, for women older than 40 years, such as the patient described, blastocyst transfer does not significantly improve success rates.

In women younger than 40 years with blastocyst transfer, an associated higher rate of implantation would be expected to allow for reduction in the number of embryos transferred while increasing the pregnancy rate. This, in turn, would be expected to result in fewer high-order multiple gestations while perhaps leading to increased numbers of twin gestations. When blastocyst transfer is compared with traditional day 3 transfer of cleavage-stage embryos, a number of interesting facts emerge. Comparing day 3 transfers of approximately 3 cleavage-stage embryos and day 5 transfers of 2 blastocysts in women younger than 40 years, it appears that pregnancy rates are not significantly different. Implantation rates also are similar. Importantly, however, the incidence of high-order multiple gestations (triplets or greater) is reduced to near 0 with blastocyst transfer of 2 embryos while the incidence of twins appears to be similar to that observed with day 3 transfer of cleavage-stage embryos.

Generally, blastocyst transfer offers some significant improvement in the outcomes that can be expected with IVF. Although cycle cancellation rates may be higher with blastocyst transfer because of poor embryo viability in culture, implantation rates are expected to be higher than day 3 transfer of cleavage-stage embryos. The use of blastocyst transfer does reduce the incidence of high-order multiple gestations with a transfer limited to 2 blastocysts but should be expected to result in similar, if not higher, rates of twin gestations. Blastocyst transfer does not appear to be a panacea for the increased risk of failure observed with IVF in older women.

American Society for Reproductive Medicine. Blastocyst production and transfer in clinical assisted reproduction. ASRM Committee Opinion. Birmingham (AL): ASRM; 2001.

American Society for Reproductive Medicine. Guidelines on number of embryos transferred. ASRM Committee Opinion. Birmingham (AL): ASRM; 1999.

Blake D, Proctor M, Johnson N, Olive D. Cleavage stage versus blastocyst stage embryo transfer in assisted conception (Cochrane Review). In: The Cochrane Library, Issue 2, 2004. Chichester, UK: John Wiley & Sons, Ltd.

Gorrill MJ, Sadler-Fredd K, Patton PE, Burry KA. Multiple gestations in assisted reproductive technology: can they be avoided with blastocyst transfers? Am J Obstet Gynecol 2000;184:1471–5; discussion 1475–7.

Thornton KL. Advances in assisted reproductive technologies. Obstet Gynecol Clin North Am 2000;27:517–27.

Toledo AA, Wright G, Jones AE, Smith SS, Johnson-Ward J, Brockman WW, et al. Blastocyst transfer: a useful tool for reduction of high-order multiple gestations in a human assisted reproduction program. Am J Obstet Gynecol 2000;183:377–9; discussion 380–2.

65

Use of bisphosphonates and other agents in osteoporosis

A 34-year-old woman, gravida 1, para 1, has a history of pelvic pain secondary to endometriosis. Over the past 8 years, she has been treated with multiple 6-month courses of gonadotropin-releasing hormone (GnRH) agonist for recurrent pelvic pain. With each GnRH agonist treatment, she had good pain relief. Within 3–4 months, however, her pain had returned. Laparoscopy 1 year ago showed stage II pelvic endometriosis. Dual-energy X-ray absorptiometry indicates a T-score of −2.6 at the spine and −2.1 at the hip. She desires conservation of her reproductive function. With respect to her bone health, the most appropriate medical management of this patient is

    (A) alendronate sodium (Fosamax)
    (B) salmon calcitonin (Miacalcin)
    (C) raloxifene hydrochloride (Evista)
    (D) human parathyroid hormone 1-34 (Forteo)
*   (E) oral contraceptives

The conservative management of pelvic pain secondary to endometriosis can be difficult and requires long-term monitoring and planning. Although GnRH agonists are highly effective in inducing hypoestrogenism and relieving pelvic pain, the response to therapy can be short in duration. The accompanying hypoestrogenic milieu also can result in significant bone loss of 3–4% over a 6-month period. Although recovery of bone density usually occurs during the posttreatment interval, some women are at risk for developing low bone mass after repeated and prolonged intervals of hypoestrogenism. In this patient, her low bone density T-score at the spine may reflect not only the result of multiple treatment courses with GnRH agonist but also failure to attain a normal peak bone mass by age 30 years. This patient's fracture risk at age 34 years is much lower than a woman aged 65 years with the same bone density T-score because other factors, such as bone quality, overall muscle tone, balance, and propensity to fall, are different at these respective ages.

Bisphosphonates are derivatives of pyrophosphate that specifically target the skeleton and are potent inhibitors of bone remodeling. Although these compounds are effective through oral administration, gastrointestinal absorption is less than 1%, requiring that these agents be administered first thing in the morning with 6–8 oz (178–237 mL) of water, one half hour before any food or drink. Currently, 2 bisphosphonates, alendronate sodium (Fosamax) and risedronate sodium (Actonel), are approved for prevention and treatment of osteoporosis in postmenopausal women. Bisphosphonates are potent antiresorptive agents that specifically target the osteoclasts. They are capable of inducing programmed cell death of osteoclasts, a process called apoptosis.

Clinical trials of up to 10 years' duration show that alendronate is effective in increasing bone density in postmenopausal women. Bisphosphonates are deposited specifically in bone and can be recycled as new osteoclasts remodel the bony matrix. Because animal studies suggest a teratogenic effect with exposure to high doses of bisphosphonates, these compounds are relatively contraindicated in women of childbearing age, such as this patient.

Salmon calcitonin (Miacalcin) has been approved by the U.S. Food and Drug Administration (FDA) for treatment of postmenopausal not premenopausal osteoporosis. This hormone can be delivered by intranasal administration on a daily basis. Antibody formation in a significant proportion of patients has been found with long-term use and may be responsible for its reduced long-term efficacy. Calcitonin should not be a consideration for this patient.

The synthetic steroid compounds called selective estrogen receptor modulators, such as raloxifene hydrochloride (Evista), have been shown to have antiresorptive properties in bone. These compounds bind to the α and β types of estrogen receptor with varying degrees of receptor affinities and appear to demonstrate estrogenic actions in some tissues (bone and liver) and antiestrogenic actions in others (endometrium and breast). The effects of raloxifene on endometriosis has not been evaluated. Clinical trials have demonstrated that raloxifene is effective in the treatment of postmenopausal osteoporosis. However, the use of raloxifene in reproductive-aged women has not been extensively evaluated and would lead to increases in hot flushes.

Human parathyroid hormone 1-34 (Forteo) is a new FDA-approved agent for treatment of severe osteoporosis. It is given as a daily injection subcutaneously at a dose of 20 µg per day using a special injection pen delivery system. Its use has been limited to a 2-year treatment period. It is the only anabolic agent approved for the treatment of severe postmenopausal osteoporosis. Clinical trials indicate a 6–8% increase per year in bone mass at the spine with an overall fracture reduction rate of 65% and 53% at the spine and hip sites, respectively. There has been no reported clinical experience in premenopausal women with human parathyroid hormone 1-34.

The use of oral contraceptives in this patient would be potentially effective in reducing pelvic pain and controlling the progression of endometriosis. Moreover, in observational studies, oral contraceptive users have been shown to have higher bone mass than nonusers. Oral contraceptives are the best choice for this patient.

Black DM, Thompson DE, Bauer DC, Ensrud K, Musliner T, Hochberg MC, et al. Fracture risk reduction with alendronate in women with osteoporosis: the Fracture Intervention Trial. FIT Research Group. J Clin Endocrinol Metab 2000;85:4118–24.

Chesnut CH 3rd, Silverman S, Andriano K, Genant H, Gimona A, Harris S, et al. A randomized trial of nasal spray salmon calcitonin in postmenopausal women with established osteoporosis: the prevent recurrence of osteoporotic fractures study. PROOF Study Group. Am J Med 2000;109:267–76.

Ettinger B, Black DM, Mitlak BH, Knickerbocker RK, Nickelsen T, Genant HK, et al. Reduction of vertebral fracture risk in postmenopausal women with osteoporosis treated with raloxifene: results from a 3-year randomized clinical trial. Multiple Outcomes of Raloxifene Evaluation (MORE) Investigators. JAMA 1999;282: 637–45.

Hornstein MD, Surrey ES, Weisberg GW, Casino LA. Leuprolide acetate depot and hormonal add-back in endometriosis: a 12-month study. Lupron Addback Study Group. Obstet Gynecol 1998;91:16–24.

McClung MR, Geusens P, Miller PD, Zippel H, Bensen WG, Roux C, et al. Effect of risedronate on the risk of hip fracture in elderly women. Hip Intervention Study Group. N Engl J Med 2001;344:333–40.

National Osteoporosis Foundation. Physician's guide to prevention and treatment of osteoporosis. Belle Mead (NJ): Excerpta Medica, Inc; 1998.

Neer RM, Arnaud CD, Zanchetta JR, Prince R, Gaich GA, Reginster JY, et al. Effect of parathyroid hormone (1-34) on fractures and bone mineral density in postmenopausal women with osteoporosis. N Engl J Med 2001;344:1434–41.

66

Continued bone loss with or following hormone therapy

A 70-year-old woman who has been taking combination hormone therapy (HT) for 15 years decides to discontinue therapy after hearing the results of the Women's Health Initiative study. Her baseline bone mineral density (BMD) showed T-scores of -2 in the lumbar vertebrae and -0.8 in her proximal femur. Dual-energy X-ray absorptiometry (DXA) 2 years ago showed improved T-scores for both the lumbar vertebrae and proximal femur. In discussing expectations for maintaining bone health and preventing fractures in this patient, you tell her that following discontinuation of therapy she will experience the most rapid bone loss in

* (A) year 1
  (B) year 3
  (C) year 5
  (D) year 10

One of the changes associated with estrogen deficiency is the acceleration of bone loss in the years following menopause, which can lead to osteoporosis. During the first 5–7 years after menopause, most women experience rapid bone loss. At this time, up to 20% of expected bone loss in a woman's lifetime may occur, increasing fracture risk.

Osteoporosis is a major public health problem in the United States, which is diagnosed in an estimated 8 million women at any one time. An additional 22 million women are estimated to have low bone mass, or osteopenia. Bone fractures are a major consequence of osteoporosis and account for approximately 1.5 million fractures annually in the United States alone.

Most bone loss is asymptomatic. Individuals may be unaware that they have osteoporosis until their bones become so weakened that a sudden bump or fall causes a fracture or a vertebral collapse. According to the Centers for Disease Control and Prevention, 93% of estrogen-deficient women with osteoporosis are unaware of their condition when diagnosed.

Currently, the most effective method for diagnosing osteoporosis in asymptomatic patients is through use of DXA, which measures the ability of bone to absorb radiation. Although standard X-rays can confirm fractures, they can detect bone loss only when at least 30% of bone mass is already lost. A DXA scan can diagnose osteoporosis before the loss of bone structure and bone strength. Typically, DXA results are reported as BMD in grams per square centimeter, and that number is compared with a reference range from young adults (T-score), which represents the number of standard deviations below the mean. A T-score of -1 represents a 10% loss; in this patient, a T-score of -2 represents a 20% loss of bone mass compared with the mean of young adults and is consistent with a diagnosis of osteopenia in the lumbar vertebrae. A T-score of -0.8 is normal.

Appendix C shows the risk factors for osteoporosis. Each standard deviation decrease in spine vertebrae bone mass increases the risk of spine fracture by 190%; each standard deviation decrease in hip bone mass increases the risk of hip fracture by 240%. For postmenopausal women with no additional risk factors, the National Osteoporosis Foundation recommends therapy for those with T-scores at or less than -2. If at least 1 additional risk factor is present, treatment should be initiated at or below a T-score of -1.5. This patient's baseline BMD at age 55 years showed osteopenia; a recommendation to begin therapy would be appropriate for her T-score of -2.

Many studies have documented the positive effects of HT on bone mass, and there is clear evidence that such therapy prevents bone loss. Although HT is believed to enhance bone mass better in the initial years after menopause, it can increase bone mass even when started long after menopause.

The Postmenopausal Estrogen/Progestin Interventions trial, a multicenter study of more than 900 women whose average age was 52 years, found that estrogen alone and the combination of estrogen and progestin was associated with an increase in BMD at the spine of nearly 5% of the women over a 3-year period. Similar results were seen at the femoral neck in this patient after 2 years of therapy; her T-score was normal for the lumbar vertebrae and for the proximal femur.

Bone loss is rare in many women taking standard doses of HT. With discontinuation of therapy, bone loss does ensue, and it is expected that a patient's BMD would decrease on average 4.5% at the spine and 2.4% at the trochanter during the first year. In a 3-year prospective study conducted in 498 women aged 65–77 years taking combined HT, discontinuation of the therapy resulted in rapid bone loss. Most of the bone loss occurred during the first year after cessation of HT, with little change during the second year.

This patient should be counselled about the potential risks of fracture associated with a decrease in BMD. Appropriate interventions should be initiated to decrease her future fracture risk.

Gallagher JC, Rapuri PB, Haynatzki G, Detter JR. Effect of discontinuation of estrogen, calcitriol, and the combination of both on bone density and bone markers. J Clin Endocrinol Metab 2002;87:4914–23.

Greenspan SL, Emkey RD, Bone HG, Weiss SR, Bell NH, Downs RW, et al. Significant differential effects of alendronate, estrogen, or combination therapy on the rate of bone loss after discontinuation of treatment of postmenopausal osteoporosis. A randomized, double-blind controlled trial. Ann Intern Med 2002;137:875–83.

Guthrie JR, Ebeling PR, Hopper JL. Barrett-Connor E, Dennerstein L, Dudley EC, et al. A prospective study of bone loss in menopausal Australian-born women. Osteoporos Int 1998;8:282–90.

Lindsay R, Cosman F. Pathophysiology of bone loss. In: Lobo RA, ed. Treatment of the postmenopausal women: basic and clinical aspects. 2nd ed. Philadelphia (PA): Lippincott Williams & Wilkins; 1999. p. 305–14.

Melton LJ III, Atkinson EJ, O'Fallon WM, Wahner HW, Riggs BL. Long-term fracture prediction by bone mineral assessed at different skeletal sites. J Bone Miner Res 1993;8:1227–33.

67
Gonadotropin-releasing hormone agonist and antagonist

An 18-year-old woman with acute myelogenous leukemia is scheduled to undergo high-dose chemotherapy and total body irradiation for a bone marrow transplant in 5 days. Her hematologist requests advice regarding the best approach to conserve ovarian function and to reduce the likelihood of vaginal bleeding during the anticipated chemotherapy-induced pancytopenia. The patient has regular menstrual cycles, and her last menstrual period began 6 days ago. She is not using contraceptives. The most appropriate treatment regimen for this patient is

(A) gonadotropin-releasing hormone (GnRH) agonist
(B) depot medroxyprogesterone acetate
(C) combination oral contraceptives
* (D) gonadotropin-releasing hormone antagonist
(E) transposition of the ovaries

Gonadotropin-releasing hormone is a decapeptide that is secreted by GnRH neurons located principally in the mediobasal hypothalamus. During the menstrual cycle, these neurons depolarize in concert resulting in "pulses" of GnRH at a frequency of 60–120 minutes to stimulate pituitary secretion of luteinizing hormone (LH) and follicle-stimulating hormone (FSH) and downstream ovarian follicular development. Gonadotropin-releasing hormone has a short half-life in the peripheral circulation of less than 5 minutes. If exogenous GnRH is administered in a continuous infusion (ie, more than 10 days), LH and FSH secretion is suppressed because of the phenomenon of down-regulation of the GnRH receptor. Synthetic analogs of GnRH have been designed to change the biologic activity of the native compound. These changes include:

1. Substitution of an amino acid in the 6th position from an L-amino acid to a D-amino acid of this decapeptide, which results in resistance to enzymatic degradation and a prolonged half-life.
2. Elimination of the 10th amino acid, which results in greater binding affinity of the analog for the GnRH receptor.
3. Substitution of an amino acid in the third position, which results in an analog that can bind to the GnRH receptor but will not activate downstream calcium channel-mediated events that result in LH and FSH secretion. This substitution is critical for GnRH antagonists.

A number of GnRH agonists are available for clinical use in the United States, including leuprolide acetate (Lupron), goserelin (Zoladex), triptorelin pamoate (Trelstar), buserelin acetate (Suprefact), and nafarelin (Synarel). These analogs can be administered by subcutaneous, intramuscular, intravenous, or in depot formulations. The major clinical indications for GnRH agonists include treatment of precocious puberty, endometriosis, uterine myomas, controlled ovarian hyperstimulation, prostate cancer, and other sex-steroid-associated disorders. Administration of GnRH agonists will result in an initial flare response characterized by an increased secretion of LH and FSH for 10–14 days before downregulation and suppression of LH and FSH secretions. The duration of the flare response can be reduced if GnRH agonists are administered during the luteal phase.

Two GnRH antagonists are available in the United States: 1) ganirelix acetate (Antagon) and 2) cetrorelix (Cetrotide). The GnRH antagonists directly compete with native GnRH for the GnRH receptor binding sites and, because of the antagonist's increased binding affinity and longer half-life, will effectively displace endogenous GnRH. Thus, LH and FSH secretion is rapidly suppressed within hours of GnRH antagonist administration. Because depot formulations of the GnRH antagonists are not yet available, clinical indications for use of GnRH antagonists have been limited to controlled ovarian hyperstimulation for the purposes of in vitro fertilization.

In young reproductive-aged patients who require chemotherapy for treatment of malignant disease, there is a high incidence of premature ovarian and testicular failure caused by accelerated loss in germ cells. Animal studies suggest that pretreatment with complete suppression of gonadotropin secretion can reduce the gonadotoxic impact of chemotherapy on germ cell loss. In this patient, who is in the follicular phase of the menstrual cycle, use of a GnRH agonist would result in a flare response with increased secretion of LH and FSH during the period of chemotherapy. To achieve rapid suppression of LH and FSH, a GnRH antagonist would be more appropriate.

Depot medroxyprogesterone acetate, combination oral contraceptives, and danazol (Danocrine) are less effective for the suppression of LH and FSH secretion. However, all 3 of these compounds would be effective in reducing endometrial development and help to induce sustained amenorrhea. How effective any or all of these agents is in preserving future fertility in women is unclear. The use of these agents has not been approved by the U.S. Food and Drug Administration for such indications. Transposition of the ovaries can be used in patients who will undergo pelvic radiation therapy but will not alter the gonadotoxic effect of systemic chemotherapy.

Behre HM, Klein B, Steinmeyer E, McGregor GP, Voigt K, Nieschlag E. Effective suppression of luteinizing hormone and testosterone by single doses of the new gonadotropin-releasing hormone antagonist cetrorelix (SB-75) in normal men. J Clin Endocrinol Metab 1992;75: 393–8.

Blumenfeld Z. Preservation of fertility and ovarian function and minimalization of chemotherapy associated gonadotoxicity and premature ovarian failure: the role of inhibin-A and -B as markers. Mol Cell Endocrinol 2002;187:93–105.

Koch Y, Baram T, Hazum E, Fridkin M. Resistance to enzymic degradation of LH-RH analogues possessing increased biological activity. Biochem Biophys Res Commun 1977;74:488–91.

Shapiro DB. An overview of GnRH antagonists in infertility treatments. Introduction. Fertil Steril 2003;80(suppl 1):S1–7; discussion S32–4.

68
Complications of hysterosalpingography

A 25-year-old woman, gravida 3, para 0, with history of polycystic ovary syndrome, comes in for evaluation of recurrent miscarriages. The patient reports a history of irregular menstrual cycles ranging in length from 35 to 90 days. She undergoes hysterosalpingography (HSG) on day 8 of her cycle to evaluate the uterine cavity after 3 days of light flow. After injection of dye, an intrauterine filling defect is noted as shown (Fig. 68-1). A pregnancy test result is positive. The most important complication to discuss with the patient is

* (A) spontaneous abortion
  (B) fetal anomalies from radiation
  (C) pelvic infection
  (D) hemorrhage
  (E) intrauterine adhesions

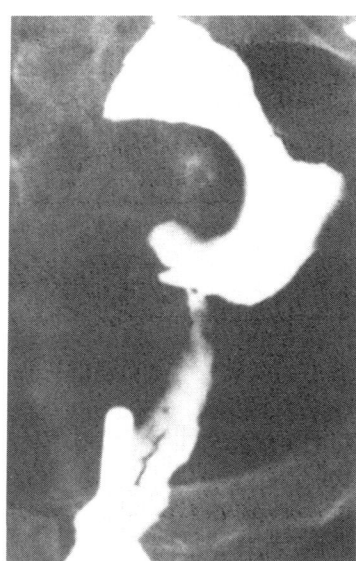

FIG. 68-1. Intrauterine pregnancy. (Justesen P, Rasmussen F, Anderson PE. Inadvertently performed hysterosalpingography during early pregnancy. Acta Radiol Diagn [Stockh] 1986;27:712.)

Hysterosalpingography remains an invaluable diagnostic tool in the evaluation of infertility and gynecologic disorders. It is one of the most common tests performed during the infertility evaluation. Through radiologic injection of contrast dye under fluoroscopy, HSG is used to assess abnormalities of the uterine cavity, tubal disease and patency, and defects in the endocervical canal.

The HSG is performed during the first half of the menstrual cycle, 2–5 days after cessation of menstrual flow. In patients with regular menses, this decreases the likelihood that patients are pregnant and that the endometrial lining is thin to prevent a false-positive tubal blockage during the passage of contrast dye. In rare cases, an undiagnosed pregnancy may be present when HSG is performed. A study conducted on 6,225 women who underwent HSG showed that 4 women who were pregnant at the time of the procedure had oligomenorrhea, metrorrhagia, or an unusual bleeding pattern considered to be a menstrual period. To reduce the likelihood of this complication, patients who have a history of irregular cycles, amenorrhea, or the possibility of an ongoing pregnancy should consider a pregnancy test before the procedure.

Hysterosalpingography carried out in a patient with an unrecognized ongoing pregnancy may result in miscarriage, infection, or bleeding. Evidence is lacking in the medical literature, however, to show the specific incidences of these outcomes. One study showed that the risk of miscarriage was 50% after HSG was performed on pregnant patients. Patients who did have ongoing pregnancies did not have an increase in complications related to pregnancy and birth.

Patients are not at risk for miscarriage, or their fetuses for congenital abnormalities, if pregnancy occurs within the month following the HSG. A study to evaluate radiation exposure in normal and abnormal hysterosalpingograms showed low exposure risk when a dose of 1 rad per minute was used.

The clinical scenario presents a pregnancy that was exposed to contrast dye and fluoroscopic radiation during HSG. The past menstrual history is suspect because of irregular menstrual cycles, and a pregnancy test could have identified this information before the procedure. After the pregnancy is exposed, there is an increased risk of miscarriage, although there is no increased risk for infants with congenital anomalies. No greater risk has been observed in these cases for pelvic infection, bleeding complications, or intrauterine adhesions. In addition, the contrast dye does not pose a higher risk than fluoroscopic radiation. For pregnancies diagnosed at HSG, therapeutic abortion is not recommended.

Goldenberg RL, White R, Magendantz HG. Pregnancy during the hysterogram cycle. Fertil Steril 1976;27:1274–6.

Heard MJ, Carson SA. Hysterosalpingography: a clinical update. Female Pat 2001;26(4):29–31, 35, 39–40.

Justesen P, Rasmussen F, Anderson PE Jr. Inadvertently performed hysterosalpingography during early pregnancy. Acta Radiol Diagn (Stockh) 1986;27:711–3.

Van Der Weiden RM, Van Zijl J. Radiation exposure of the ovaries during hysterosalpingography. Is radionuclide hysterosalpingography justified? Br J Obstet Gynaecol 1989;96:471–2.

69
Male infertility and hypergonadotropic hypogonadism

A 25-year-old man with azoospermia receives a diagnosis of Klinefelter's syndrome and is found to have immature spermatozoa on testicular biopsy. In vitro fertilization (IVF) with intracytoplasmic sperm injection (ICSI) is performed, and his wife becomes pregnant. A 16-week amniocentesis is most likely to find a fetus with which one of the following karyotypes?

   (A) 47,XXY
   (B) 45,X
* (C) Normal karyotype
   (D) 47,XYY
   (E) Trisomy 21

Klinefelter's syndrome is diagnosed in 1 in every 500 newborn males and 1 in 30 infertile men. It is the most common cause of hypergonadotropic hypogonadism in males and accounts for nearly 15% of all cases of azoospermia. Ninety percent of these men have a 47,XXY karyotype. Mosaicism, usually 46,XY/47,XXY, is found in the remainder of patients. The pathologic gonadal process associated with an extra X chromosome begins as early as childhood and progresses with time. It involves a gradual hyalinization and fibrosis of the seminiferous tubules. Eventually, there is a near total loss of germ cells in 99% of men. The same process appears to similarly affect Leydig cell function. As the testes become more hyalinized and fibrotic, androgen production decreases.

Although most males with Klinefelter's syndrome initiate the pubertal process, testosterone levels are rarely higher than the lower limit for normal adults. Puberty usually is not spontaneously completed. These males, if left untreated, have small genitalia; decreased pubic, axillary, facial, and body hair; increased adiposity in a feminine distribution often accompanied by gynecomastia; and decreased muscle mass. They are taller than predicted by parental height because of the extra X chromosome and delayed epiphyseal closure secondary to hypogonadal androgen production and subsequent conversion to estrogen.

A number of behavioral and psychologic problems have been previously reported for males with Klinefelter's syndrome, including specific learning disabilities and poor school performance. A number of these tendencies have disappeared with the early use of androgen therapy during the adolescent years. In addition to completing the physical maturation of puberty, androgen therapy has been associated with improved self-esteem and greater ability for concentration and focus during learning and work. Androgen therapy also has shown a reduced tendency toward depression.

Although the practice of androgen therapy has greatly changed the phenotype of Klinefelter's syndrome, even more impressive has been the outcome of assisted reproductive technology (ART) in treating the infertility for some of these men. Although virtually all of the nonmosaic men with Klinefelter's syndrome have azoospermia, rare mosaic men have a few spermatozoa in the ejaculate. Until the hyalinization of the seminiferous tubules is complete, rare immature and mature sperm may be found in the testes in either of the forms of Klinefelter's syndrome. In contrast to Turner's syndrome, for which 1% of patients will spontaneously conceive, only a few males with Klinefelter's syndrome have been reported to achieve a spontaneous pregnancy and fewer of these men have had paternity proved. With the advent of ICSI, it was hypothesized that for men with rare sperm in the ejaculate or the testes, pregnancy might be possible by IVF. What was not known was the proportion of the immature or mature spermatozoa that were abnormal and that would result in a child with a sex chromosome aneuploidy if injected into an oocyte.

Most of the mature sperm studied by fluorescent in-situ hybridization for both mosaic and nonmosaic men with Klinefelter's syndrome are normal (Table 69-1). More than 90% of the sperm obtained from men with mosaic Klinefelter's syndrome have been chromosomally normal (ie, haploid). For nonmosaic men studied, the highest percentage of abnormal testicular mature sperm identified has been 25%. These studies have been reassuring and have allowed ART centers to proceed with IVF and ICSI for couples with Klinefelter's syndrome, with preliminary outcomes being similarly reassuring. A total of 11 pregnancies have been reported for mosaic males at the time of writing. These pregnancies have occurred in the first 2 attempts for the couples and consisted of 3 sets of twins, 1 set of triplets, and 7 singletons. Only 1 of these 16 fetuses at midgestation was aneuploid (ie, a 47,XXY fetus of triplets), and the remaining 15 infants were delivered as either 46,XX or 46,XY. The first delivery for a male with nonmosaic Klinefelter's syndrome was of 46,XX and 46,XY twins. Patients with Turner's syndrome who became pregnant spontaneously have been reported to deliver children with trisomy 21. Despite the fact that it is debated whether Turner's syndrome has a true predisposition to trisomy should they rarely become pregnant spontaneously, none of the children born to men with Klinefelter's syndrome have trisomy. Although the children delivered from each of these pregnancies have all been normal, the numbers are limited, and the outcomes could certainly change as a larger number of couples are treated.

A couple that today presents for counseling to discuss their reproductive options when the man has Klinefelter's syndrome has more opportunities available. Although it would appear from these early reports that most infants born to men with Klinefelter's syndrome by IVF with ICSI will be karyotypically normal, what is not yet known is the percentage of men at different ages of presentation for these services who will have viable sperm in their testes. Given that the hyalinization process is progressive with time, it would seem logical that the sooner the testes were biopsied (ie, the younger the man), the better would be this chance. However, this remains to be proved. For those who have had IVF, it appears that implantation rates are very normal in addition to the fact that the infants are nearly all chromosomally normal. No doubt, preimplantation genetic diagnosis should be offered if available, as should prenatal diagnosis.

TABLE 69-1. Results of 2-Color Fluorescence In-Situ Hybridization of 202 Sperm From a Patient With Mosaic Klinefelter's Syndrome

Presumed Karyotype	No. of Sperm (%)
23,X	102 (50)
23,Y	85 (42)
24,XY*	10 (5)
24,XX*	4 (2)
24YY*	0 (0)
25,XXY*	1 (0.5)

*Abnormal karyotype.

Reprinted from Fertility & Sterility, Vol 69, Kruse R, Guttenbach M, Schartmann B, Schubert R, van der Ven H, Schmid M, et al, Genetic counseling in a patient with XXY/XXXY/XY mosaic Klinefelter's syndrome: estimate of sex chromosome aberrations in sperm before intracytoplasmic sperm injection, 482, Copyright 1998, with permission from Elsevier.

Kruse R, Guttenbach M, Schartmann B, Schubert R, van der Ven H, Schmid M, et al. Genetic counseling in a patient with XXY/XXXY/XY mosaic Klinefelter's syndrome: estimate of sex chromosome aberrations in sperm before intracytoplasmic sperm injection. Fertil Steril 1998;69:482–5.

Poulakis V, Witzsch U, Diehl W, de Vries R, Becht E, Trotnow S. Birth of two infants with normal karyotype after intracytoplasmic injection of sperm obtained by testicular extraction from two men with nonmosaic Klinefelter's syndrome. Fertil Steril 2001;76:1060–2.

Ron-El R, Raziel A, Strassburger D, Schachter M, Bern O, Friedler S. Birth of healthy male twins after intracytoplasmic sperm injection of frozen-thawed testicular spermatozoa from a patient with nonmosaic Klinefelter syndrome. Fertil Steril 2000;74:832–3.

70

Diagnosis of gonadotropin-secreting tumors

A 27-year-old woman presents with a 5-month history of daily headaches, irregular vaginal bleeding, and pelvic pain. She had been taking low-dose combination oral contraceptives for 3 years and stopped them 6 months ago. Vaginal ultrasonography reveals bilateral multicystic ovaries, with the right ovary measuring 69 mm × 43 mm (Fig. 70-1) and the left ovary measuring 56 mm × 51 mm. She has a basal serum follicle-stimulating hormone (FSH) level of 10 mIU/mL, prolactin level of 8 ng/mL, and thyroid-stimulating hormone (TSH) level of 1.6 μU/mL. Her serum estradiol level is 840 pg/mL. The next step in the management of this patient is

(A) ultrasound-guided aspiration of the cysts
(B) surgical excision of the cysts
* (C) magnetic resonance imaging (MRI) of the sella turcica
(D) thyrotropin-releasing hormone (TRH) stimulation test
(E) administration of combination oral contraceptives

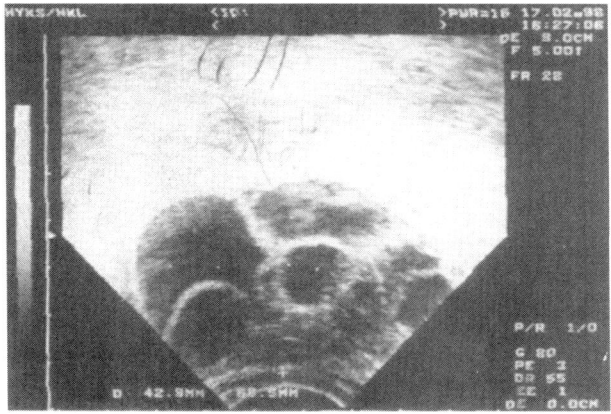

FIG. 70-1. Transvaginal ultrasound examination of the ovary showing a multicystic ovary measuring 69 mm × 49 mm. (Välimäki MJ, Tiitinen A, Alfthan H, Paetau A, Poranen A, Sane T, et al. Ovarian hyperstimulation caused by gonadotroph adenoma secreting follicle-stimulating hormone in 28-year-old woman. J Clin Endocrinol Metab 1999;84:4205.)

This patient presented with irregular menses and pelvic pain in association with enlarged multicystic ovaries. In addition, there were normal circulating concentrations of FSH, prolactin, and TSH and markedly elevated levels of estradiol. This is an enigmatic presentation. However, the data suggest the possibility of gonadotropin stimulation of the ovaries. Had the luteinizing hormone (LH) level been measured as well, it is highly likely that this level would have been suppressed, as would have been expected for FSH. Normally, both LH and FSH levels would be expected to be undetectable (<2 mIU/mL) with this presentation. Attention should focus on the pituitary gland and evaluation of the patient for a pituitary tumor secreting FSH. Thus, the next step in management is MRI of the sella turcica. In this case, a nonprolactin-secreting macroadenoma would be expected.

This pituitary tumor also is likely to produce FSH. Gonadotropin-secreting pituitary adenomas make up approximately 40% of identified macroadenomas. Moreover, the vast majority of so-called "nonfunctioning" tumors secrete either the α-subunit common to FSH, LH, TSH, or gonadotropin when studied in vitro. If α-subunit had been measured by immunoassay, it is likely that it would have been significantly elevated even if FSH levels were in the normal range.

Particularly rare in this case is the presence of a gonadotropin-producing tumor in a young woman that causes ovarian hyperstimulation. Only a few such cases have been reported in the literature. Most gonadotropin-secreting tumors have been identified in older men. Large quantities of gonadotropins and their subunits are rarely secreted, and such tumors do not cause a consistently recognizable clinical syndrome. Diagnosis of tumors that secrete intact FSH or LH is even more difficult in postmenopausal women who normally have elevated levels of gonadotropins and ovaries unable to respond to the gonadotropin. There is little point in aspirating the many cysts present or in excising them without identifying and treating the cause.

It is reasonable to perform a TRH stimulation test but only after first performing an MRI study to determine that there is a tumor. Paradoxically, intact gonadotropin levels, the α-subunit, and β-subunit of LH typically increase in individuals with gonadotrope tumors in response to TRH; such increases would be expected in this patient.

Administration of combination oral contraceptives is not warranted in this patient. It will not cause regression of the ovarian cysts. Resection of the pituitary adenoma is

71

Hypothyroidism and hyperprolactinemia

A 25-year-old nulligravid woman presents with lethargy, constipation, cold intolerance, and breast discharge. On physical examination, her pulse rate is 55 beats per minute, and she has spontaneous bilateral galactorrhea. Her prolactin level is 67 ng/mL, and she has a thyroid-stimulating hormone (TSH) level of 15 µU/mL. The hormone responsible for prolactin elevations and galactorrhea in this patient is

(A) insulinlike growth factor-I
* (B) thyrotropin-releasing hormone (TRH)
(C) free thyroxine (T_4)
(D) TSH
(E) vasopressin

Although a distinct prolactin-releasing factor has been identified in various birds, such a factor has not been identified in humans. It is believed that TRH corresponds to prolactin-releasing factor in humans. Gonadotropin-releasing hormone, vasopressin, and other hormones have been reported to induce the release of prolactin in vitro, but any role in human physiology is still unclear.

The thyroid axis is stimulated by the hypothalamic factor TRH and inhibited by somatostatin and dopamine. The thyroid hormones, triiodothyronine and free T_4, regulate TSH levels by suppression of TRH secretion by reducing the number TRH receptors. Thyrotropin-releasing hormone also stimulates prolactin secretion directly in the pituitary gland. Small doses of TRH are capable of increasing the secretion of TSH and also can increase prolactin levels, indicating a physiologic role for TRH in the control of prolactin secretion. This is the reason why primary hypothyroidism can be associated with galactorrhea. Cessation of galactorrhea with the administration of thyroid hormone provides strong circumstantial evidence to support the conclusion that TRH is a stimulant of prolactin secretion.

The fact that this patient's basal prolactin level is less than 100 ng/mL also suggests that she does not have a prolactinoma. However, pituitary tumors do occur in this setting.

Bole-Feysot C, Goffin V, Edery M, Binart N, Kelly PA. Prolactin (PRL) and its receptor: actions, signal transduction pathways and phenotypes observed in PRL receptor knockout mice. Endocr Rev 1998;19:225–68.

De Greef WJ, Voogt JL, Visser TJ, Lamberts SW, van der Schoot P. Control of prolactin release induced by suckling. Endocrinology 1987;121:316–22.

72

Informed consent for donor eggs

A 44-year-old Chinese-American woman is considering using an oocyte donor because of her age. The preferable age of the donor is

    (A) 17 years
    (B) 20 years
*   (C) 26 years
    (D) 35 years
    (E) 38 years

The American Society for Reproductive Medicine (ASRM) has developed guidelines for oocyte donation to assist clinicians, patients, and donors in making an informed decision. Because of the recipient's ethnic background, it may be difficult to find an anonymous Chinese-American or Asian oocyte donor. The recipient may need to recruit a known oocyte donor by contacting local ethnic social groups or by placing advertisements.

The ASRM recommends that donors be preferably between the ages of 21 and 34 years. Younger donors could donate, but they should have attained their state's age of legal majority before they consider oocyte donation. In this particular clinical setting, the 17-year-old and 20-year-old donors are less desirable because they may not be able to make informed decisions concerning their donations. Donors younger than 21 years may not have had children, and they may regret their decision if they should subsequently become infertile. Donors who are between ages 21 and 34 years are more suitable candidates. On the basis of age, the 26-year-old woman would be a better donor because she should have a lower incidence for spontaneous abortion than a 35-year-old woman. Oocyte donors older than 34 years have an increased risk of having either a spontaneous abortion or a chromosomally abnormal infant. Because of this possibility, the ASRM recommends that recipients be specifically informed of the donor's age if the donor is older than 34 years.

Although proven fertility is not a requirement, donors with a prior history of conceiving and delivering a healthy infant are more desirable than women who have not conceived. The ASRM further recommends that the oocyte donor attend a counseling session and undergo a genetic and psychologic evaluation before she donates her oocytes. They also recommend that oocyte donors receive some monetary compensation. This amount should reflect the time, inconvenience, risks, and the physical and emotional demands associated with oocyte donation. The amount should not be excessive to minimize the possibility of inducement of the donor and the "suggestion that payment is for the oocytes themselves." Payment also should be received regardless of outcome of the oocyte donation. Follow-up information concerning a donor's experience with oocyte donation indicates that although their donation often is altruistically motivated, most would not donate if compensation were not provided.

Financial incentives in recruitment of oocyte donors. The Ethics Committee of the American Society for Reproductive Medicine. Fertil Steril 2000;74:216–20.

Guidelines for oocyte donation. American Society for Reproductive Medicine. Fertil Steril 2002;77(suppl 5):S6–8.

Klock SC, Stout JE, Davidson M. Psychological characteristics and factors related to willingness to donate again among anonymous oocyte donors. Fertil Steril 2003;79:1312–6.

73
Fertility drugs and ovarian cancer

A 28-year-old woman, gravida 1, para 1, gave birth 1 year ago after conceiving in her fifth cycle of clomiphene citrate (Clomid, Serophene). She currently is breastfeeding. She does not have a family history of ovarian cancer but remains concerned about an increased risk of ovarian cancer because of her use of clomiphene. The best next step is annual

   (A) serum CA 125 level testing
* (B) pelvic examination
   (C) transvaginal ultrasonography
   (D) pulsed Doppler study of the ovaries

The answer to the question of whether an association exists between fertility drugs and ovarian cancer is that it seems doubtful. In 1992, the authors of a collaborative analysis pooled and reanalyzed the data from 12 case–control studies involving 2,197 cases of ovarian cancer and 8,893 controls. They claimed that the association of ovulation induction agents and ovarian cancer increased 27 times in infertile women when compared with fertile controls. Pregnancy, lactation, and the use of oral contraceptives were associated with a reduction in the risk of ovarian cancer. The study was criticized because of the lack of a suitable control group because nulligravidity and infertility are established risk factors for ovarian cancer. Additionally, only 3 of the case–control studies appeared to contain data on the past use of fertility drugs.

Several years later, a large cohort study was reported of 10,358 women who underwent in vitro fertilization (IVF) between 1978 and 1992, with and without exposure to fertility drugs. The exposed group (n = 5,564) received ovarian stimulation by fertility drugs to induce multiple follicle formation, while the unexposed group (n = 4,794) underwent natural cycle IVF without ovarian stimulation by fertility drugs. Follow-up was limited and ranged from 1 to 15 years. Rates of ovarian cancer were not different from the general population. When the exposed patients were compared with the unexposed patients, the relative risk of ovarian cancer was 1.45 (95% confidence interval, 0.28–7.55).

Even in the reports that suggest an association between fertility drugs and ovarian cancer, once an infertile woman conceives, any hypothesized risk is negated.

Although there is no consensus on the optimal care of infertile women previously exposed to fertility drugs who fail to conceive, annual pelvic examinations are recommended. Thirty-one percent of reproductive endocrinologists surveyed recommended that close surveillance of nulligravid women with refractory infertility should occur. Unfortunately, the optimal mode of follow-up has not been determined.

Annual serum CA 125 and transvaginal ultrasonography lack adequate sensitivity and specificity to be used as screening tools even in persistently infertile women. Color and pulsed Doppler ultrasonography can reveal the vascularity of an adnexal mass. Blood flow information is indicative of a tumor's angiogenic intensity but cannot serve as a definitive diagnostic marker for cancer. At present, there is no evidence to suggest that anything more than annual examinations are needed.

Houmard BS, Seifer DB. Infertility treatment and informed consent: current practices of reproductive endocrinologists. Obstet Gynecol 1999;93:252–7.

Ness RB, Cramer DW, Goodman MT, Kjaer SK, Mallin K, Mosgaard BJ, et al. Infertility, fertility drugs, and ovarian cancer: a pooled analysis of case-control studies. Am J Epidemiol 2002;155:217–24.

Schelling M, Braun M, Kuhn W, Bogner G, Gruber R, Gnirs J, et al. Combined transvaginal B-mode and color Doppler sonography for differential diagnosis of ovarian tumors: results of a multivariate logistic regression analysis. Gynecol Oncol 2000;77:78–86.

Venn A, Watson L, Lumley J, Giles G, King C, Healy D. Breast and ovarian cancer incidence after infertility and in vitro fertilisation. Lancet 1995;346:995–1000.

Whittemore AS, Harris R, Itnyre J. Characteristics relating to ovarian cancer risk: collaborative analysis of 12 US case-control studies. II. Invasive epithelial ovarian cancers in white women. Collaborative Ovarian Cancer Group. Am J Epidemiol 1992;136:1184–203.

74

Use of donor sperm

A 28-year-old woman whose spouse has long-term diabetes mellitus wishes to undergo donor sperm insemination because of male factor infertility. The couple requested the use of a known sperm donor. The spouse's medical history is negative except for smoking, and he has fathered 2 children in the past. The couple has requested processing of fresh sperm for insemination rather than freezing sperm to increase the chance for pregnancy and overall success. The most commonly recommended test for screening candidates for donor insemination is

    (A) genetic testing for inheritable disease
*   (B) screening for sexually transmitted diseases (STDs)
    (C) psychologic testing
    (D) urine drug screen

Artificial donor insemination is a common practice today that can overcome male factor infertility in the childless couple. Guidelines for screening of donors have been set forth by the American Society for Reproductive Medicine (ASRM). Particular concern has been placed on the screening for STDs, particularly human immunodeficiency virus (HIV). As of 2003, ASRM revised its guidelines for use of semen in donor insemination and stated that the use of fresh semen was no longer an acceptable standard of practice for sperm donation.

Donor insemination is performed for a variety of indications to overcome male factor infertility. For example, donor sperm is useful in cases of oligospermia, failed vasectomy reversal, cancer treatment, history of genetic abnormalities, or noncorrectable erectile dysfunction, or for single women who desire fertility.

Couples or single women who have chosen to proceed with donor insemination should undergo a complete medical evaluation along with a psychologic evaluation and recommended testing for STDs, including HIV. This includes not only the female recipient but also the husband or partner as well. Current recommendations for STD testing are shown in Box 74-1.

Selection of candidates for sperm donation requires a thorough evaluation to maintain high quality and acceptable success rates. Main features for selection include normal semen parameters, good health, and no significant history of genetic abnormalities. In addition, donors should be younger than 50 years to decrease the risk of additional autosomal mutations that increase with age.

A standard medical and genetic history with physical examination should be completed on all donors. It is important to identify individuals who may be excluded because of high-risk behavior, such as those with history of homosexual contact, intravenous drug users, and those at increased risk for HIV or other STDs. If there is any past history of genital herpes, genital warts, or chronic hepatitis, the candidates also should be excluded. Donors should be rescreened every 6 months to ensure that there is no new evidence of STD transmission.

Once a candidate is selected as a sperm donor, he should be counseled about the need for additional STD screening, and he should be compensated for his time and expense. A consent to donate should be obtained from the donor in which he relinquishes future legal rights to offspring produced as well as certifies to the accuracy of the medical history that precludes any STDs in the past. Records should be kept on all donors to protect future medical–legal status and in case information related to the donor is needed by an anonymous request to the recipient or resulting offspring.

The most important aspect of donor insemination is that all specimens be frozen and quarantined for at least 180 days before use. This is necessary because STDs, and most importantly HIV, may be present and not detectable by laboratory assays. Follow-up verification of negative test results will allow the specimens to be released for use. Although this process may appear complex, there were some reported cases of HIV transfer before quarantine.

BOX 74-1

Laboratory Screening of Potential Semen Donors for Sexually Transmitted Diseases Should Include

- Serologic testing for syphilis
- Hepatitis B surface antigen
- Urethral cultures for *Neisseria gonorrhea* and *Chlamydia trachomatis*
- Serum antibody testing for cytomegalovirus
- Initial screen for human immunodeficiency virus (HIV), to be repeated in 180 days

Data from The American Society for Reproductive Medicine. Guidelines for sperm donation. Fertil Steril 2002;77(suppl 5):2–5.

This case scenario outlines a donor insemination case using a friend who is healthy with a history of fertility. Even though the couple wishes to proceed with fresh semen for insemination, it is paramount that this donor be carefully evaluated and screened and his sperm frozen and quarantined for at least 6 months. At that time, his sperm can be released after he is retested for STDs and proved to be negative. There is no binding legal contract that has been established between the 2 parties (couple and friendly donor), and the risk of potential medicolegal problems is high. The lack of screening for STDs is very important but quarantine of sperm is of utmost importance. In addition, there is a risk of transmission of genetic disease, but this can be ascertained during the initial medical history. Chronic smoking in the donor does not cause birth defects, but it is a factor in infertility and should be avoided in the donor population. Donor banks are used frequently for obtaining samples. However, clinics also may screen potential candidates and safely perform inseminations based on the present recommendations for care.

Quarantine of frozen sperm and STD testing are paramount to maintain specimens that are low risk for transmittable infection. Following recommended guidelines for screening will help maintain healthy donors and recipients, increase pregnancy rates, and lead to safe deliveries.

Barratt CL, Chauhan M, Cooke ID. Donor insemination—a look to the future. Fertil Steril 1990;54:375–87.

Nachtigall RD. Donor insemination and human immunodeficiency virus: a risk/benefit analysis. Am J Obstet Gynecol 1994;170:1692–6; discussion 1696–8.

75

Evaluation of premature thelarche

A 20-month-old child is referred for evaluation of premature breast development. Physical examination demonstrates Tanner stage II–III breast development (Fig. 75-1), absent pubic hair, and prepubertal genitalia. She is in the 65th percentile for height and weight measurements. The most appropriate next step in management is

    (A) bone age imaging of the hand and wrist
*   (B) observation and follow-up in 6 months
    (C) gonadotropin-releasing hormone (GnRH) challenge test
    (D) magnetic resonance imaging (MRI) of the head

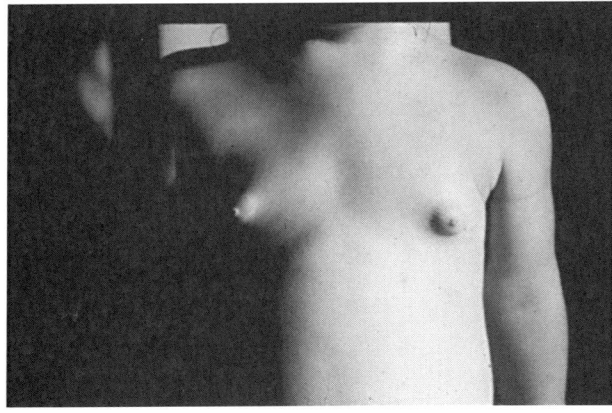

FIG 75-1. A 20-month-old infant showing Tanner stage II–III breast development.

Classical premature thelarche is a benign state that likely represents ovarian responses in the upper 2.5 percentile of the infant population to the normal and dynamic changes within the hypothalamic–pituitary–ovarian circuit. As such, the breast development is an isolated pubertal event limited to the normal period when gonadotropin levels increase during infancy and often will regress with suppression of the arcuate nucleus (ie, GnRH and, in response, follicle-stimulating hormone [FSH] and luteinizing hormone [LH]) that follows sometime between ages 2 and 4 years. The initial evaluation requires a thorough physical examination, assessment of the child's growth status, and, for most children as presented here, close follow-up only. Further evaluation is necessary because the possibility of progression to true precocious puberty or an autonomous estrogen-secreting tumor cannot be ruled out.

Shortly after birth, gonadotropin levels increase in both male and female infants to levels as high as 10–20 mIU/mL (Fig. 75-2; see color plate). In male infants, LH levels are higher than FSH levels, and, until disappearance of the fetal Leydig cells, testosterone will be produced and secreted at levels in the lower male adult range (ie, 150–250 ng/ml). In contrast, for female infants, FSH levels are higher than LH levels. Although it is not uncommon to find follicular stimulation at this time accompanied by ovarian cysts and minimal estrogen secretion, significant estrogen production is rare because LH levels are lower than FSH levels. Luteinizing hormone is required at the theca cells to produce the androgen precursors for estrogen production in the granulosa cells of the follicle. Ultimately, suppression of GnRH occurs centrally and is followed by a decrease in FSH and LH levels during the middle childhood years in all infants. Although recent evidence demonstrates that GnRH suppression is not complete or absolute at this time and the transition to puberty at the level of the arcuate nucleus is more gradual than previously thought, the very low levels of estrogen secreted during the middle childhood years are insufficient for producing an identifiable physical change.

Isolated precocious thelarche usually occurs before age 2 years during the time when gonadotropin levels are high (Fig. 75-2; see color plate). It is thought to represent the rare physiologic response to the increase of gonadotropin levels at a time when the FSH/LH ratio remains prepubertal (ie, FSH level > LH level). Because the subsequent maturational processes within the hypothalamic–pituitary–ovarian circuit progress normally, breast development for such children will stop at the time gonadotropin levels normally decrease, if not before. It is estimated that up to 90% of patients who present with some breast development before age 2 years will demonstrate a physical regression to the prepubertal breast. Close observation usually is all that is required for these children and is indicated in this case.

Patients with atypical isolated precocious thelarche often present between ages 2 and 8 years, after gonadotropin levels should have decreased. Some of them have a very slow progression to true precocious puberty, while for many others, breast regression is minimal, if at all. A small portion of these children will have a variant of true precocious puberty. Some may have isosexual precocity related to estrogen production from an ovarian tumor, most commonly the granulosa cell tumor. Because true precocious puberty may be more incipient for them, it is prudent for clinicians to have a lower threshold for initiation of a workup in this age group. Other patients with atypical precocious thelarche may present before age 2 years with signs or symptoms suspicious of true precocity or an estrogen secreting ovarian tumor. Evidence of rapidly advancing skeletal or physical growth, the appearance of other pubertal landmarks (ie, pubic hair or vaginal bleeding), or symptoms of pain or a central nervous system (CNS) disturbance should prompt a more aggressive and earlier evaluation.

Although bone age measurements are necessary to confirm the suspicion of abnormally fast skeletal growth, the GnRH challenge test has been shown to usually differentiate isolated precocious thelarche from true precocity. Girls with isolated premature thelarche will demonstrate a predominant FSH response to a GnRH bolus; true precocious puberty is associated with a predominant LH response. The presence of an LH predominant response should prompt the full workup for true precocious puberty, including imaging of the head (eg, MRI) for CNS tumors. Any suspicion of abnormal autonomous estrogen secretion from the ovary should prompt further investigation, including ovarian ultrasonography and measurement of estradiol levels.

Larriuz-Serrano MC, Perez-Cardona CM, Ramos-Valencia G, Bourdony CJ. Natural history and incidence of premature thelarche in Puerto Rican girls aged 6 months to 8 years between 1990 and 1996. P R Health Sci J 2001;20:13–8.

Palmert MR, Boepple PA. Variation in the timing of puberty: clinical spectrum and genetic investigation. J Clin Endocrinol Metab 2001;86:2364–8.

Stanhope R. Premature thelarche: clinical follow-up and indication for treatment. J Pediatr Endocrinol Metab 2000;13(suppl 1):827–30.

76
Luteal phase support

A 29-year-old pregnant woman, 5 weeks from her last menstrual period, documented on her calendar, presents with sharp abdominal pain. She undergoes a left ovarian cystectomy for a bleeding corpus luteum. The woman begins progesterone therapy immediately after the laparoscopy. To reduce the likelihood of a spontaneous abortion, progesterone supplementation should be continued through which week of gestation?

   (A) 6
* (B) 10
   (C) 14
   (D) 18
   (E) 22

In the first trimester of pregnancy, progesterone is produced initially from the corpus luteum and then primarily from the placenta. As the pregnancy progresses through the first trimester, the secretion of progesterone by the corpus luteum remains constant and the placental contribution to the total circulating level of progesterone increases. At approximately 7 weeks from the last menstrual period (LMP), the production of progesterone from the placenta is sufficient to maintain the fetus without the added support of the corpus luteum. This transition has been coined the "luteal-placental shift" and the fetal-placental unit now becomes independent of progesterone production by the corpus luteum. In a classic study, removal of the corpus luteum before 7 weeks from the LMP led to a decrease in circulating progesterone concentration and spontaneous abortion. In pregnancies where luteectomy occurred more than 7 weeks after the LMP, these pregnancies did not abort and were maintained because of increased production of progesterone by the placenta replacing the contribution of the corpus luteum.

The transition from the corpus luteum to the placenta as the major source of circulating progesterone is a gradual one. It begins after the seventh week of gestation and continues through the tenth week of gestation. Traditionally, progesterone-in-oil is administered daily by intramuscular injection to replace the luteal source after removal of the corpus luteum. However, vaginal preparations of progesterone may be given. Because of individual variation in the placental production of progesterone, clinicians often will supplement through the tenth week of gestation to ensure adequate circulating levels of progesterone.

Csapo AI, Pulkkinen MO, Wiest WG. Effects of luteectomy and progesterone replacement in early pregnant patients. Am J Obstet Gynecol 1973;115:759–65.

Nakajima ST, Nason FG, Badger GJ, Gibson M. Progesterone production in early pregnancy. Fertil Steril 1991;55:516–21.

Speroff L, Glass RH, Kase NG. Clinical gynecologic endocrinology and infertility. 6th ed. Baltimore (MD): Lippincott Williams & Wilkins; 1999. p. 276–7.

77

Vaginoplasty versus Frank method for müllerian aplasia

An 18-year-old woman requests information about the creation of a functional vagina. An ultrasonogram has documented absence of a uterus, cervix, and vagina. Physical examination reveals mature Tanner stage V breast and pubic hair development and a blind vagina with 3 cm depth. The least invasive approach that has the greatest likelihood for creating a functional vagina for this patient is

    (A) use of a split thickness skin graft around a vaginal mold in the potential space
    (B) coitus every other day
    (C) laparoscopic placement of a vaginal expander
*   (D) use of a firm dilator by the patient over several months

The complete absence of the vagina is a rare gynecologic condition with a reported incidence of 1 in 4,000–10,000 female births. The most common condition associated with absence of the upper two thirds of the vagina is known as müllerian agenesis or aplasia. A patient with this condition will have an otherwise normal female phenotype and normal ovarian function.

There are several treatment options for creation of a functional vagina that will allow for sexual intercourse. Historically, one of the most commonly used procedures (McIndoe technique) involved the surgical dissection of the potential space between the rectum and the bladder, placement of a mold covered with a split thickness skin graft into the newly created space, followed by consistent use of a vaginal dilator until regular coitus was possible. Although this technique has an extremely high success rate, it requires general anesthesia, creation of a split thickness skin graft, and results in postoperative pain following the procedure.

The least invasive means of achieving a functional vaginal opening involves the use of serial vaginal dilators with pressure applied by the patient for at least 20 minutes 3 times per day. This pressure can be applied by the patient (Frank method) or by using the force of gravity and the patient's own weight (Ingram method). The latter method involves the woman sitting on a bicycle seat while using progressively larger dilators. For most patients, the Ingram technique is easier than the Frank method. These methods do not subject the woman to general anesthesia, the potential complications of abdominal surgery, or the issues of narcotic pain management. In addition, these methods have been shown to produce a functional vagina allowing for satisfactory sexual intercourse over the course of several months even in cases of a flat perineum.

Sexual intercourse is a valuable means of maintaining a functional vaginal length and width following creation of a neovagina. It may be difficult for sexual intercourse alone to create a functional vagina in cases where only a perineal dimple existed previously.

A technique has been developed and commonly used in Europe for expanding vaginal length using a traction device, the Vechietti procedure. The ability to approach the rectovesical peritoneal potential space and, thus, the perineum abdominally has led to the development of this approach via laparotomy or laparoscopy. Once the potential space has been created, a wire suture, needle, and perineal holding device can be placed through the perineal skin under direct visualization and palpation and the wire suture brought up to the symphysis pubis and anchored in place via a traction device. Progressive upward traction can be applied allowing for invagination, followed by a regular regimen of dilators or coitus. Although this method has reported high success rates, it also requires general anesthesia, intraabdominal surgery with its potential complications, and management of postoperative pain.

Frank RT. The formation of an artificial vagina without operation. Am J Obstet Gynecol 1938;35:1053–5.

Ingram JM. The bicycle seat stool in the treatment of vaginal agenesis and stenosis: a preliminary report. Am J Obstet Gynecol 1981;140:867–73.

Pratt JH. Vaginal atresia corrected by the use of small and large bowel. Clin Obstet Gynecol 1972;15:639–49.

Rock JA. Surgery for anomalies of the mullerian ducts. In: Rock JA, Thompson JD, eds. Te Linde's operative gynecology. 8th ed. Philadelphia (PA): Lippincott-Raven, 1997. p. 687–729.

Veronikis DK, McClure GB, Nichols DH. The Vecchietti operation for constructing a neovagina: indications, instrumentation, and techniques. Obstet Gynecol 1997;90:301–4.

78

Testing for thyroid dysfunction

A 33-year-old woman comes in for evaluation of primary infertility. She is in good health with normal menstrual cycles. The initial evaluation reveals that follicle-stimulating hormone and luteinizing hormone concentrations are normal. Her serum prolactin level is 31 ng/mL. Her thyroid-stimulating hormone (TSH) level is 4 µU/mL and free thyroxine (T_4) level is 1.1 ng/dL. The most appropriate next diagnostic test for this patient is

* (A) triiodothyronine (T_3) concentration
* (B) repeat TSH concentration
* (C) thyrotropin-releasing hormone (TRH) stimulation test
* (D) pituitary magnetic resonance imaging (MRI)
* (E) thyroid ultrasonography

Subclinical hypothyroidism is defined as a mild elevation of TSH levels in conjunction with normal serum free T_4 concentrations and lack of overt clinical manifestations of hypothyroidism. The prevalence of subclinical hypothyroidism ranges from 10% to 20%, depending on the population. The presence of thyroid antibodies identifies a subset of patients who are at risk of progressing to overt hypothyroidism. More frequent thyroid screening is required in these patients.

Although the diagnostic criteria and treatment modalities for overt hypothyroidism are well known, the literature on assessment and treatment of patients with subclinical hypothyroidism is markedly less extensive. The precise pathophysiology, natural history, prevalence, risks and long-term outcome of subclinical hypothyroidism are unknown. Patients with subclinical hypothyroidism may have vague, nonspecific symptoms of hypothyroidism, but attempts to identify the patients on the basis of specific, thyroid-related signs and symptoms have not been successful. Thus, this disorder can only be diagnosed on the basis of laboratory test results. Advances in the development of ultrasensitive TSH assays has led to reassessment of the normal range, with a reduction of the upper limit of normal to 2.5 µU/mL.

A number of causes of high serum TSH concentrations do not properly fit the definition of subclinical hypothyroidism, such as

* A period of recovery from nonthyroidal illness
* A large pulse of TSH secretion, especially late in the evening
* Assay variability
* Adrenal insufficiency
* Medications, eg, metoclopramide or domperidone (Motilium)
* Thyroid-stimulating hormone-secreting pituitary adenomas

Therefore, minimal elevations in serum TSH concentrations must be confirmed by repeat testing before the diagnosis of subclinical hypothyroidism can be accepted.

Triiodothyronine levels are not useful in the diagnosis of hypothyroidism because they are frequently normal in mild hypothyroidism. Patients show minimal or no signs of hypothyroidism because a normal T_3 level maintains their metabolic status.

The TRH stimulation test was a useful diagnostic test during the era of first-generation TSH assays. Because first-generation TSH assays had a functional sensitivity within the euthyroid range and could not be used to assess thyrotoxicosis, the TRH stimulation test was useful. Patients with thyrotoxicosis had blunted or absent responses to TRH administration, whereas patients with hypothyroidism had exaggerated responses. Third-generation TSH assays have made TRH testing unnecessary in patients with an intact pituitary–thyroid axis. The response of TSH to TRH administration is proportional to the basal serum TSH concentration, even in patients with nonthyroidal illness. Nevertheless, the TRH stimulation test may continue to have some utility in the assessment of patients with untreated central hypothyroidism in whom the response to TRH administration may not be proportional to basal levels and may be blunted or delayed.

Tumors of the pituitary gland are best diagnosed with MRI, which offers better resolution than other radiologic modalities for identifying soft tissue changes. However, in this case, it is important to make the diagnosis of a thyroid abnormality before evaluating the patient with an MRI. Hyperprolactinemia and anovulation may be associated with primary hypothyroidism. Enlargement of the pituitary gland is frequently seen in long-standing primary hypothyroidism. Because TRH secretion is increased in primary hypothyroidism and TRH stimulates prolactin release, prolactin levels may be elevated in individuals with hypothyroidism.

In the case of a nodular or cystic thyroid, ultrasonography provides the best anatomic representation of the thyroid gland. With the use of high-resolution (7.5–10 MHz) probes, modern ultrasound machines provide excellent spatial resolution and allow nodules as small as 2 mm to be detected and biopsied.

Some authors have recommended treatment for most patients with subclinical hypothyroidism, in large part because unrecognized symptoms may improve and correction of abnormal serum lipid concentrations may be cardioprotective. The fundamental clinical question is whether a patient in whom the only abnormality is an elevated serum TSH level requires thyroid hormone therapy. Three randomized trials have addressed this question. In 2 of 3 trials, approximately one half of the patients who received levothyroxine had fewer hypothyroid symptoms when assessed by standardized scoring instruments and had improved psychometric test scores. Because this is a patient with infertility, it is critical to adequately replace thyroid hormone to ensure normal neurologic development of the fetus in any ensuing pregnancy. In treating women with hypothyroidism, it also is important to maintain TSH levels in the normal range because too much treatment can lead to accelerated bone loss.

Ayala AR, Danese MD, Ladenson PW. When to treat mild hypothyroidism. Endocrinol Metab Clin North Am 2000;29:399–415.

Haddow JE, Palomaki GE, Allan WC, Williams JR, Knight GJ, Gagnon J, et al. Maternal thyroid deficiency during pregnancy and subsequent neuropsychological development of the child. N Engl J Med 1999;341:549–55.

Haggerty JJ Jr, Garbutt JC, Evans DL, Golden RN, Pedersen C, Simon JS, et al. Subclinical hypothyroidism: a review of neuropsychiatric aspects. Int J Psychiatry Med 1990;20:193–208.

McDermott MT, Ridgway EC. Subclinical hypothyroidism is mild thyroid failure and should be treated. J Clin Endocrinol Metab 2001;86:4585–90.

Nystrom E, Caidahl K, Fager G, Wikkelso C, Lundberg PA, Lindstedt G. A double-blind cross-over 12-month study of L-thyroxine treatment of women with "subclinical" hypothyroidism. Clin Endocrinol (Oxf) 1998;29:63–75.

79

Biochemical hyperthyroidism and osteoporosis

A 48-year-old Asian woman, gravida 2, para 2, comes in for her annual examination. Over the past 2 years, her menstrual cycles have decreased from every 28–30 days to every 21–23 days. A decade ago, Hashimoto's thyroiditis was diagnosed, and her thyroid gland was ablated by radioactive iodine. Since then, she has used levothyroxine sodium (Synthroid), and her only symptom has been low back pain. On physical examination, her height has decreased by 0.05 m (2 in.) to 1.6 m (5 ft 2 in.), her weight is 56.7 kg (125 lb), blood pressure level is 122/74 mm Hg, and pulse rate is 88 beats per minute. She appears to be clinically euthyroid, and the remainder of her physical examination is unremarkable. Laboratory studies show a thyroid-stimulating hormone (TSH) level of 0.04 µU/mL and total thyroxine (T_4) level of 14 µg/dL. In addition to the Pap test and mammography, the most appropriate step in her management would be

    (A) day 3 follicle-stimulating hormone (FSH) level test
    (B) estradiol level test
*   (C) dual-energy X-ray (DXA) scan
    (D) thyroid antibodies screen

In patients taking thyroid hormone therapy, it is important to monitor the circulating concentration of TSH and T_4 at least on an annual basis. Although the conversion of T_4 to free triiodothyronine appears to be fairly constant for most individuals, the variation in the bioavailability of T_4 can be significant between different drug batches from the same manufacturer and from different manufacturers. In addition, changes in estrogen levels during estrogen therapy can alter thyroglobulin binding protein levels and the subsequent metabolism of T_4. These factors can result in biochemical hypothyroidism or hyperthyroidism.

Some patients may experience weight changes, insomnia, fatigue, or constipation. In many cases, there are no definitive clinical signs or symptoms, and the patient appears to be clinically euthyroid. On physical examination, the patient may have a normal pulse rate between 60–90 beats per minute, absence of fine tremors, and normal deep tendon reflexes, with no delay in the relaxation component. Thus, it is important to assess thyroid status biochemically. In this patient, her TSH level is very low because of increased circulating levels of T_4, which have caused biochemical hyperthyroidism. Patients who have long-standing hyperthyroidism experience accelerated bone turnover with an increased risk of decreased bone mineral density (BMD).

In patients who are of slight build, thin, or of Asian or Caucasian ethnicity, it is important to screen for a decrease in BMD. In the present patient, there also is a 0.05 m (2 in.) decrease in overall height as determined by a stadiometer. This measurement tool for height is accurate, reproducible, and inexpensive. A reduction in height could be caused by subclinical vertebral fractures or a decrease in lumbar BMD. This patient also may have nonspecific symptoms of low back pain or may show a change in her posture.

A DXA scan is the criterion standard in making the diagnosis of osteopenia (T-score less than -1 from the young adult mean) or osteoporosis (T-score less than -2.5 from the young adult mean). It is the most important of the listed tests for this patient. Bone density also provides an accurate estimate of fracture risk. For example, a T-score less than -1 at the lumbar spine or hip is associated with approximately a 2-fold increased risk in fracture.

A day 3 FSH has been used as a measure of ovarian reserve in patients who are about to undergo in vitro fertilization procedures. Its predictive value as a marker for onset of menopause is unreliable because of the pulsatile nature of FSH secretion. Serum estradiol levels also are highly variable. During the transition to menopause, estradiol levels may be low, normal, or high; therefore, its predictive value is unreliable. In this patient, thyroid antibody screening may remain positive in light of her previous history of Hashimoto's thyroiditis. However, this test will not help in the management of the patient's underlying biochemical hyperthyroidism. Flexible sigmoidoscopy is recommended as part of the preventive screening strategy for colon cancer and is indicated in patients at age 50 years.

Arafah BM. Increased need for thyroxine in women with hypothyroidism during estrogen therapy. N Engl J Med 2001;344:1743–9.

Ben-Shlomo A, Hagag P, Evans S, Weiss M. Early postmenopausal bone loss in hyperthyroidism. Maturitas 2001;39:19–27.

Cummings SR, Black DM, Nevitt MC, Browner W, Cauley J, Ensrud K, et al. Bone density at various sites for prediction of hip fractures. The Study of Osteoporotic Fractures Research Group. Lancet 1993;341:72–5.

Marshall D, Johnell O, Wedel H. Meta-analysis of how well measures of bone mineral density predict occurrence of osteoporotic fractures. BMJ 1996;312:1254–9.

National Osteoporosis Foundation. Physician's guide to prevention and treatment of osteoporosis. Belle Mead (NJ): Excerpta Medica, Inc; 1998.

Tannenbaum C, Clark J, Schwartzman K, Wallenstein S, Lapinski, R, Meier D, et al. Yield of laboratory testing to identify secondary contributors to osteoporosis in otherwise healthy women. J Clin Endocrinol Metab 2002;87:4431–7.

80

Changes in perimenopause

A 45-year-old woman nonsmoker presents with menorrhagia over the past 6 menstrual cycles; however, last month she skipped a cycle. A pregnancy test result is negative, and endometrial biopsy shows a proliferative endometrium. The patient also has occasional hot flushes, night sweats, and irritability. She requests hormonal intervention to manage her hot flushes and control her bleeding. Of the following therapies, the most appropriate method to manage the patient's signs and symptoms is

    (A) combined hormone therapy
    (B) sequential hormone therapy
* (C) low-dose combination oral contraceptives
    (D) monthly 10-day course of medroxyprogesterone acetate
    (E) transdermal estradiol patch

The time before the last menstrual cycle is most commonly referred to as the menopausal transition (formerly perimenopause), with a median age of onset of 47.5 years. In 1966, the World Health Organization defined perimenopause as the 2–8 years preceding menopause, which has a median age of 51.3 years. Menopausal transition is characterized by changing hormone levels. Estrogen levels may be low, normal, or high. Gonadotropin levels may be elevated or in the normal range. Progestin levels may suggest ovulation or at other times be low. For many women, one of the first symptoms of perimenopause is menstrual cycle irregularity, with occasional skipped cycles. Other common symptoms are hot flushes, night sweats, fatigue, irritability, and insomnia. Compared with younger women, perimenopausal women have been found to have shorter follicular phases and a shorter menstrual cycle, with elevated follicle-stimulating hormone (FSH) levels. Luteinizing hormone levels and overall mean estrone conjugate urinary excretion also are elevated, and luteal phase pregnanediol excretion is diminished. A comparative clinical study found increased FSH levels in women aged 43–47 years compared with women aged 19–38 years. The elevated FSH levels are caused by a lack of restraint of inhibin A and inhibin B, with inhibin B reduction before ovulation and inhibin A reduction after ovulation. Inhibin A also is believed to play an endocrine role in maintaining elevated FSH levels in older reproductive-aged women. A random FSH level will be of little value because of fluctuating levels.

Perimenopausal women who receive combination or sequential hormone therapy or medroxyprogesterone acetate may continue to experience abnormal bleeding. A monthly 10-day course of medroxyprogesterone acetate may be used in an attempt to control bleeding. During the perimenopausal transition, erratic release of FSH may result in excess production of ovarian estrogen, which will not be controlled by cyclic progestins. Studies suggest that medroxyprogesterone acetate in dosages of 20 mg per day can reduce the incidence of vasomotor symptoms by 75–90%, but is not a proven method of reliable contraception and may adversely affect the lipid profile.

The transdermal estradiol patch alone is not appropriate because of the risk of endometrial hyperplasia. In addition, the levels of estrogen available will not be sufficient to suppress sporadic follicular development, with resulting irregular bleeding.

Previously, oral contraceptives were not recommended for women aged 35 years or older because of concerns regarding increased cardiovascular risks. Current epidemiologic data on contemporary low-dose combination oral contraceptives (ie, preparations containing 20–35 µg of ethinyl estradiol) suggest there is no significantly increased cardiovascular risk unless the woman smokes or she has hyperlipidemia, familial thrombophilia, poorly controlled diabetes mellitus, or untreated hypertension. Low-dose oral contraceptives would be appropriate for this patient because they promote cyclic menses by suppressing follicular development, contain sufficient estrogen to control hot flushes, and provide endometrial protection as well as contraception. The risk of developing ovarian and endometrial carcinoma also is reduced. Some women may experience vasomotor symptoms during the placebo week.

McKinlay SM, Brambilla DJ, Posner JG. The normal menopause transition. Maturitas 1992;14:103–15.

Santoro N, Adel T, Skurnick JR. Decreased inhibin tone and increased activin A secretion characterize reproductive aging in women. Fertil Steril 1999;71:658–62.

Santoro N, Brown JR, Adel T, Skurnick JH. Characterization of reproductive hormonal dynamics in the perimenopause. J Clin Endocrinol Metab 1996;81:1495–501.

Shaaban MM. The perimenopause and contraception. Maturitas 1996; 23:181–92.

Soules MR, Sherman S, Parrott E, Rebar R, Santoro N, Utian W, et al. Executive summary: stages of reproductive aging workshop (STRAW). Fertil Steril 2001;76:874–8.

81
Dysmenorrhea

A healthy 20-year-old woman has a 2-year history of dysmenorrhea with pain that is moderately severe the first 3 days of her 5-day menses. Ibuprofen provides some relief. Her menstrual cycles are regular but with heavy flow. Pelvic ultrasonography is negative. She would like to attempt pregnancy in 6 months but requests treatment to decrease the number of bleeding days, relieve pain during menses, and provide reliable contraception with few side effects. The best therapy for her is

* (A) cyclic oral contraceptives
* (B) continuous oral contraceptives
* (C) gonadotropin-releasing hormone (GnRH) agonist
* (D) depot medroxyprogesterone acetate
* (E) progestin-only pill

Primary dysmenorrhea is a condition associated with ovulatory menstrual cycles, in which prostaglandins, produced during the late luteal phase, cause myometrial contractions and pain. Other symptoms associated with dysmenorrhea (ie, headache, nausea, diarrhea, and backache) can be explained by the release of prostaglandin compounds into the systemic circulation. Women with primary dysmenorrhea have greater prostaglandin production than asymptomatic women. The bulk of endometrial prostaglandin production occurs during the first 48 hours of menses, and this is the time of greatest menstrual discomfort. Nonsteroidal antiinflammatory agents (prostaglandin inhibitors) are effective in reducing symptoms of dysmenorrhea in most women, but additional therapy is required in approximately 15% of women with dysmenorrhea.

In an epidemiologic study of 19-year-old Swedish women, dysmenorrhea was reported in 72% of the women, and 15% reported discomfort that limited daily activity and was not improved by analgesics. Dysmenorrhea was found to be significantly less common in oral contraceptive users. Oral contraceptives may produce an atrophic and decidualized endometrium, which is associated with decreased prostaglandin synthesis. They offer a safe and effective choice for the treatment of dysmenorrhea because they decrease pain and menstrual flow and induce cycle regularity when taken as prescribed.

A recent randomized trial examined a group of women who took standard cyclic low-dose oral contraceptives (20 μg ethinyl estradiol/100 μg levonorgestrel, 3 weeks on and 1 week off) for 6 months and compared them with continuous users of the same low-dose pill given without any hormone-free days for 6 months. Although both groups had high levels of satisfaction, women in the continuous use group reported significantly fewer bleeding days that required protection (18 days versus 38 days), bloating (0.7 days versus 11 days), and menstrual pain (2 days versus 13 days). Continuous oral contraceptives are the best choice to treat this patient. Results may vary between studies because of variances between new and prior use.

A newly approved 4-month extended use contraceptive, Seasonale, uses 84 days of continuous ethinyl estradiol/levonorgestrel, followed by a 7-day pill-free interval. Reducing the frequency of hormone withdrawal is likely to decrease the incidence of hormone withdrawal symptoms (headache, dysmenorrhea, hypermenorrhea, premenstrual symptoms) and lead to improved tolerability. The breakthrough bleeding rate has been shown to be greater with this drug than with continuous oral contraceptives. A recent study has found that patients with hormone withdrawal symptoms prefer a treatment regimen with extended use of active pills and a shortened hormone-free interval.

Total duration of extended use has not been well defined and has ranged from 6 weeks to 1 year. Continuous oral contraceptives have been reported to be effective for the treatment of dysmenorrhea secondary to endometriosis. During 2 years of continuous oral contraceptives for endometriosis, there was a significant decrease in endometriosis-associated pain and dysmenorrhea reported, with 80% of subjects satisfied or very satisfied with the continuous oral contraceptives. Breakthrough bleeding with continuous oral contraceptives remains a significant problem for some women.

Secondary dysmenorrhea is associated with a variety of pathologic conditions, of which endometriosis may be the most common. It occurs in 7–10% of all women, in 38% of infertile women, and in more than 70% of women with chronic pelvic pain. The pain may be caused by inflammation of the endometriotic lesions and stimulation of local nerve fibers. For women with normal gynecologic findings suggestive of mild disease, oral contraceptives may be most effective in reducing pain. If a trial of oral contraceptives for 3–6 months does not produce significant relief, other agents, such as depot medroxyprogesterone acetate, danazol (Danocrine), or GnRH-agonist, may be necessary.

Depot medroxyprogesterone acetate can be very effective in the treatment of endometriosis and dysmenorrhea. As with oral contraceptives, it produces a state of pseudopregnancy and a thin decidualized endometrium. There are problems with breakthrough bleeding in approximately 40% of patients during the first 3–6 months. Other side effects include weight gain, fluid retention, and depression. Many patients will experience amenorrhea, which typically results in relief from dysmenorrhea and pain. For patients who desire fertility soon, depot medroxyprogesterone acetate is not the first choice because resumption of ovulation is unpredictable and may take 6 months or longer after the last injection.

A long-acting GnRH-agonist may create pseudomenopause for the treatment of endometriosis. This creates a state of hypoestrogenism similar to menopause and, thus, patients have amenorrhea. Endometriotic lesions, fibroids, and adenomyosis all shrink dramatically; thus, it is very effective for secondary dysmenorrhea. Freedom from pain may be accompanied by vasomotor symptoms, urogenital atrophy, and bone loss. An average 3–4% decrease in trabecular bone may occur during 6 months of therapy. The possible side effects of GnRH-agonist may be worse than minor dysmenorrhea. Therefore, GnRH-agonist should not be used as the first choice for this patient.

American College of Obstetricians and Gynecologists. Medical management of endometriosis. ACOG Practice Bulletin 11. Washington, DC: ACOG; 1999.

Andersch B, Milsom I. An epidemiologic study of young women with dysmenorrhea. Am J Obstet Gynecol 1982;144:655–60.

Anderson FD, Hait H. A multicenter, randomized study of an extended cycle oral contraceptive. Contraception 2003;68:89–96.

Dawood MY, Ramos J, Khan-Dawood FS. Depot leuprolide acetate versus danazol for treatment of pelvic endometriosis: changes in vertebral bone mass and serum estradiol and calcitonin. Fertil Steril 1995;63: 1177–83.

Kwiecien M, Edelman A, Nichols MD, Jensen JT. Bleeding patterns and patient acceptability of standard or continuous dosing regimens of a low-dose oral contraceptive: a randomized trial. Contraception 2003; 67:9–13.

Robinson JC, Plichta S, Weisman CS, Nathanson CA, Ensminger M. Dysmenorrhea and use of oral contraceptives in adolescent women attending a family planning clinic. Am J Obstet Gynecol 1992;166: 578–83.

Sulak PJ, Kuehl TJ, Ortiz M, Shull BL. Acceptance of altering the standard 21-day/7-day oral contraceptive regimen to delay menses and reduce hormone withdrawal symptoms. Am J Obstet Gynecol 2002; 186:1142–9.

Vercellini P, Frontino G, De Giorgi O, Pietropaolo G, Pasin R, Crosignani PG. Continuous use of an oral contraceptive for endometriosis-associated recurrent dysmenorrhea that does not respond to a cyclic pill regimen. Fertil Steril 2003;80:560–3.

82

Serum human chorionic gonadotropin levels

A 28-year-old woman, gravida 2, comes in for evaluation of oligomenorrhea. She had a normal uncomplicated vaginal delivery 10 months ago and continues to bottle-feed her infant. Her laboratory results include a serum human chorionic gonadotropin (hCG) level of 48 mIU/mL and normal thyroid-stimulating hormone and prolactin levels. Repeat hCG tests 3 and 10 days later show levels of 52 mIU/mL and 49 mIU/mL, respectively. Urine pregnancy test results remain negative. The most likely diagnosis is

(A) hydatidiform mole
(B) choriocarcinoma
* (C) "phantom" hCG
(D) ectopic gestation
(E) intrauterine gestation

Most commonly, serial quantitative serum hCG values that plateau raise concern about ectopic gestation. Serial hCG values should double every 2–3 days in an intrauterine pregnancy. In both ectopic and intrauterine pregnancies, urine pregnancy test results will be positive. Gestational trophoblastic neoplasia (GTN) is the term now commonly applied to choriocarcinoma and related tumors (ie, hydatidiform mole, invasive mole, and choriocarcinoma). A woman with a hydatidiform mole presents with markedly elevated serum hCG levels and a positive urinary pregnancy test result. A single hCG level is nondiagnostic. With the widespread use of ultrasonography to assess early pregnancy and bleeding, many molar pregnancies are detected early in gestation when the most common clinical presentation is that of a threatened abortion with painless vaginal bleeding.

Metastatic GTN is a disease that occurs outside the uterus. Poor prognosis is characterized by serum hCG values higher than 40,000 mIU/mL, brain or liver metastasis, long duration from last pregnancy, and a pregnancy that is term.

Low-level serum hCG quantitative values with or without a preceding pregnancy present a rare but important clinical challenge and therapeutic dilemma. Physicians have mistakenly treated reproductive-aged women with chemotherapy or extirpative surgery for choriocarcinoma when in reality no true disease was present. In such cases, heterophilic antibodies in the blood cause false positive or "phantom" hCG titers, which fail to decrease significantly after treatment.

Most hCG assays in use today are sandwich assays in which 2 animal antibodies are raised against hCG: 1) the capture antibody, which is in solid phase and 2) the tracer antibody, which is in liquid phase, and usually is labeled with some identifier, such as an enzyme. The patient's blood is added to the assay system and binds to both antibodies in the solid and liquid phase. The tracer antibody complex becomes immobilized and the quantity is directly proportional to the amount of hCG in the woman's serum. Approximately 1–5% of the general population is estimated to have heterophilic antibodies that bridge the gap between the capture and the tracer antibody and, thus, give false-positive levels. These antibodies bind human as well as animal antibodies (eg, human antimouse immunoglobulin G) and give a false-positive level in the sandwich assay. The antibodies used in most immunoassays are raised from different animal sources.

Box 82-1 indicates how phantom hCG may be distinguished from true hCG. It has been recommended that current protocols for the diagnosis and treatment of choriocarcinoma be modified to include a compulsory urine test for hCG.

BOX 82-1

Ways in Which Phantom Serum Human Chorionic Gonadotropin Can Be Distinguished From True Human Chorionic Gonadotropin

- There is a lack of immunoreactivity in the urine, because the heterophilic antibodies due to their large size are not excreted in the urine and result in complete absence of positivity in a parallel urine.
- There is no quantitative decrease in human chorionic gonadotropin (hCG) levels in parallel when serum is diluted (eg, if the sample is diluted by 50%, the hCG level should decrease accordingly).
- Phantom hCG also can be confirmed by the finding of widely (more than 4-fold) variable results in different commercial hCG tests.

Boscato LM, Stuart MC. Heterophilic antibodies: a problem for all immunoassays. Clin Chem 1988;34:27–33.

Cole LA. Phantom hCG and phantom choriocarcinoma. Gynecol Oncol 1998;71:325–9.

Rotmensch S, Cole LA. False diagnosis and needless therapy of presumed malignant disease in women with false-positive human chorionic gonadotropin concentrations. Lancet 2000;355:712–5.

83

Risk of in vitro fertilization in Turner's syndrome

In counseling patients on the use of donor oocytes, it is important to inform them of a substantially increased risk of maternal death during pregnancy if their ovarian failure is associated with

    (A) premature menopause at age 35 years
    (B) natural menopause at age 50 years
    (C) bilateral oophorectomy for stage IV endometriosis
*   (D) Turner's syndrome
    (E) fragile X gene premutation

Women with ovarian failure now have available the alternative treatment of becoming pregnant and giving birth to a child through the use of donor oocytes. For most women who have premature menopause before age 40 years or even natural menopause at or around age 50 years or those who lose ovarian function for an identified cause (eg, those with oophorectomy for benign ovarian disease; autoimmune ovarian failure; and some genetic disorders, such as fragile X gene premutation), becoming pregnant with donor oocytes does not pose any significant risks to them that would not have occurred had they become pregnant spontaneously with a singleton pregnancy. In contrast, for one condition, Turner's syndrome, disturbing evidence demonstrates a potentially high risk of becoming pregnant; and, for a few other conditions there may be reason for some concern.

An increasing body of data suggests that patients with Turner's syndrome have unique and significant cardiovascular risks. Such risks appear to be compounded by the increased cardiovascular demands of pregnancy and this results in a maternal mortality rate as high as 2%. Numerous reports exist on patients with Turner's syndrome who developed aortic dilation, dissection, and rupture in the nonpregnant state. Risk factors for this occurrence include presence of bicuspid aortic valve, with or without aortic stenosis, regurgitation, or both; the presence of coarctation of the aorta or its prior repair; and systemic hypertension. However, 10% of patients with aortic dissection or rupture have no identifiable risk factors. Postmortem histopathologic examination of the vessels of these patients has demonstrated the presence of cystic medial necrosis, the identical finding associated with vessel dilation and dissection in patients with Marfan syndrome.

That pregnancy poses additional risks to some patients with cardiovascular anomalies is well known. Increases in stroke volume occur throughout the pregnancy and in cardiac output beginning in the midtrimester and continuing through the immediate postpartum period. For patients with Marfan syndrome, mortality rates associated with these risks of pregnancy range from 5% for patients with a normal aorta to as high as 50% for those with an involved aorta. Ovarian failure in patients with Turner's syndrome might be considered a natural protective mechanism, which prevents these potential increased risks of pregnancy. Not all patients with Turner's syndrome, however, exhibit ovarian failure at puberty. Although virtually all will ultimately lose ovarian function prematurely, 15% initiate puberty, 5% menstruate for variable periods, and 1% may become spontaneously pregnant.

Although the low frequency of serious maternal complications for patients with Turner's syndrome who become pregnant spontaneously is reassuring, a small number of patients with Turner's syndrome who have become pregnant with donor oocytes are known to have developed dilation and dissection of the ascending aorta. A review of the literature and survey of all U.S. donor oocyte programs showed 4 maternal deaths in the United States for an estimated 200 donor oocyte pregnancies in patients with Turner's syndrome. This seemingly high maternal mortality rate is a cause for concern and has resulted in reexamination of the practice of offering oocyte donation to these patients.

National organizations, such as the American Society for Reproductive Medicine, have developed practice guidelines that address the issue of oocyte donation whereas further information is being collected. Presently, extensive counseling is the most important part of the care of patients who seek oocyte donation as an option. Although death may be avoided in patients who are aware of this syndrome and, therefore, are not misdiagnosed when aortic dissection occurs, screening for cardiac risk factors before pregnancy and at regular intervals throughout pregnancy is essential for those who elect to proceed with in vitro fertilization in hopes of becoming pregnant. Death has been reported even in patients who do not have identified risk factors (eg, hypertension, bicuspid aortic valves, or coarctation) and even in patients for whom dissection is recognized and timely surgery performed.

In addition to Turner's syndrome, other causes of ovarian failure may pose additional concerns should pregnancy be achieved through oocyte donation. For some women whose ovarian failure occurs after treatment for malignancies, pregnancy may be a relative contraindication because of the risk of recurrence increased by the pregnant state. For women who undergo donor oocyte because of age-related infertility that occurs during the fifth decade of life or natural menopause after age 40 years, studies have demonstrated that some pregnancy complications occur at a higher rate (eg, hypertensive disorders of pregnancy and preeclampsia, gestational diabetes mellitus, and small-for-gestational age infants). Associated with the high donor oocyte pregnancy rates are the high rates of multiple gestation. Recent Centers for Disease Control and Prevention data have demonstrated that in the year 2000, 40% of pregnancies in women aged 50 years and older were multiple gestations. This might imply that combination of age and multiple pregnancies would compound the risks of pregnancy. Overall, however, if the women are healthy, pregnancy has proved to be reasonably safe for women even into their early 50s.

An understanding of the risks of pregnancy to the woman is essential for the physician who is counseling couples who want to receive oocyte donation. However, many additional issues are important. One important issue is the risk for passing on a genetic condition to the next generation if a sister is used as a known donor. For example, premutations of the fragile X gene (*FMR-1* gene) cause ovarian failure; further expansion of this premutation causes fragile X syndrome. This premutation in the *FMR-1* gene is associated with a 21-fold greater risk of developing premature ovarian failure. It is found in 2% of sporadic ovarian failure and 14% of familial cases. Therefore, a woman with premature ovarian failure who uses her sister as a known oocyte donor needs to be screened to rule out this etiology. Should the sister also carry the premutation, expansion of the trinucleotide repeat mutation could continue and lead to a son with fragile X syndrome.

Beauchesne LM, Connolly HM, Ammash NM, Warnes CA. Coarctation of the aorta: outcome of pregnancy. J Am Coll Cardiol 2001;38:1728–33.

Garvey P, Elovitz M, Landsberger EJ. Aortic dissection and myocardial infarction in a pregnant patient with Turner syndrome. Obstet Gynecol 1998;91:864.

Karnis MF, Zimon AE, Lalwani SI, Timmreck LS, Klipstein S, Reindollar RH. Risk of death in pregnancy achieved through oocyte donation in patients with Turner syndrome: a national survey. Fertil Steril 2003;80:498–501.

Lin AE, Lippe B, Rosenfeld RG. Further delineation of aortic dilation, dissection, and rupture in patients with Turner syndrome. Pediatrics 1998;102:e12.

Nagel TC, Tesch LG. ART and high risk patients! Fertil Steril 1997;68: 748–9.

Weytjens C, Bove T, van Der Niepen P. Aortic dissection and Turner's syndrome. J Cardiovasc Surg (Torino) 2000;41:295–7.

84

Diagnosis of nonprolactin secreting pituitary tumor

A 37-year-old woman, gravida 1, para 1, presents with amenorrhea and galactorrhea of 2 years' duration. She reports that she has experienced increasingly severe frontal headaches over this period. Initial laboratory studies reveal serum follicle-stimulating hormone (FSH) level of 21 mIU/mL, prolactin level of 46 ng/mL, and thyroid-stimulating hormone (TSH) level of 2.6 µU/mL. The best next step in the management is

    (A) pituitary function testing
    (B) formal visual field testing
    (C) pelvic ultrasonography
*   (D) magnetic resonance imaging (MRI) of the sella turcica
    (E) treatment with a dopamine agonist

The evaluation and management of amenorrhea and galactorrhea requires measurement of basal TSH levels to rule out primary hypothyroidism and basal prolactin levels to determine if hyperprolactinemia is present. The presence of amenorrhea requires the measurement of basal FSH levels to rule out ovarian failure. In ovulating women, FSH levels generally range from 2 mIU/mL to 10 mIU/mL except during the preovulatory gonadotropin surge. However, this patient is unlikely to be ovulatory because she has amenorrhea. Her FSH level is unusually high for her age, and she has mild hyperprolactinemia. Thus, the next best step in her management is an MRI of the sella turcica.

Given these unusual findings, it is likely that the MRI would show a macroadenoma (Fig. 84-1). The data suggest that the neoplasm is not a prolactinoma and that the hyperprolactinemia results from inadequate dopamine suppression produced by stalk compression by the pituitary mass. Another possibility is compression of lactotropes by the tumor itself, resulting in the mild hyperprolactinemia. It is the discrepancy between the size of the tumor and the mild elevation in prolactin levels that suggests this is not a prolactinoma.

The increased FSH level suggests that this macroadenoma may be producing gonadotropins. Gonadotrope adenomas most frequently secrete intact FSH, followed in decreasing order of frequency by intact luteinizing hormone (LH), free α-subunit of LH, and free β-subunit of LH. Gonadotropin levels frequently are in the normal range. The elevations tend to be small and can be mistaken for the elevations seen in mild primary hypogonadism. The elevations in FSH usually do not produce a clinical syndrome, but this is not always the case, and ovarian hyperstimulation has been reported. Gonadotrope adenomas are sometimes referred to as null cell adenomas because they were originally thought to be nonsecreting tumors. Immunohistochemical methods have been used to document gonadotropin secretion in some patients.

Evaluation for secretion of other anterior pituitary tumors is warranted when a macroadenoma is present or when there is a disparity between basal prolactin levels and the size of the tumor, as in this case. Because the prolactin level is only 46 ng/mL in this patient, measurement of corticotropin, growth hormone, and LH levels in the basal state are warranted as is pituitary function testing. This is not the next step, however, and should be performed only after presence of a pituitary (or hypothalamic) tumor is documented. Intact gonadotropin levels and the α- and β-subunits of LH frequently increase paradoxically in response to a thyrotropin-releasing hormone stimulation test in individuals with gonadotrope adenomas.

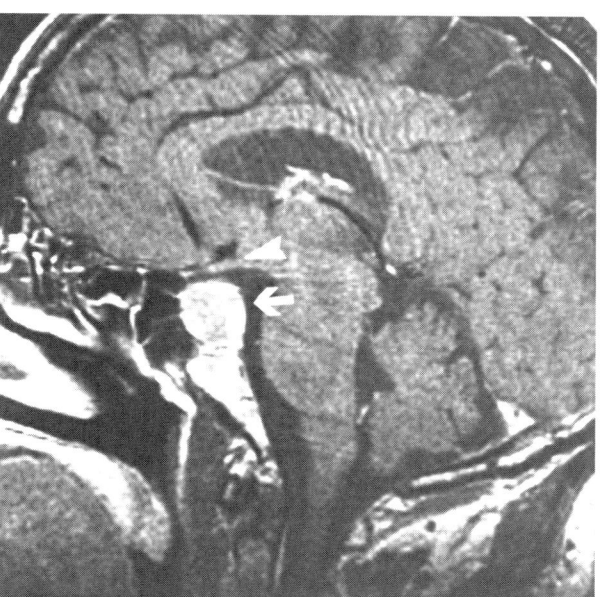

FIG. 84-1. Lateral magnetic resonance imaging view showing an enlarged pituitary gland (arrow) and normal optic chiasm (arrowhead).

Formal visual field testing is always indicated in patients with macroadenomas. However, this test also is not warranted until documentation of the tumor by MRI.

Although gynecologists commonly perform pelvic ultrasonography in the office, there is no reason to do so in the absence of any abnormal findings. If enlarged adnexa are detected on pelvic examination or if the patient experiences bilateral pelvic pain, it might be reasonable to proceed with ultrasonography because cases of ovarian hyperstimulation in the presence of gonadotropin adenomas have been reported.

A trial of a dopamine agonist is not indicated just because this patient has hyperprolactinemia. Complete evaluation is warranted first. Therapy with a dopamine agonist would be expected to reduce prolactin levels but might not affect tumor size.

The management of gonadotrope adenomas depends on the size, location, and symptoms of the tumor. If the tumor is a microadenoma (less than 10 mm in diameter on MRI) and the patient is asymptomatic, observation is the most appropriate approach. The MRI should be repeated if symptoms develop, and visual field examination and MRI should be carried out annually. If a nonprolactin-secreting adenoma causes the typical symptoms seen in this patient (headache, galactorrhea, amenorrhea, as well as visual disturbances), or is larger than 10 mm, surgical therapy is warranted. The transsphenoidal approach is preferred. Recurrence is common. Although a dopamine agonist would not be appropriate in this patient before definitive diagnosis, gonadotrope adenomas sometimes respond to a dopamine agonist or to octreotide acetate (Sandostatin), which inhibits secretion of growth hormone. A trial of these agents may be warranted in this patient before surgery.

Bremner WJ, Huhtaniemi I, Amory JK. Pituitary gonadotropins and their disorders. In: Becker KL, ed. Principles and practice of endocrinology and metabolism. 3rd ed. Philadelphia (PA): Lippincott Williams and Wilkins; 2001. p. 170–7.

Itskovitz-Eldor J, Kol S. Disorders of the pituitary gonadotroph. In: Adashi EY, Rock JA, Rosenwaks Z. Reproductive endocrinology, surgery, and technology. Vol. 2. Philadelphia (PA): Lippincott-Raven; 1996. p. 1279–301.

Leese G, Jeffreys R, Vora J. Effects of cabergoline in a pituitary adenoma secreting follicle-stimulating hormone. Postgrad Med J 1997;73: 507–8.

Warnet A. The role of octreotide (Sandostatin) in non-growth hormone, non-thyroid-stimulating hormone-, and non-prolactin-secreting adenomas. Metabolism 1992;41(suppl 2):59–61.

85

Lifestyle factors and fertility

A sedentary 32-year-old woman with body mass index of 28 kg/m^2 consumes daily 1 glass of wine and 3 cups of coffee; she smokes 1 pack of cigarettes per day. She requests your advice regarding the lifestyle modification that would most improve her success with in vitro fertilization (IVF). The change in lifestyle that would likely lead to the highest success rate in her use of IVF would be to

(A) initiate an exercise program
(B) reduce caffeine intake
(C) initiate a low-fat diet
* (D) stop smoking
(E) reduce alcohol consumption

A variety of factors affect IVF success. There has been much discussion of the role of lifestyle in fertility, but very few long-term studies have addressed the impact of lifestyle on IVF treatment success. Researchers that have observed an association between fertility outcomes and lifestyle changes usually have found those connections in relation to smoking habits. It is well established that smokers have an increased risk for premature menopause, limited ovarian reserve, and osteoporosis compared with nonsmokers. A 30% reduction in pregnancy rates after IVF was observed when smokers were compared with nonsmokers. Multiple studies have shown up to a 40% reduction in the number of oocytes retrieved in smokers compared with nonsmokers in assisted reproductive technology (ART) cycles. Women who have smoked at some time in their lives are 2–3 times less likely to become pregnant by ART than women who have never smoked. Most studies of men have found no statistically significant effects of smoking on achieving a pregnancy or on pregnancy outcome. In men, smoking is associated with lower sperm count and reduced motility. The potential theoretical adverse effect of passive smoking on women has not been thoroughly investigated. Compelling evidence exists that smoking in the years before couples undergo ART

86

Sheehan's syndrome

A 25-year-old woman presents with marked weakness and fatigue. Her last pregnancy 8 months ago was complicated by a postpartum hemorrhage with a blood loss of 2,000 mL, and she required a transfusion of 4 units of blood. She also experienced profound hypotension as a result of the blood loss. She has amenorrhea despite the discontinuation of oral contraceptives 3 months ago. In this clinical scenario, the hormone that is most likely preserved is

    (A) prolactin
    (B) follicle-stimulating hormone (FSH)
*   (C) vasopressin
    (D) adrenocorticotropic hormone (ACTH)
    (E) thyroid-stimulating hormone (TSH)

After a severe postpartum hemorrhage with hypovolemia, the pituitary gland may become necrotic, leading to the development of Sheehan's syndrome. In normal uncomplicated pregnancies, the pituitary enlarges because of hyperplasia of the lactotropes and is more sensitive to changes in blood flow. A sudden decrease in blood flow can lead to complete pituitary necrosis or partial necrosis with preservation of pituitary function. Often an orderly progression of events occurs. Initially, prolactin production decreases leading to a failure to lactate. If Sheehan's syndrome is caused by an acute decrease in arterial blood pressure, symptoms may be acute and include sudden onset of severe headache, nausea, and vomiting. Symptoms may be similar to those associated with a subarachnoid hemorrhage. If the blood supply to the pituitary gland is only marginally affected, the patient may be relatively asymptomatic until she is exposed to a severe infection or surgery, leading to an adrenal crisis.

In most cases, gonadotropins (FSH and luteinizing hormone [LH]) are affected leading to hypogonadism and menstrual disturbances. If the patient's pubic hair was shaved before delivery, these areas may fail to regrow because of the lack of adrenal androgen production necessary for pubic hair growth. There is a similar loss of existing pubic and axillary hair. Menses may be absent to very infrequent because of an absence of episodic FSH and LH release from the pituitary gland. Patients will experience associated vasomotor symptoms, dyspareunia, atrophic vaginitis, and eventual osteopenia. If growth hormone production is affected, patients can present with symptoms of fatigue, decreased muscle mass, and quality of life.

Other manifestations of Sheehan's syndrome include the development of secondary adrenal insufficiency leading to symptoms of weakness, fatigue, hypoglycemia, or dizziness. The diagnosis is suspected when cortisol and ACTH levels are low, and they do not increase after an insulin tolerance test. In some cases, thyroid function may be normal and in others it may be reduced with low TSH levels. Depending on the degree of anterior pituitary necrosis, some patients may have varying presentations. In a few cases, a return to normal fertility has been reported.

87

Use of antiestrogens

In the anovulatory woman, the principal site of action for clomiphene citrate (Clomid, Serophene) is the

(A) uterus
(B) ovary
(C) anterior pituitary gland
(D) posterior pituitary gland
* (E) hypothalamus

Clomiphene citrate is a nonsteroidal orally active antiestrogen, which has different mechanisms of action depending on the baseline ovulatory status of the woman. Its principal mechanism of action is to bind to hypothalamic estrogen receptors. Because of its slow metabolism, it occupies the hypothalamic receptors for a prolonged period, eventually leading to a reduction in the total number of hypothalamic estrogen receptors. As the drug binds to the hypothalamic receptors, the receptors are internalized within the hypothalamic cells where some receptors are degraded. After the drug is metabolized, there are functionally less hypothalamic estrogen receptors available for binding. Because of the reduction in the number of hypothalamic estrogen receptors and the prolonged binding of the drug, negative feedback to the hypothalamus is decreased, which results in increased secretion of gonadotropin-releasing hormone (GnRH).

When clomiphene citrate is administered to normally cycling women, one hypothesis is that there is a presumed increase in GnRH pulse frequency, leading to an increase in follicle-stimulating hormone (FSH) and the luteinizing hormone (LH) pulse frequency but not pulse amplitude. When clomiphene citrate is administered to an ovulatory woman, the action is modified and there is an increase in GnRH pulse amplitude leading to increased FSH and LH pulse amplitude because GnRH pulse frequency is already increased in an ovulatory women. Because of the long half-life of clomiphene citrate, only 51% of the oral dose is excreted within 5 days, and zuclomiphene, the active form of clomiphene citrate, can be detected in the circulation up to 1 month after the administration of a single 50 mg tablet. The long half-life of the drug is secondary to enterohepatic circulation. The half-life also is responsible for the development of tolerance to a given dose, thus leading to the requirement for higher doses of clomiphene citrate. Because of its antiestrogenic action, clomiphene citrate is associated with side effects of decreased cervical mucus and endometrial thickness. These negative side effects increase with dose and length of time of drug administration.

American College of Obstetricians and Gynecologists. Ovulation induction. In: Precis: an update in obstetrics and gynecology. Reproductive endocrinology. 2nd ed. Washington, DC: ACOG; 2002. p. 136–41.

Mikkelson TJ, Kroboth PD, Cameron WJ, Dittert LW, Chungi V, Manberg PJ. Single-dose pharmacokinetics of clomiphene citrate in normal volunteers. Fertil Steril 1986;46:392–6.

Speroff L, Glass RH, Kase NG. Clinical gynecologic endocrinology and infertility. 6th ed. Baltimore (MD): Lippincott Williams & Wilkins; 1999. p. 1098–100.

Yen SS, Jaffe RB, Barbieri RL. Reproductive endocrinology. 4th ed. Philadelphia (PA): WB Saunders; 1999. p. 567–8.

88
Postpartum thyroiditis

A 23-year-old woman, gravida 1, para 1, with type 1 diabetes mellitus, presents with fatigue, palpitations, and dizziness at 3 months postpartum. On examination, she has a resting pulse rate of 90 beats per minute and a slightly enlarged tender thyroid gland. Laboratory studies reveal a serum thyroid-stimulating hormone (TSH) level less than 0.1 µU/mL and a free thyroxine level of 2.6 ng/dL. The most likely explanation for this woman's symptoms is

    (A) depression
    (B) multinodular goiter
* (C) thyroiditis
    (D) Graves' disease
    (E) thyroid papillary carcinoma

Thyroid dysfunction is common in young women. Perhaps most common after delivery, especially in a woman with type 1 diabetes mellitus, as in this case, is postpartum thyroiditis. The occurrence of transient hyperthyroidism, transient hypothyroidism, or transient hyperthyroidism followed by transient hypothyroidism is typical of postpartum thyroiditis. Although most women are euthyroid 1 year after delivery, significant numbers eventually develop permanent hypothyroidism. The prevalence of postpartum thyroiditis has ranged from 1.1% to 16.7% in various studies but is increased approximately 3-fold in women with type 1 diabetes mellitus.

Why thyroiditis is so common postpartum is apparently related to the immune changes that normally occur during pregnancy. Immune function is suppressed only to increase again during the postpartum period. Typically, autoimmune disorders, such as rheumatoid arthritis, Graves' disease, and myasthenia gravis, decrease in severity during pregnancy only to become exacerbated postpartum.

The presence of thyroid autoantibodies in serum is strongly associated with postpartum thyroiditis. At delivery, more than one half of women who subsequently develop postpartum thyroiditis already have antibodies present. Similarly, the presence of antithyroid peroxidase antibodies also predicts development of postpartum thyroiditis. In fact, it appears that even the presence of antibodies during pregnancy is as predictive, but it is not clear that screening all pregnant women is cost-effective. Some clinicians have suggested that women with type 1 diabetes mellitus should be routinely tested for thyroid antibodies because the incidence is so great in these women.

In addition to measuring thyroid antibodies, a radioactive iodine or technetium uptake may help make the diagnosis because it is low in the thyrotoxic phase of postpartum thyroiditis. The low uptake presumably reflects destruction of thyroid follicles. This phase, however, is always transient and typically resolves in approximately 1 month. Moreover, a scan is not indicated in a breast-feeding woman.

To date, no studies have assessed the benefit of treating the hyperthyroid phase of postpartum thyroiditis. Still, it seems reasonable to treat symptomatic women who have thyrotoxicosis with β-blockers, with the understanding that the treatment will only be of short duration. The treatment of individuals who have hypothyroidism with postpartum thyroiditis is controversial. Most clinicians will treat postpartum women with symptomatic hypothyroidism. Whether or not to treat asymptomatic women, and, if so, for how long is unresolved. It would seem reasonable to treat even asymptomatic women who attempt pregnancy or who have elevated TSH levels. Therapy may be continued until childbearing is complete, when the thyroid hormone can be stopped, and the patient can be evaluated for persistent hypothyroidism.

It has been suggested that there may be an increased incidence of postpartum depression in patients who have positive thyroid autoantibodies. However, results of studies are inconsistent. Depression may be a finding in this case, but it is not a likely cause of the patient's symptoms. Multinodular goiter, Graves' disease, and thyroid papillary carcinoma can occur in the postpartum period, but thyroiditis is far more likely.

Lazarus JH. Thyroid dysfunction: reproduction and postpartum thyroiditis. Semin Reprod Med 2002;20:381–8.

Solomon BL, Fein HG, Smallridge RC. Usefulness of antimicrosomal antibody titers in the diagnosis and treatment of postpartum thyroiditis. J Fam Pract 1993;36:177–82.

Stagnaro-Green A. Clinical review 152: Postpartum thyroiditis. J Clin Endocrinol Metab 2002;87:4042–7.

Terry AJ, Hague WM. Postpartum thyroiditis. Semin Perinatol 1998;22:497–502.

89

Oral contraceptives and preexisting conditions

A 34-year-old woman had a spontaneous vaginal delivery 5 months ago and now requests a reliable method of contraception as soon as possible. Her pregnancy was complicated by severe preeclampsia. She is currently bottle-feeding her infant. Physical examination is unremarkable except for a blood pressure reading of 150/100 mm Hg. She is not compliant in taking her antihypertensive medications. The method of long-term reversible contraception that would be most cost-effective for this patient is

(A) combined oral contraceptives
(B) transdermal patch
(C) vaginal ring
* (D) intrauterine device (IUD)
(E) progestin-only pill

Several studies have shown the risks for adverse cardiovascular events in women who have hypertension while using combined hormonal contraception. The largest study to examine this evidence was the World Health Organization Collaborative Study of Cardiovascular and Steroid Hormone Contraception. This study included cases with deep vein thrombosis, ischemic and hemorrhagic stroke, as well as acute myocardial infarction in 21 centers in 17 countries. The odds ratio for ischemic and hemorrhagic stroke was found to range from 3.1 to 10.7 for combined oral contraceptive users with a history of hypertension, compared with nonusers with no history of hypertension.

A 12-fold risk for acute myocardial infarction was observed among oral contraceptive users with hypertension, compared with nonusers with hypertension. To date, only one study has evaluated venous thromboembolism with regard to oral contraceptive use and hypertension, and it found no significant risk in this patient population.

A meta-analysis of drug treatment studies estimated that for every 7.5 mm Hg increase in diastolic blood pressure, the incidence of stroke is increased by 46% and the incidence of myocardial infarct by 29%. Therefore, among women with a history of hypertension, the balance of the evidence suggests that a high risk of cardiovascular events, including stroke and acute myocardial infarction, may be expected in patients who take combined oral contraceptives. There currently are no data on the use of the transdermal patch or the vaginal ring in patients with chronic hypertension. Because both methods have no first pass effect through the liver, theoretically, there should be less effect on blood pressure. At this time, all combined hormonal contraceptives should be used with caution in patients who have untreated or poorly controlled chronic hypertension. There appears to be no increased risk for oral contraceptive use in women with well-controlled hypertension.

No studies have shown an increased risk of stroke, acute myocardial infarction, or venous thromboembolism among progestin-only pill users or progestin-type contraceptives. Because the progestin-only pill has a higher failure rate compared with the IUD and requires patient compliance, this pill would not be the best choice for this patient. The IUD would be the most appropriate method of contraception for this noncompliant patient. The parity of the patient should not be the primary consideration in the choice to use an IUD. The patient's desire for future fertility is not a contraindication for IUD use.

Acute myocardial infarction and combined oral contraceptives: results of an international multicentre case-control study. WHO Collaborative Study of Cardiovascular Disease and Steroid Hormone Contraception. Lancet 1997;349:1202–9.

American College of Obstetricians and Gynecologists. The use of hormonal contraception in women with coexisting medical conditions. ACOG Practice Bulletin 18. Washington, DC: ACOG; 2000.

Curtis KM, Chrisman CE, Peterson HB. Contraception for women in selected circumstances. WHO Programme for Mapping Best Practices in Reproductive Health. Obstet Gynecol 2002;99:1100–12.

Venous thromboembolic disease and combined oral contraceptives: results of international multicentre case-control study. World Health Organization Collaborative Study of Cardiovascular Disease and Steroid Hormone Contraception. Lancet 1995;346:1575–82.

90

Management of abnormal uterine bleeding

A 44-year-old woman, who smokes 1 pack of 20 cigarettes per day, has a history of heavy menstrual periods. Her menstrual periods are regular, last 8 days, and are heavy for 5 days with intermittent passage of small clots. Evaluation to date has included saline infusion ultrasonography, which shows slightly enlarged anterior–posterior diameter and a normal endometrial cavity. Pap test and cervical culture results are negative. Endometrial biopsy showed secretory endometrium. She has no immediate interest in fertility. The most appropriate treatment for this patient is

    (A) cyclic oral contraceptives (OCs)
    (B) leuprolide acetate (Lupron) for 3–6 months
    (C) depot medroxyprogesterone acetate
*   (D) levonorgestrel intrauterine system

The endometrium represents one of the most active tissues in the human body, with the functionalis layer experiencing complete regeneration every 28 days. Growth is primarily regulated by estrogen and progesterone, the secretion of which can elicit the secretion of the necessary growth factors for embryo implantation, or whose withdrawal causes orderly shedding in preparation for the next ovulation. Endometrial tissue breakdown involves a series of enzymes known as metalloproteinases that degrade the collagen, gelatins, fibronectin, laminin, and other components of extracellular matrix and basement membrane. Dysregulation of this process by inadequate or excessive exposure of the endometrium to the sex steroid hormones can cause departure from the expected growth factor and enzyme regulation and disrupt cyclical monthly menses. Anovulatory states, in which the regular monthly menstrual cycle is disturbed, predispose to heavy or irregular bleeding.

Menorrhagia is defined as excessive or prolonged uterine bleeding that occurs at regular intervals, or more strictly the loss of at least 80 mL of blood per menstrual cycle or bleeding that lasts for more than 7 days. The diagnosis of abnormal uterine bleeding should be made after taking a medical history to help categorize it as ovulatory or anovulatory. Anovulatory bleeding often is associated with irregular or sporadic ovulation as may occur at the extremes of the reproductive years, with hyperandrogenic anovulation (polycystic ovary syndrome) or other endocrine dysfunction. For ovulatory menorrhagia, as seen in this patient, uterine cavity evaluation is indicated. Menorrhagia can occur secondary to polyps, fibroids, and adenomyosis.

In a recent study of 433 perimenopausal women with abnormal uterine bleeding, saline infusion ultrasonography revealed no endometrial thickening, polyp, or fibroid in nearly 80% of women. Thus, most women with abnormal bleeding may benefit from some sort of medical therapy rather than surgical intervention. Patients with focal anatomic lesions often are treated with hysteroscopy and lesion removal with high success. The patient described has regular periods now and is ovulatory. The thickened anterior-posterior diameter of the uterus on ultrasound may be normal, or associated with adenomyosis, but no endometrial defects are described. She is a good candidate for medical therapy, but consideration should be given to her smoking history.

The levonorgestrel intrauterine system is a system which is designed to release levonorgestrel at a rate of 20 µg per day over a period of nearly 5 years. It is an extremely effective contraceptive and has recently been shown to be very effective in the treatment of menorrhagia. Typically, during the first 3 months of use, women will experience some irregular spotting, but at 6 months there is nearly 50% amenorrhea which remains stable at 12 and 24 months. Oligomenorrhea is typical in 25% of women. Use of the levonorgestrel intrauterine system in women with menorrhagia is effective in 3 out of 4 women in whom previous medical therapies have failed. Several recent studies have compared the levonorgestrel intrauterine system with endometrial ablation. Both endometrial ablation and the levonorgestrel intrauterine system have similar rates of satisfaction, reduction in uterine bleeding, and amenorrhea at 1 year. A recent meta-analysis suggests that the levonorgestrel intrauterine system offers the most effective treatment for menorrhagia. The evidence indicates this is the best approach for treating this patient.

Oral contraceptives are effective for reduction of menstrual blood flow. The combination of exogenous estrogen and progestin results in a stable endometrium that often is free of bleeding for months at a time. Cyclical monthly therapy (3 weeks on, 1 week off) reduces menstrual volume in the average cyclical user compared with spontaneous menses. Oral contraceptives also can be taken continuously, which can result in further freedom of menses. One common way to prescribe continuous administration is 63 active pills followed by 7 placebos (3 packs of active pills with 1 week off). However, there are few data to support continuous oral contraceptives for the treatment of menorrhagia. This often avoids the breakthrough bleeding associated with longer courses. Oral contraceptives are contraindicated in smokers older than 35 years and, thus, are not the best choice in this patient.

Depot medroxyprogesterone acetate can be effective for control of abnormal bleeding because 40% of users have amenorrhea at the end of 1 year. Most users have irregular or prolonged bleeding during the first 3 months, making this method less desirable than many others for cycle control.

Leuprolide acetate (Lupron) is a gonadotropin-releasing hormone agonist that profoundly suppresses pituitary secretion of luteinizing hormone and follicle-stimulating hormone, leading to a state of ovarian rest and profound hypoestrogenism in most users. This causes atrophy of the uterine blood supply and of the endometrium. Amenorrhea is the result in most users. This state of pseudomenopause does have side effects. Vasomotor symptoms often are quite severe, and bone loss from estrogen deficiency is significant after 6 months of use. Leuprolide should not be used for more than 6 months without providing add-back.

Fraser IS. Vaginal bleeding patterns in women using once-a-month injectable contraceptives. Contraception 1994;49:399–420.

Hidalgo M, Bahamondes L, Perrotti M, Diaz J, Dantas-Monteiro C, Petta C. Bleeding patterns and clinical performance of the levonorgestrel-releasing intrauterine system (Mirena) up to two years. Contraception 2002;65:129–32.

Irvine GA, Campbell-Brown MB, Lumsden MA, Heikkila A, Walker JJ, Cameron IT. Randomized comparative trial of the levonorgestrel intrauterine system and norethisterone for treatment of idiopathic menorrhagia. Br J Obstet Gynaecol 1998;105:592–8.

Marjoribanks J, Lethaby A, Farquhar C. Surgery versus medical therapy for heavy menstrual bleeding. Cochrane Database Syst Rev 2003;(2):CD003855.

Monteiro I, Bahamondes L, Diaz J, Perrotti M, Petta C. Therapeutic use of levonorgestrel-releasing intrauterine system in women with menorrhagia: a pilot study (1). Contraception 2002;65:325–8.

91

Bowel injury during endoscopy

A 33-year-old woman comes to the emergency department with intermittent severe cramping abdominal pain with associated nausea 72 hours after an operative laparoscopy for removal of an 8 cm × 8 cm right ovarian dermoid cyst. She is afebrile, and her abdomen is distended and tender precluding a satisfactory examination. The best way to evaluate her for bowel injury is

  (A) colonoscopy
* (B) computerized axial tomography (CAT) scan of the abdomen
  (C) flat plate and upright abdominal X-ray
  (D) upper gastrointestinal series with small bowel follow-through

Operative laparoscopy allows the surgeon to perform a wide variety of procedures using minimally invasive techniques. It is possible to remove adnexal masses and solid tumors, such as leiomyomata, via accessory ports. To remove such masses, it usually is necessary to use 10 mm or greater accessory ports. Any time accessory ports are used, the risks for intraoperative injury or postoperative complications increase. Common injuries related to trocar insertion include vascular trauma, direct puncture injury to intraabdominal or pelvic viscera, postoperative wound hematoma or infection, and bowel injury or herniation through any of the port sites used for the procedure. Herniation of the bowel can lead to bowel obstruction, strangulation of the bowel, and eventual bowel infarction and perforation.

Laparoscopic-related incisional hernias are extremely uncommon; in one survey, they were estimated to occur at a rate of 21 per 100,000 cases. The most common site for occurrence of such hernias is the umbilical port (76%), and more than 80% were associated with ports 10 mm or greater. However, incisional hernias have been reported with the use of ports as small as 5 mm, especially when the port is replaced multiple times. The involvement of the bowel in these hernias is even less common (20%) with the more common finding of omentum within these hernias. When bowel involvement does occur, symptoms usually become evident within the first 1–2 weeks following surgery. Symptoms range from colicky pain; a palpable mass at the incisional site that may or may not be tender; nausea, with or without vomiting; a rigid abdomen; or high fevers.

The patient, who presents with severe intermittent cramping and nausea, may have several possible etiologies for those symptoms. Some of the possibilities include viral gastrointestinal syndromes, medication-related sensitivities, residual carbon dioxide peritoneal irritation, urinary tract infection, pelvic peritonitis, bowel or other visceral injury, and incisional hernia with or without bowel involvement.

The surgeon evaluating this patient should be concerned primarily with complications directly related to the procedure. Colonoscopy, although useful in the diagnosis of intraluminal pathology of the large bowel, will be of extremely limited value in this case because of the greater likelihood of external injury to either small or large bowel.

Recent literature has noted the utility of ultrasonography and particularly CAT scan with contrast in diagnosing bowel herniation or bowel obstruction (Fig. 91-1). This technology allows the surgeon to more accurately and noninvasively evaluate the more serious causes of abdominal pain and nausea than standard flat plate and upright films, which will not diagnose cases of incisional hernia that involve the bowel with or without bowel obstruction.

The patient who has the typical signs and symptoms of a bowel obstruction will present with a very tender distended abdomen with absent or high-pitched bowel sounds. She may have low or high-grade fevers and changes in complete blood count with elevations in white blood cell count. Flat plate and upright radiographs of the abdomen will identify distended loops of small bowel and even air fluid levels in cases of ongoing bowel obstruction. If bowel obstruction is suspected, the initial treatment is hospitalization with intravenous hydration and bowel decompression. Confirmation of small bowel obstruction can be further made by performing an upper gastrointestinal series with small bowel follow through. Although both flat plate and upright films of the abdomen and upper gastrointestinal tract with small bowel follow through are extremely valuable in making the diagnosis of ileus and bowel obstruction, they will not address the diagnosis of early herniation unless the bowel has become strangulated with resultant obstruction or infarction.

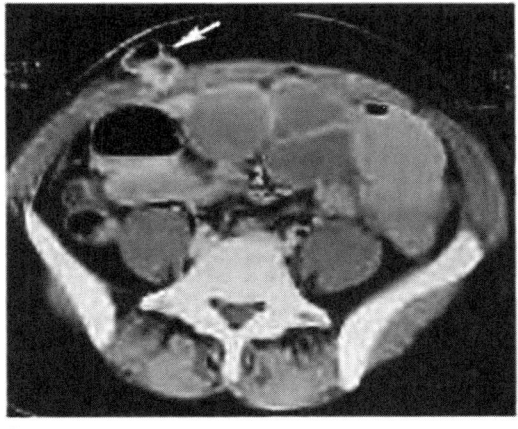
A

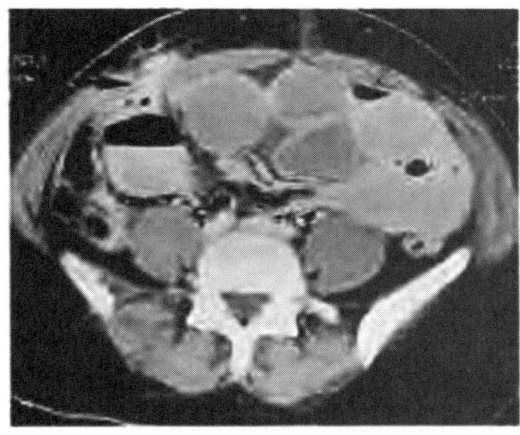
B

FIG. 91-1. A. Axial computed tomography of the abdomen with oral and intravenous contrast medium shows multiple loops of dilated small bowel with air-fluid levels. There is a loop of small bowel seen herniated out of the peritoneum into the soft tissues of the anterior abdominal wall (arrow). **B.** A more cranial image shows a decompressed segment of small bowel reentering the abdomen, confirming the site of obstruction (arrow). (Bemporad JA, Zreik TG, Brink JA. Laparoscopic hernias: two case reports and a review of the literature. J Comput Assist Tomogr 1999;23:88. Copyright 1999 Lippincott Williams and Wilkins.)

Kurtz BR, Daniell JF, Spaw AT. Incarcerated incisional hernia after laparoscopy. A case report. J Reprod Med 1993;38:643–4.

Maglinte DD, Reyes BL, Harmon BH, Kelvin FM, Turner WW Jr, Hage JE, et al. Reliability and role of plain film radiography and CT in the diagnosis of small-bowel obstruction. AJR Am J Roentgenol 1996;167:1451–5.

Montz FJ, Holschneider CH, Munro MG. Incisional hernia following laparoscopy: a survey of the American Association of Gynecologic Laparoscopists. Obstet Gynecol 1994;84:881–4.

Wicks A, Voyvodic F, Scroop R. Incisional hernia and small bowel obstruction following laparoscopic surgery: computed tomography diagnosis. Australas Radiol 2000;44:331–2.

92 Treatment of macroadenoma

A 29-year-old woman, gravida 1, para 1, gave birth 18 months ago and breastfed her infant for 16 months. For the past 8 weeks, she has attempted to wean the infant, but her breasts continue to engorge and leak. She mentions that she has not slept well during breastfeeding and has "pressure-type" headaches that are relieved with ibuprofen. She has had amenorrhea since the delivery. Physical examination is significant for bilateral galactorrhea, decreased rugation of the vaginal mucosa, and normal visual fields by confrontation. Laboratory studies indicate a prolactin level of 240 ng/mL, thyroid-stimulating hormone (TSH) level of 2.3 µU/mL, follicle-stimulating hormone (FSH) level of 2.4 mIU/mL, thyroxine (T_4) level of 9.2 µg/dL, and growth hormone (GH) level of less than 1 ng/mL. A computed tomography (CT) scan of the pituitary with contrast reveals a 19-mm lesion in the left anterior pituitary gland without distortion of the optic chiasm. The most appropriate next step in the management of this patient is

(A) observation
* (B) bromocriptine mesylate (Parlodel)
(C) oral contraceptives
(D) pituitary irradiation
(E) transsphenoidal hypophysectomy

The most common space-occupying lesion within the sella turcica is the pituitary adenoma. Prolactin-secreting adenomas are the most common pituitary microadenomas with approximately 20% considered to be macroadenomas (ie, tumors greater than 10 mm in diameter). The annual incidence of all pituitary adenomas is approximately 2 cases per 100,000. The pituitary tumors in which there are no increases in serum levels of anterior pituitary hormones are called nonfunctioning pituitary adenomas. Among the larger pituitary macroadenomas, the most common are the nonfunctioning pituitary adenomas followed by macroprolactinomas.

Macroadenomas lead to clinical symptoms because of their enhanced release of pituitary hormones or from space-occupying effects resulting in visual field defects, pressure-type headaches, or subsequent compression of normal endocrine functioning areas. This patient has hypogonadotropic hypogonadism (ie, low FSH level), which is the most frequently observed clinical endocrine dysfunction. The hypogonadism may be related to compression of the pituitary stalk, which inhibits delivery of dopamine to the anterior pituitary gland indirectly and causes an elevation in prolactin levels or direct hypersecretion of prolactin from the macroadenoma, as seen in this patient. If the macroadenoma compresses and destroys normal functioning anterior pituitary gland tissue, adrenal failure caused by decreased secretion of adrenocorticotropic hormone (ACTH) or secondary hypothyroidism can occur. In this latter case, the TSH level may be low or undetectable whereas the free T_4 level will be low.

The diagnosis of macroadenomas is made with radiologic imaging techniques, such as magnetic resonance imaging (MRI) or CT scan, and by endocrine evaluation. Generally, the MRI or CT scan will determine if the optic chiasm is compromised whereas Goldman perimetry visual fields testing will determine the degree of visual compromise. However, confrontational visual fields testing is unreliable. For individuals who present with endocrine disturbances in conjunction with a macroadenoma, endocrine testing will help document the degree of pituitary insufficiency and possible hyposecretion of pituitary hormones. One endocrine test for GH, ACTH, and prolactin secretion is the insulin tolerance test in which insulin is given intravenously (0.05–0.15 units/kg) to induce hypoglycemia and activate counter-regulatory hormone secretion, which leads to activation of the sympathetic system and increases in ACTH and cortisol, GH, and prolactin secretion. This test should be closely supervised with 50% glucose readily available for intravenous administration if symptomatic hypoglycemia occurs.

For prolactin-secreting macroadenomas, a trial with a dopamine agonist such as bromocriptine mesylate (Parlodel), 10–30 mg per day in divided doses, or cabergoline (Dostinex), 0.25–1 mg twice per week, often is effective in reducing tumor size and reversing the space-occupying effects in a relatively short period and is the correct choice in this patient. For nonprolactin macroadenomas, surgical resection often is the treatment of choice. In the unusual patient in whom the tumor has extended into the cavernous sinus or other brain structures where total resection is not possible, postoperative radiation often is used. Radiation to the pituitary gland usually will result in eventual development of a hypopituitary state. During medical treatment, sequential monitoring of tumor size should be considered. If too much radiation is delivered to the optic chiasm, fibrosis and eventual blindness may occur.

For patients with prolactin microadenomas who become pregnant, clinical monitoring is necessary to determine if the adenoma increases in size during pregnancy. Visual disturbances, increased nausea, and headaches may suggest pituitary enlargement requiring MRI evaluation. These patients usually will respond to reinstitution of bromocriptine therapy.

Pituitary apoplexy is more commonly seen with macroadenomas than with microadenomas. This medical emergency is characterized by acute infarction of the pituitary gland. Patients will experience sudden onset of severe retro-orbital headache and visual disturbances, which may be followed by lethargy or loss of consciousness. These symptoms can mimic other neurologic emergencies, such as cavernous sinus thrombosis, basilar artery occlusion, or ruptured aneurysm. Pituitary apoplexy will require emergency radiologic imaging to pinpoint the actual diagnosis.

The use of oral contraceptives in this patient is contraindicated. The higher pharmacologic doses of estrogen in oral contraceptives may cause additional enlargement of the macroadenoma.

Feldkamp J, Santen R, Harms E, Aulich A, Modder U, Scherbaum WA. Incidentally discovered pituitary lesions: high frequency of macroadenomas and hormone-secreting adenomas—results of a prospective study. Clin Endocrinol (Oxf) 1999;51:109–13.

Katznelson L, Alexander JM, Klibanski A. Clinical review 45: Clinically non-functioning pituitary adenomas. J Clin Endocrinol Metab 1993;76:1089–94.

St-Jean E, Blain F, Comtois R. High prolactin levels may be missed by immunoradiometric assay in patients with macroprolactinomas. Clin Endocrinol (Oxf) 1996;44:305–9.

Vance ML. Hypopituitarism. N Engl J Med 1994;330:1651–62.

93

Management of fibroids in infertile women

A 28-year-old nulligravid woman comes in for evaluation of an enlarged uterus and inability to conceive. She has a normal bleeding pattern and has documented that she is ovulatory by ovulation kits. Her husband has a normal semen analysis. A recent ultrasound examination documented the presence of 3 uterine leiomyomata. Her primary care physician told her that she would require further evaluation to determine if the fibroids will interfere with her ability to conceive. The next step in evaluation is

    (A) sonohysterography
    (B) laparoscopy
    (C) hysteroscopy
*   (D) hysterosalpingography (HSG)

The most common uterine neoplasms are leiomyomata (fibroids), which occur 3–9 times more frequently in African-American women than in Caucasian women, suggesting a genetic predisposition in some individuals. In a study of 1,364 randomly selected urban health plan members aged 35–49 years who were screened for fibroid tumors by ultrasonography, 51% of premenopausal women with no previous diagnosis had ultrasound evidence of uterine fibroid tumors, with the tumors developing in African-American women at an earlier age than in white women (odds ratio, 2.9; 95% confidence interval, 2.5–3.4).

Uterine leiomyomata are benign proliferations of smooth-muscle cells and fibrous connective tissue that can occur singly or multiply and range from 1–2 mm to greater than 20 cm in size. Most are asymptomatic and generally do not require intervention or investigation unless they appear to be interfering with the ability to conceive, as in this patient.

For patients with infertility, HSG is the screening procedure of choice for evaluation of the uterine cavity, is the least invasive method, and has low complication rates. With HSG, information about tubal architecture and patency also can be obtained to determine the degree of fallopian tube occlusion. This type of tubal detail would not be apparent on a sonohysterogram. If fallopian tubes are patent, the test can increase 3-month cycle fecundity, with tubal lavage providing a therapeutic effect. In patients with evidence of lower genital tract infection or an allergy to contrast media that contain iodide, HSG should be avoided.

Hysteroscopy can diagnose intrauterine pathology, allowing concurrent treatment, and is more sensitive than HSG for detecting intrauterine synechiae, endometrial polyps, and submucous myomas. Although this patient has 3 leiomyomata detected by ultrasonography, she has no history of abnormal bleeding and, thus, would be unlikely to have an intracavitary lesion. In addition, hysteroscopy does not provide any information about the fallopian tubes.

Laparoscopy in conjunction with chromotubation can be used to diagnose tubal disease and would allow concurrent ablation of endometriosis or lysis of pelvic adhesions. Compared with HSG, laparoscopy has a higher complication rate, is more costly to perform, and must be done in conjunction with hysteroscopy to obtain the most complete details about the uterine cavity. Laparoscopy is not indicated in this patient unless she has an allergy to radiographic contrast media or is suspected of having endometriosis or pelvic adhesive disease.

Sonohysterography has been favorably compared with hysteroscopy in some studies that have evaluated abnormal bleeding. However, detailed visualization of fallopian tube anatomy is difficult with sonohysterography, even with infusion of saline or the use of a contrast medium.

In the absence of abnormal bleeding, which would indicate an intracavitary lesion, multiple myomectomy is not indicated. Several studies have demonstrated the benefits of preoperative HSG in the identification of submucosal myomas. This allows a more targeted surgical approach to myomectomy when indicated.

A review of the literature to determine whether leiomyomata are associated with decreased fertility rates and whether surgical removal subsequently increases fertility rates found that only fibroids with a submucosal or intracavitary component were associated with decreased reproductive outcomes. In these cases, hysteroscopic myomectomy may be beneficial.

Chan AH, Fujimoto VY, Moore DE, Martin RW, Vaezy S. An image-guided high intensity focused ultrasound device for uterine fibroids treatment. Med Phys 2002;29:2611–20.

Day Baird D, Dunson DB, Hill MC, Cousins D, Schectman JM. High cumulative incidence of uterine leiomyoma in black and white women: ultrasound evidence. Am J Obstet Gynecol 2003;188:100–7.

Fleischer AC, Vasquez JM, Cullinan JA, Eisenberg E. Sonohysterography combined with sonosalpingography: correlation with endoscopic findings in infertility patients. J Ultrasound Med 1997;16:381–4.

Pritts EA. Fibroids and infertility: a systematic review of the evidence. Obstet Gynecol Surv 2001;56:483–91.

Richmond JA. Hysterosalpingography. In: Lobo RA, Mishell DR, Paulson RJ, Shoupe D, eds. Textbook of infertility, contraception, and reproductive endocrinology. 4th ed. Malden (MA): Blackwell Science; 1997. p. 567–79.

94

Diagnosis of hypothyroidism

A 38-year-old woman is in her first trimester of pregnancy after her first in vitro fertilization cycle for unexplained infertility. She has been treated for Hashimoto's thyroiditis for 3 years. Her thyroid-stimulating hormone (TSH) levels have varied between 0.75 µU/mL and 1.5 µU/mL during the past 2 years with a maintenance dose of 50 µg of levothyroxine. A repeat TSH level obtained at the 6-week visit is 3.75 µU/mL. The most appropriate management plan for this patient is to

(A) maintain the current dosage of levothyroxine through pregnancy and repeat TSH test after delivery
* (B) increase the levothyroxine dosage and repeat the TSH test in 6 weeks
(C) maintain the current dosage of levothyroxine and repeat the TSH test in the mid-second trimester
(D) decrease the levothyroxine dosage and repeat the TSH test in 6 weeks
(E) discontinue thyroid therapy and repeat the TSH test in the mid-second trimester

Overt hypothyroidism has known adverse sequelae in the nonpregnant patient, increasing the risks for dyslipidemia, coronary artery disease, myocardial infarction, altered neuropsychiatric status including depression, and death in older individuals. Fetal death has long been associated with maternal hypothyroidism. Results of one study indicated that women with a TSH level greater than 6 µU/mL in the second trimester have 4 times the risk of fetal death compared with those with a normal TSH level. Findings of other studies have suggested that mild or subclinical hypothyroidism also may have similar adverse effects on the health of adults and developing fetuses.

That subclinical hypothyroidism is an independent risk factor for such conditions as cardiac dysfunction, hypercholesterolemia, and neuropsychiatric disorders is becoming increasingly evident. As a result, there has been a recent recommendation from The Endocrine Society to decrease the upper limit of normal for TSH values to 3 µU/mL.

The incidence of hypothyroidism varies with age and geographic distribution. In many parts of the developing world, iodine deficiency is the leading cause of hypothyroidism, and, as a result, the overall incidence of hypothyroidism is increased. In developed countries, such as the United States and the United Kingdom, autoimmune disease is the predominant cause of hypothyroidism. The largest study of the prevalence of thyroid dysfunction in an iodine replete community was reported from Northern England first in 1977 and as a 20-year follow-up in 1995. For this community, 1.4–1.9% of women at baseline had overt hypothyroidism, and subclinical hypothyroidism was identified at 4–5-fold higher than overt hypothyroid rates. The prevalence for both overt and subclinical hypothyroidism increased with age. Nearly 10% of women older than 50 years were initially found to have elevated TSH levels. Because of the prevalence and adverse outcomes for mild and overt hypothyroidism, guidelines for more frequent testing have been made by a number of national organizations in the absence of outcomes research, demonstrating a cost–benefit effect (Table 94-1).

Growing evidence suggests that the impact of this condition on brain development and subsequent mental and psychomotor performance of the child is likely significant. It has long been known that congenital hypothyroidism has a predictive association with intellectual impairment, and combined maternal and fetal iodine deficiency is associated with impaired school achievement among other neuropsychologic measures. Only recently, however, has the potential significance of mild and overt untreated maternal hypothyroidism been reported. In one study, children have been studied at various intervals during the first year of life as well as during ages 7–9 years. A range of mental, neuropsychologic, and psychomotor deficits have been described including a reduction of intelligence quotient scores by a mean of 7 points in children of women with hypothyroidism compared with the children of euthyroid controls. Such long-term deficits have been found for children of women identified to have either subclinical or overt hypothyroidism. To date, however, these results are only from observational studies. Interventional trials have not been performed to demonstrate improvement in these neurologic measures with treatment.

Although there are no recommendations for screening all pregnant women at their first prenatal visit for hypothyroidism, close follow-up at regular intervals of women with hypothyroidism who become pregnant is essential. Thyroid-stimulating hormone levels may increase by 50% or more for them during pregnancy with increases of L-thyroxine doses by an average of 30% being common. Once adjustments are made, follow-up TSH screening is vital. Given the very long half-life of L-thyroxine, retesting is not recommended until 6 weeks after dosage adjustments.

TABLE 94-1. National Guidelines for Thyroid-Stimulating Hormone Screening

Organization	Year	Guideline
American College of Physicians	1998	Selective screening in all women older than 50 years with 1 or more symptoms
U.S. Preventive Services Task Force	1996	No routine screening
American Thyroid Association	2000	All adults beginning at age 35 years and every 5 years after
American College of Obstetricians and Gynecologists	2002	Periodic assessment after age 19 years in high-risk individuals

American College of Obstetricians and Gynecologists. Reproductive endocrinology. In: Precis: an update in obstetrics and gynecology. 2nd ed. Washington, DC: ACOG; 2002.

Blazer S, Moreh-Waterman Y, Miller-Lotan R, Tamir A, Hochberg Z. Maternal hypothyroidism may affect fetal growth and neonatal thyroid function. Obstet Gynecol 2003;102:232–41.

Haddow JE, Palomaki GE, Allan WC, Williams JR, Knight GJ, Gagnon J, et al. Maternal thyroid deficiency during pregnancy and subsequent neuropsychological development of the child. N Engl J Med 1999;341: 549–55.

Pop VJ, Kuijpens JL, van Baar AL, Verkerk G, van Son MM, de Vijlder JJ, et al. Low maternal free thyroxine concentrations during early pregnancy are associated with impaired psychomotor development in infancy. Clin Endocrinol 1999;50:149–55.

Smallridge RC, Ladenson PW. Hypothyroidism in pregnancy: consequences to neonatal health. J Clin Endocrinol Metab 2001;86: 2349–53.

Stephens PA. Current issues in thyroid disease management: leading experts discuss new JAMA and JCE&M reports during Endocrine Society audioconference. Endocrine News 2004(April):17–20.

Thyroid disease in pregnancy. ACOG Practice Bulletin 37. American College of Obstetricians and Gynecologists. Obstet Gynecol 2002:100: 387–96.

Vanderpump MP, Tunbridge WM, French JM, Appleton D, Bates D, Clark F, et al. The incidence of thyroid disorders in the community: a twenty-year follow-up of the Whickham Survey. Clin Endocrinol (Oxf) 1995;43:55–68.

95
Mifepristone (Mifeprex) and pregnancy termination

A healthy 29-year-old woman, 6 weeks past her last menstrual period, has been treated for medical termination of pregnancy. On her first treatment visit, she received mifepristone (Mifeprex), and 2 days later she received misoprostol. Her bleeding had been heavy for 5 days, and now, 10 days after she received mifepristone, she reports that she continues to experience bleeding at a rate similar to a normal menstrual period, with no clotting blood but with the need to change pads every 4 hours. Office ultrasonography reveals no sac present but a 1.2-cm hyperechoic area consistent with tissue and blood. Her hematocrit concentration is 37%, her pulse rate is 90 beats per minute, and she shows no orthostatic changes with standing. The next step in management is

* (A) reassurance
* (B) dilation and curettage
* (C) repeat misoprostol
* (D) measurement of human chorionic gonadotropin (hCG) level

Mifepristone, a derivative of norethindrone, binds to the progesterone receptor with an affinity equal to progesterone but does not activate the receptor, thus acting as an antiprogestin. If given during early pregnancy, mifepristone results in trophoblastic separation, a decrease in hCG production, increased uterine prostaglandin production, and cervical softening. These events allow expulsion of the pregnancy from the uterus when a uterotonic agent, such as misoprostol, is added.

Misoprostol is a prostaglandin E_1 analog in tablet form. It is approved for use by the U.S. Food and Drug Administration (FDA) for prevention of gastric ulcers in individuals who take antiinflammatory drugs on a long-term basis and is used clinically for cervical softening for labor induction. The FDA-approved combination of mifepristone and misoprostol for termination of early pregnancy includes oral mifepristone, 600 mg, followed approximately 48 hours later by misoprostol, 400 mg orally.

Effectiveness of these medications for pregnancies of up to 49 days of gestation is approximately 96% and less than 85% if more than 49 days of gestation. Complete abortion rates generally are in the range of 90–98%. A "failure" is defined as occurring when a suction aspiration or curettage is performed for any reason. A true method failure has been defined as the presence of gestational cardiac activity on vaginal ultrasonography 2 weeks following mifepristone administration. Serum hCG levels should decrease by at least 50% within 1 week of initiation of the medication. The average time to achieve an hCG level that is no longer detectable is approximately 33 days, but it can take as long as 90 days. Measurement of hCG at this time would not be advisable for this patient. No studies have assessed the efficacy of additional doses of mifepristone, methotrexate, or misoprostol in these circumstances.

The possible side effects of this treatment include bleeding and pain, nausea, dizziness, headache, vomiting, fever and chill, and diarrhea in order of decreasing frequency of occurrence. Counseling should emphasize that the patient is likely to have bleeding and cramping that is much heavier than menses and should be compared with a miscarriage. This patient can be counseled that the soaking of 2 pads per hour for 2 consecutive hours is not a point at which intervention is necessary, but that it is time to check with a care provider. Whether it is imperative to seek emergency care depends on how the patient feels, her hematocrit level, whether the bleeding is slowing, and her geographic distance from medical facilities.

Very rarely do women who are having a medical abortion require a dilation and curettage. Overall, fewer than 1% of women who undergo a medical abortion will need emergent curettage for appreciable bleeding. Ultrasonography is sometimes done to examine the uterus. The sole purpose of the ultrasound examination is to confirm that the gestational sac is no longer present. The postabortion uterus will normally contain sonographically hyperechoic tissue that consists of blood clots and decidua. In the absence of extra bleeding, the clinician should follow such patients conservatively.

Creinin MD, Aubeny E. Medical abortion in early pregnancy. In: Paul M, Lichtenburg ES, Borgatta L, Grimes DA, Stubblefield PG, eds. A clinician's guide to medical and surgical abortion. New York (NY): Churchill Livingstone; 1999. p. 91–106.

Kahn JG, Becker BJ, MacIsaa L, Armory JK, Neuhaus J, Olkin I, et al. The efficacy of medical abortion: a meta-analysis. Contraception 2000; 61:29–40.

Spitz IM, Bardin CW, Benton L, Robbins A. Early pregnancy termination with mifepristone and misoprostol in the United States. N Engl J Med 1998;338:1241–7.

96
Congenital adrenal hyperplasia

A newborn term infant is evaluated for ambiguous genitalia. A brief physical examination reveals no palpable mass in the labioscrotal folds. The infant has a phallic structure and evidence of internal müllerian structures. Based on these findings the most likely diagnosis is

    (A) mixed gonadal dysgenesis
* (B) congenital adrenal hyperplasia (CAH)
    (C) androgen insensitivity
    (D) male pseudohermaphroditism

Congenital adrenal hyperplasia is an inherited autosomal recessive disorder that is caused by a defect in the enzymatic pathway that converts cholesterol to cortisol. The most common of these is 21-hydroxylase deficiency. The classic form causes ambiguous genitalia in the newborn female and virilization that develops slowly over time in both sexes. Careful palpation for the presence or absence of gonads can provide an important key to diagnosis. In addition, genetic evaluation with karyotype analysis and hormonal investigation will guide the clinical assessment and differentiate female from male pseudohermaphroditism.

Ambiguous genitalia presents a diagnostic challenge to the clinician that requires immediate attention to the newborn with a detailed evaluation and well-organized treatment plan. A comprehensive history and physical examination are essential when evaluating ambiguous genitalia in the newborn. A family history of other affected siblings, problems in the newborn period, or maternal ingestion of drugs during pregnancy are important. One key to diagnosis is the palpation of gonads in the inguinal regions or labioscrotal folds. If the gonads are not palpable, a diagnosis of female pseudohermaphroditism is most likely; if they are palpable, however, the diagnosis of male pseudohermaphroditism is more appropriate. Ambiguous genitalia that present with cryptorchidism may have palpable testicular tissue found in both the inguinal canal and labioscrotal folds.

The physical examination should evaluate for the presence of a vagina and internal müllerian structures. These may go unrecognized because of fusion of the labioscrotal folds. A phallic structure may be present that represents an enlarged clitoris or hypospadias. After a careful physical examination, hormonal and genetic testing will determine the correct etiology for the ambiguous genitalia. Elevation of 17-hydroxyprogesterone levels confirms the diagnosis of classical CAH, which is caused by a deficiency of 21-hydroxylase. It is important to evaluate electrolytes for salt wasting to prevent a metabolic emergency that sometimes can occur in the newborn period. Next, the karyotype is an essential part of the evaluation to aid in etiology, treatment, and sex assignment.

Standard results may take up to 4 weeks; however, the use of polymerase chain reaction to evaluate for the presence of the sex-determining region SRY on the Y chromosome usually can be reported within 1 day.

After a comprehensive clinical investigation, a more defined etiology for the cause of the ambiguous genitalia may be determined. Female pseudohermaphroditism can arise from abnormalities of the fetal adrenal gland, elevated androgen production from a maternal source (ie, ovary, adrenal, or ingestion of hormones), or excess androgen production from the placenta (eg, placental sulfatase deficiency). Causes of male pseudohermaphroditism commonly involve defective androgen action or biosynthesis. A defect in androgen sensitivity or 5α-reductase is only clinically apparent in males.

Congenital adrenal hyperplasia caused by 21-hydroxylase deficiency can occur in newborn males, but it is not the most likely etiology in this case. A more detailed physical examination may locate additional gonadal tissue and an opening to the bladder, most likely though the phallic structure that is present.

After an extensive evaluation, the physician must discuss and determine the preferred sex for rearing with the parents. Several important aspects should be taken into account: etiology of the genital abnormality, the functional anatomy of the genitalia, and the concerns of the family involved. With female pseudohermaphroditism, the sex assignment should always be declared female. Future childbearing is possible in the presence of a normal uterus and ovaries. With male pseudohermaphroditism, sex selection is not as clear, and a number of factors may influence whether a child is raised as a boy or girl (eg, possible virilization at puberty, ability to accomplish surgical reconstruction, and predicted response to endogenous or exogenous testosterone). Males with pseudohermaphroditism who are to be raised as girls should be castrated. Intraabdominal gonads that contain a Y chromosome may predispose to gonadal tumor.

A multidisciplinary approach to diagnosis and treatment of a newborn with ambiguous genitalia is necessary. The medical team should focus on all aspects of manage-

97

Ovulation induction selection of appropriate patients

A 32-year-old woman, gravida 1, para 1, wants a second opinion for secondary infertility. She conceived easily 3 years ago and had a normal term vaginal delivery. After breastfeeding for 14 months, she did not resume regular menstrual cycles. Her menstrual cycles are now at 21–42-day intervals. She reports heavy menses or vaginal spotting and occasional hot flushes. Laboratory test results show a serum prolactin level of 14 ng/mL, thyroid-stimulating hormone (TSH) level of 2.1 µU/mL, day 3 follicle-stimulating hormone (FSH) level of 32 mIU/mL, and estradiol level of 32 pg/mL. After 5 days of clomiphene citrate (Clomid, Serophene) at a dose of 100 mg per day (clomiphene challenge test), she has a day 10 FSH level of 41 mIU/mL and an estradiol level of 54 pg/mL. Her mother had natural menopause at age 45 years, and her 39-year-old sister continues to menstruate. The approach that would provide the best chance for this patient to achieve pregnancy would be

      (A) human menopausal gonadotropin (hMG)
      (B) clomiphene citrate
*   (C) donor oocytes with assisted reproductive technology (ART)
      (D) gonadotropin-releasing hormone (GnRH) agonist flare with hMG
      (E) clomiphene citrate with hMG

The evaluation of secondary infertility in this patient should focus on ovulatory abnormalities because of her history of irregular cycles. Baseline prolactin and TSH levels were normal. Her baseline FSH level was greater than 15 mIU/mL on day 3 of the menstrual cycle. With clomiphene stimulation, the FSH level increased further without an appropriate increase in the estradiol level. The data provided suggest that this individual has reached the end of her reproductive function. To evaluate her ovarian reserve, the clomiphene challenge test, a dynamic test of the hypothalamic–pituitary–ovarian axis, was performed.

Clomiphene citrate is a partial estrogen receptor antagonist and blocks the negative feedback of estrogen on the hypothalamic–pituitary–ovarian axis, leaving regulation of FSH release primarily to inhibin B. Thus, measuring FSH serum levels following a course of clomiphene citrate during the follicular phase may be a good measure in evaluation of ovarian reserve. The clomiphene challenge test is an adjunct to the day 3 FSH and estradiol testing. It consists of administration of clomiphene citrate, 100 mg daily, on cycle days 5–9 in which day 3 basal FSH and estradiol levels are measured. Follicle-stimulating hormone and estradiol levels are measured again on day 10. In a study of clomiphene challenge testing, 588 infertility couples who did not have sperm abnormalities, moderate or severe endometriosis, or pelvic adhesions, an increase in FSH levels of more than 10 mIU/mL on either day 3 or day 10 was classified as abnormal. Using these criteria, 48.5% of patients with normal clomiphene challenge test results achieved pregnancy without ART compared with 4.8% of patients with abnormal clomiphene challenge test findings. Age also was an independent variable predictive of pregnancy rate in patients with a normal clomiphene challenge test result. An alternative criterion in which the clomiphene challenge test is considered abnormal is if the sum of day 3 and day 10 FSH levels is greater than 26 mIU/mL. The time to begin to screen infertile patients with clomiphene challenge test is unclear although some have advocated screening all infertility patients older than 30 years.

At birth, there are approximately 500,000 oocytes present in the ovaries. The numbers of viable oocytes decrease with aging and is influenced by genetic factors as well as environmental exposures. The etiology for this patient's premature reduction in ovarian reserve is unclear. A reduction in ovarian reserve is related to either an increase in the rate of oocyte atresia or an overall decrease in the number of starting oocytes. These conditions appear to be genetically linked. The patient has not been exposed to radiation or chemotherapy medications, both of which have been shown to reduce ovarian reserve.

Although the clomiphene challenge test is the most common method used to assess ovarian reserve, other approaches for estimating ovarian reserve include ultrasound determination of ovarian volume, ultrasound determination of antral follicle count, and measurement of serum inhibin B levels. These tests have been shown to correlate with the clomiphene challenge test in smaller studies but must be considered experimental at this time.

In patients who present with irregular menstrual cycles, decreased ovarian reserve, and increased baseline FSH levels in the menopausal range, the use of gonadotropin stimulating drugs, such as clomiphene citrate, hMG, GnRH agonists, or combinations of these medications, will have little impact in stimulating additional follicular development because the hypothalamic–pituitary unit has already increased endogenous gonadotropin output. Moreover, it would be difficult to monitor for follicular development given the sporadic and unpredictable nature of ovulation in these patients. For patients who want to pursue pregnancy under these circumstances, an oocyte donor provides the best overall pregnancy rate.

For those couples who do not choose oocyte donation, estrogen therapy (ET) may be instituted for treatment of intermittent hypoestrogenism in this age group. Because ET at this dose usually does not suppress FSH and intermittent ovulation, spontaneous pregnancy has been reported in patients with these types of disorders.

Klein NA, Battaglia DE, Fujimoto VY, Davis GS, Bremner WJ, Soules MR. Reproductive aging: accelerated ovarian follicular development associated with a monotropic follicular development associated with a monotropic follicle-stimulating hormone rise in normal older women. J Clin Endocrinol Metab 1996;81:1038–45.

Loumaye E, Billion JM, Mine JM, Psalti I, Pensis M, Thomas K. Prediction of individual response to controlled ovarian hyperstimulation by means of a clomiphene citrate challenge test. Fertil Steril 1990; 53:295–301.

Navot D, Rosenwaks Z, Margalioth EJ. Prognostic assessment of female fecundity. Lancet 1987;2:645–7.

Scott RT, Leonardi MR, Hoffmann GE, Illions EH, Neal GS, Navot D. A prospective evaluation of clomiphene citrate challenge test screening of the general infertility population. Obstet Gynecol 1993;82:539–44.

Scott RT, Opsahl MS, Leonardi MR, Neal GS, Illions EH, Navot D. Life table analysis of pregnancy rates in a general infertility population relative to ovarian reserve and patient age. Hum Reprod 1995;10:1706–10.

98
Prevention of adhesions

A 22-year-old nulligravid woman presents with a history of severe dysmenorrhea for the past 6 months. On physical examination, you find a markedly retroverted, fixed uterus with significant nodularity on the uterosacral ligaments and bilateral adnexal fullness. You perform operative laparoscopy for extensive endometriosis with severe peritoneal adhesions, complete obliteration of the cul-de-sac, and bilateral endometriomas. The best method to prevent postoperative adhesions in this patient is

    (A) intraperitoneal dexamethasone
    (B) lactated Ringer's solution with heparin
*   (C) oxidized regenerated cellulose (Interceed)
    (D) oral indomethacin (Indocin)
    (E) 32% dextran 70 (Hyskon)

The prevention of pelvic adhesions postoperatively continues to be a major challenge for gynecologic surgeons. Pelvic adhesions can be the result of inflammation, infection, endometriosis, or surgical trauma. Meticulous and atraumatic surgical technique continues to be the most important step in the prevention of postoperative pelvic adhesions, given the limited number of effective agents available for their prevention. Theoretically, postoperative adhesions can be reduced through the use of either physical or liquid barriers to prevent 2 surfaces damaged in the course of a surgical procedure from being in contact with each other.

Most of the agents used to reduce postoperative adhesions have been found to be effective in animal models of adhesion formation. Oxidized regenerated cellulose (Interceed) is the best-studied agent to prevent adhesion formation and has been shown to reduce the incidence of pelvic adhesion formation, both new and reformation, following laparoscopic surgery and laparotomy. It would, therefore, be the best choice at this time for this patient. This agent becomes a gel shortly after placement on a surgically traumatized pelvic surface. The gel reduces the formation of fibrin bridges between tissue surfaces and, thus, makes the chance of adhesion formation less likely. The material is resorbed within a few weeks as it is metabolized into glucose and glucuronic acid. Interceed has been demonstrated to reduce adhesion formation in women in well-controlled randomized prospective studies. In one study of 66 women with bilateral adnexal adhesions, the use of Interceed on the adnexa of one side resulted in a 39% reduction of postoperative adhesion scores compared with the contralateral side without the membrane. The use of Interceed also has been reported to decrease by 2-fold the number of adnexal adhesions found at laparoscopy. Similar findings have been reported after ovarian surgery. However, no studies have reported improved fecundity or pain reduction as an outcome.

There is evidence that bioabsorbable membrane/antiadhesive (Seprafilm) is effective in preventing adhesion formation in women following myomectomy. To date, however, no data are available for the prevention of pelvic adhesions after laparoscopic surgery for endometriosis, and no studies have reported improvement in fecundity as an outcome. Studies have reported that expanded polytetrafluoroethylene (Gore-Tex) may be superior to Interceed in preventing adhesion formation at sites other than the pelvis. Its usefulness is limited because of the need for suturing the material at the surgical sites and subsequent later removal, which exposes the patient to a greater surgical risk and repeated operations.

There currently are no control trials that have shown that the installation of intraperitoneal dexamethasone or crystalloid solution, either in the form of normal saline or Ringer's lactate, decreases the formation of postoperative adhesions or improves fertility. Although studies have reported that indomethacin (Indocin) reduces inflammation postoperatively, to date no clinical trial has shown evidence of prevention of adhesions. The installation of 32% dextran 70 (Hyskon) has been used extensively in gynecologic surgery, but the results of clinical trials have been mixed. Two large human trials suggested a beneficial action, while 2 others were unable to substantiate this claim.

The efficacy of Interceed(TC7)* for prevention of reformation of postoperative adhesions on ovaries, fallopian tubes, and fimbriae in microsurgical operations for fertility: a multicenter study. Nordic Adhesion Prevention Study Group. Fertil Steril 1995;63:709–14.

Farquhar C, Vandekerckhove P, Watson A, Vail A, Wiseman D. Barrier agents for preventing adhesions after surgery for sub-fertility (Cochrane Review). In: The Cochrane Library, Issue 2, 2004. Chichester, UK: John Wiley & Sons Ltd.

99

Complications of endometrial ablation

A 42-year-old woman, gravida 2, para 2, with congestive heart failure and iron deficiency anemia has severe menorrhagia from a 3 cm submucosal myoma. A hysteroscopic resection and endometrial ablation is scheduled. The optimal intraoperative management would involve which type of electrosurgical resectoscope and distention medium?

	Electrosurgical resectoscope	Distention medium
* (A)	bipolar	normal saline
(B)	bipolar	1.5% glycine
(C)	monopolar	normal saline
(D)	monopolar	1.5% glycine
(E)	monopolar	3% sorbitol

Compared with thermal balloon and cryodestructive endometrial ablation, hysteroscopic approaches have increased intraoperative complication rates. In this patient, the presence of a submucosal fibroid excludes any nonhysteroscopic approach to ablation. Monopolar or bipolar thermal delivery devices used in hysteroscopy may be unaffected, assisted, or deterred by the distention media used to fill the uterine cavity.

The electrosurgical approach to hysteroscopy was originally limited to the monopolar resectoscopic loop and a nonconductive, hypo-osmotic distention media. For operative hysteroscopy, gynecologists adopted the use of

100

Risks of intracytoplasmic sperm injection

A 32-year-old man with normal gonadotropin levels has severe oligospermia on multiple semen analyses. He and his wife request information about intracytoplasmic sperm injection. You counsel the couple that with the following condition 100% of male children will be affected.

* (A) Y chromosome microdeletion
   (B) Mutation in the cystic fibrosis transmembrane conductance regulator gene
   (C) Premature testicular failure
   (D) Congenital bilateral absence of the vas deferens

Analysis of 2 semen samples is recommended before categorizing a man as having oligospermia (ie, less than 20 million sperm/mL). Approximately 5–15% of men with azoospermia (ie, no sperm in ejaculate) or severe oligospermia (ie, less than 2–3 million sperm/mL) have chromosomal abnormalities. Microdeletions of the Y chromosome are detected in 10–15% of men with azoospermia and 3–10% of men with oligospermia. These microdeletions are too small to be detected by a routine karyotype but can be identified with gene probes along the Y chromosome.

Most deletions occur in nonoverlapping regions of the long arm of the Y chromosome (*Yq11*) that contain multiple genes important for spermatogenesis. These regions have been designated *AZFa, AZFb,* and *AZFc*. Deletions in these areas provide prognostic information. For example, sperm retrieval from testicular biopsy in men with azoospermia with the *AZFa* and *AZFb* region deletions is extremely poor. Sons of affected individuals will inherit the microdeletion and may be infertile. Although a Y chromosomal microdeletion is not known to be associated with other health problems, few data regarding the phenotypes of sons of affected men are available. Balanced translocations and sex chromosome anomalies may occur in men with azoospermia. The most common sex chromosome abnormality detected in men with nonobstructive azoospermia is Klinefelter's syndrome (47,XXY).

Approximately 10–15% of men with azoospermia have congenital bilateral absence of the vas deferens. Two thirds of the men with congenital bilateral absence of the vas deferens will have documented mutations of the cystic fibrosis transmembrane conductance regulator gene. Unilateral obstruction is not associated with oligospermia and may go unrecognized unless it is associated with other genital abnormalities.

Premature testicular failure is reflected by hypergonadotropic gonadal failure with elevated serum gonadotropin levels, low testosterone concentrations, and azoospermia. Severe oligospermia does not predispose

101

Evaluation of chronic pelvic pain

A 25-year-old nulligravid woman seeks nonsurgical management of her pelvic pain. She describes the pain as persistent lower abdominal pain that increases in severity immediately preceding and following menses. She has been treated in the past with antibiotics, cyclic oral contraceptives, and nonsteroidal antiinflammatory drugs (NSAIDs); however, none has resolved her pain. You suspect she has endometriosis, and you have chosen not to perform laparoscopy. Based on your clinical suspicion of endometriosis and her desire to avoid surgery, the best medication to prescribe to relieve her pelvic pain is

* (A) gonadotropin-releasing hormone (GnRH) agonist
* (B) danazol (Danocrine)
* (C) continuous oral contraceptives
* (D) depot medroxyprogesterone acetate

Endometriosis is common in women of reproductive age, with the mean age of diagnosis being 25–29 years. Medical management is an appropriate first therapeutic step for a symptomatic young woman suspected of having endometriosis.

Gonadotropin-releasing hormone agonists are derived from the decapeptide hormone, GnRH. Pituitary gonadotropin secretion is suppressed during treatment with a GnRH agonist and results in induction of a pseudoprepubertal state, characterized by low serum gonadotropin and estradiol concentrations. Depending on the extent of the disease, GnRH agonist therapy can improve symptoms of endometriosis in up to 90% of patients. An initial 6-month course of GnRH agonist therapy is recommended. After a 6-month course of therapy, ovarian function usually returns to normal within 6–12 weeks. Long-term treatment is not recommended unless addback progestin or estrogen plus progestin are used because of the risk of osteoporosis from the hypoestrogenic state induced during therapy with a GnRH agonist.

In a randomized, double-blind, controlled trial, women aged 18–45 years with moderate to severe pelvic pain of at least 6 months' duration underwent extensive, noninvasive diagnostic testing and laboratory evaluation, including pelvic ultrasonography, complete blood count, erythrocyte sedimentation rate, and endocervical cultures. Women who had clinically suspected endometriosis received either leuprolide acetate, 3.75 mg per month, or placebo for 3 months. Posttreatment laparoscopy was used to evaluate the accuracy of the clinical diagnosis of endometriosis. At 12 weeks, the 49 women who received leuprolide acetate had clinically and statistically significant mean improvements from baseline in all pain measures, which also were significantly greater than that reported by the 46 women in the placebo group. Laparoscopically confirmed endometriosis was found in 78% of the leuprolide group and 87% of the placebo group, confirming the success of empiric use of depot leuprolide for treating patients with chronic pelvic pain and clinically suspected endometriosis.

Importantly, the addition of add-back therapy to treatment with a GnRH agonist reduces or eliminates side effects and allows the best opportunity for continued therapy. This makes GnRH agonist the best choice for this patient.

Danazol (Danocrine) is an orally active synthetic steroid. Acting as an androgen, it induces pituitary suppression, resulting in a state of hypoestrogenemia.

Danazol also directly inhibits ovarian steroidogenesis, displaces estrogen from its receptor, and inhibits hepatic synthesis of sex hormone-binding globulin. In women with endometriosis, danazol improves symptoms in 66–100% of patients; however, up to 66% discontinue therapy because of its androgenic side effects, which include oily skin, acne, hirsutism, and deepening of the voice. In addition, anabolic effects, such as weight gain, and hypoestrogenemic effects, such as breast atrophy and hot flushes, are common symptoms. There is no way to eliminate these side effects short of discontinuing therapy, and this makes danazol a poor choice for this patient.

Although most clinicians start patients on oral contraceptives as first-line therapy for chronic pelvic pain caused by suspected endometriosis, there are no data from randomized, placebo-controlled trials regarding its use. In patients with endometriosis-associated pain, high-dose preparations of combination oral contraceptives have been shown to be effective. Only low-dose oral contraceptives are currently available. There are no data to support their ability to relieve pain in women with endometriosis. In addition, data are lacking to show continuous oral contraceptives are better than cyclic oral contraceptives. Thus, continuous oral contraceptives would not be an appropriate choice for this patient. The use of oral contraceptives in combination with NSAIDs, which have not previously provided relief for this patient, also is not supported by the data.

High doses of progestins suppress pituitary gonadotropin secretion, causing decreased ovarian estrogen production. Complete resolution of pain in as many as 50% of women with endometriosis has been reported with administration of depot medroxyprogesterone acetate, with partial relief in an additional 15% of women. A significant incidence of headache, fluid retention, and weight gain is associated with high progestin doses that often lead to noncompliance or discontinuation of therapy. There is no option but to discontinue progestin therapy should these side effects arise, and, thus, depot medroxyprogesterone acetate is not the best choice for this patient.

Use of the long-acting progestin, depot medroxyprogesterone acetate, also can result in prolonged disturbance of normal hypothalamic–pituitary–ovarian function. Long-term use also has been associated with reduced bone mineral density. Abnormal bleeding or spotting is a persistent side effect and can occur in up to 40% of patients taking high-dose progestin therapy for endometriosis.

Guarnaccia MM, Olive DL. Diagnosis and management of endometriosis. In: Carr BR, Blackwell RE, eds. Reproductive medicine. 2nd ed. Stamford (CT): Appleton and Lange; 1998. p. 641–63.

Ling FW. Randomized controlled trial of depot leuprolide in patients with chronic pelvic pain and clinically suspected endometriosis. Pelvic Pain Study Group. Obstet Gynecol 1999;93:51–8.

Martin DC, Ling FW. Endometriosis and pain. Clin Obstet Gynecol 1999;42:664–86.

Vercellini P, Cortesi I, Crosignani PG. Progestins for symptomatic endometriosis: a critical analysis of the evidence. Fertil Steril 1997;68: 393–401.

Vercellini P, Trespidi L, Colombo A, Vendola N, Marchini M, Crosignani PG. A gonadotropin-releasing hormone agonist versus a low-dose oral contraceptive for pelvic pain associated with endometriosis. Fertil Steril 1993;60:75–9.

102
Indicators for future fractures

A 55-year-old postmenopausal woman has a lateral chest X-ray that shows 2 prior vertebral crush fractures. She is 1.68 m (5 ft 6 in.) tall, weighs 41 kg (110 lb), and smokes 8 cigarettes per day. A dual-energy X-ray absorptiometry scan of her femur shows a bone mineral density (BMD) of 0.723 mg/cm^2 (T score –1.3, Z score –0.4) (Fig. 102-1; see color plate). Her mother died at age 70 years, 3 months after a hip fracture. Given this patient's history, her greatest risk factor for a future fracture is

    (A) low bone mass
* (B) previous vertebral fractures
    (C) smoking history
    (D) weight
    (E) family history

The epidemiology of vertebral fractures, when compared with that of hip fractures, is less well established. This is mainly because there is no universally accepted definition of vertebral fracture, and, because of their asymptomatic nature, a large proportion of such fractures escape clinical recognition. Only approximately one third of women with vertebral fractures observed on X-rays receive medical attention and only 10% require hospital admission. One quarter of vertebral fractures result from traumatic falls, and the remainder occur as a result of daily activity.

The National Osteoporosis Foundation has established guidelines for BMD testing. All women older than 65 years, and women younger than 65 years who have 1 or more risk factors for osteoporosis other than menopause, should be screened. Smoking, body weight less than 57.6 kg (127 lb), a first-degree relative with an osteoporotic fracture, and a personal history of a fracture as an adult are all considered risk factors for future osteoporotic fracture. In the patient described, many of those risk factors are present. It is important to recognize that an individual with any previous adult fracture from any cause carries the highest risk for future osteoporotic fracture at any site.

Women who have osteopenia are thought to have approximately a 2-fold increase in fracture rate compared with women who have normal BMD. Each standard deviation decrease in lumbar BMD is associated with approximately a 2-fold increase in spine fracture risk. However, having evidence of a previous fracture, even if clinically asymptomatic, places this patient at a 4-fold greater risk for future fracture. This increased risk exists regardless of BMD so that vertebral fractures that occur atraumatically represent underlying bone fragility not measured by BMD. This patient with 2 vertebral crush fractures by definition has severe osteoporosis.

Efforts to identify other risk factors for future vertebral fractures remain inconsistent and vary between men and women. In women, other risk factors that have been reported for vertebral fractures include late menarche, early menopause, short duration of fertility, low consumption of diary products, reduced physical activity, and family history of hip fracture. Few of these risk factors are potent and some may only be associated with severe vertebral deformities.

Cooper C, Atkinson EJ, O'Fallon WM, Melton LJ III. Incidence of clinically diagnosed vertebral fractures: a population-based study in Rochester, Minnesota, 1985–1989. J Bone Miner Res 1992;7:221–7.

Cummings SR, Nevitt MC, Browner WS, Stone K, Fox KM, Ensrud KE, et al. Risk factors for hip fractures in white women. Study of Osteoporotic Fractures Research Group. N Engl J Med 1995;332:767–73.

Incidence of vertebral fracture in Europe: results from the European Prospective Osteoporosis Study (EPOS). J Bone Miner Res 2002;17:716–24.

National Osteoporosis Foundation. Physician's guide to prevention and treatment of osteoporosis. Belle Mead (NJ): Excerpta Medica; 1998.

Siris ES, Miller PD, Barrett-Connor E, Faulkner KG, Wehren LE, Abbott TA, et al. Identification and fracture outcomes of undiagnosed low bone mineral density in postmenopausal women: results from the National Osteoporosis Risk Assessment. JAMA 2001;286:2815–22.

Wu F, Mason B, Horne A, Ames R, Clearwater J, Liu M, et al. Fractures between the ages of 20 and 50 years increase women's risk of subsequent fractures. Arch Intern Med 2002;162:33–6.

103

Management of androgen insensitivity syndrome

A 16-year-old adolescent with no history of sexual activity is being evaluated for primary amenorrhea. On physical examination, she has Tanner stage IV breast development, Tanner stage II pubic hair, a 2 cm vaginal pouch, no visible cervix, and no palpable uterus or ovaries. Laboratory analysis reveals a follicle-stimulating hormone level of 8.3 mIU/mL, testosterone level of 811 ng/dL, and a 46,XY karyotype. The next step in management for this patient is

    (A) breast augmentation
    (B) estrogen therapy
    (C) vaginoplasty
*   (D) psychologic counseling

The incidence of complete androgen insensitivity has been estimated to be as high as 1 in 20,000. In some series, it is the third most frequent cause of primary amenorrhea after gonadal dysgenesis and müllerian agenesis. The diagnosis of androgen insensitivity syndrome in an adolescent or adult usually is not difficult. Typically, the patient is a phenotypic female seen for primary amenorrhea and found to have little or no axillary and pubic hair, no uterus, a 46,XY karyotype, and serum testosterone concentration characteristic of normal adult men (Figs. 103-1 and 103-2; see color plates).

The internal genitalia are characterized by absence or near absence of all structures except the testes, which may be located in the abdomen, in the inguinal canal, or in the labia majora. A lack of androgen tissue receptors results in scant pubic and axillary hair. These patients are taller than normal women with average height 172 cm (67.7 in.). Many patients have a small vaginal pouch, the embryonic remnant of the prostatic utricle, which can be lengthened with the aid of vaginal dilators, sexual intercourse, or by surgical creation of a neovagina.

Women with androgen insensitivity have a female body habitus secondary to peripheral aromatization of androgens to estrogens. The breast development appears normal because they lack androgen antagonism at the level of the breast. These patients typically have a paucity of glandular tissue and small pale areolae. Nevertheless, there is rarely a need for breast augmentation.

Estrogen treatment is indicated when gonadectomy is performed after puberty or at the time of expected puberty if gonadectomy is performed prepubertally. Psychologic development is feminine, including typical maternal instincts.

Nonsurgical approaches to the creation of a vagina, such as use of progressively larger dilators, are used more commonly today than in the past. Such methods are felt to be at least as successful as vaginoplasty and are not associated with surgical complications.

Most patients report satisfactory outcome after vaginoplasty, as well as normal libido and ability to achieve orgasm. A vaginoplasty should not be attempted until the patient is ready to become sexually active. Lack of use of the newly created vagina will result in agglutination, scarring, and obliteration of the vaginal canal.

Opinions differ as to how much and when women with androgen insensitivity should be told about their diagnosis. Most recommend that women be informed about the diagnosis and appropriate education be provided gradually, based on the age and maturity of the patient. Such disclosure prevents the unfortunate event of the patient learning the diagnosis inadvertently. Consent for surgical treatment, such as gonadectomy, requires full disclosure. It can be devastating emotionally for a patient to discover that her chromosomal and gonadal sex are not consistent with the phenotypic sex, and severe psychiatric problems can arise. Psychologic counseling is recommended and disclosure must be individualized, usually after consultation with the family and development of a support network.

The testes have the histologic appearance of undescended testes with a normal or increased number of Leydig cells and no spermatogenesis. Because patients with complete androgen insensitivity have a normal pubertal growth spurt, they feminize at the time of expected puberty, and any gonadal tumors in these patients do not develop until after puberty, gonadectomy should be delayed until sexual maturation is complete. Testicular tumors rarely develop before age 20 years in patients with androgen insensitivity syndrome.

Goodall J. Helping a child to understand her own testicular feminisation. Lancet 1991;337:33–5.

Sultan C, Lumbroso S, Paris F, Jeandel C, TerouanneB, Belon C, et al. Disorders of androgen action. Semin Reprod Med 2002;20:217–28.

Wisniewski AB, Migeon CJ, Meyer-Bahlburg HF, Gearhart JP, Berkovitz GD, Brown TR, et al. Complete androgen insensitivity syndrome: long-term medical, surgical, and psychosexual outcome. J Clin Endocrinol Metab 2000;85:2664–9.

104

Intracytoplasmic sperm injection for male infertility

An infertile couple is contemplating in vitro fertilization (IVF) after previous failed therapies. They have heard about the use of intracytoplasmic sperm injection (ICSI) in assisted reproductive technology (ART) but do not know if it is indicated in their case. The most appropriate indication for use of ICSI during IVF is

* (A) sperm count of 5 million per mL
* (B) sperm motility of 50%
* (C) semen volume of 0.5 cc
* (D) strict morphology of 8% normal sperm

The ICSI procedure involves injection of a single human sperm into the cytoplasm of a mature egg with the use of a microinjection technique. The procedure was first successfully used in Belgium in 1992, and it is now the preferred technique for severe male factor infertility. In the past, the only options for these patients were IVF with decreased rates and child adoption.

In the infertile couple who is considering IVF where there are no female factors, a low sperm count (less than 20 million/mL) may be a criterion for ICSI in some patients (Appendix E). The procedure can be done with ejaculated, epididymal, or testicular sperm for a variety of urologic indications, such as ejaculatory duct obstruction, failed vasectomy reversal (vasoepididymostomy or vasovasostomy), congenital bilateral absence of the vas deferens, and extensive scarring from herniorrhaphy repair or previous infection. In addition to male factor issues, ICSI also may be indicated for previous failed fertilization, unexplained infertility, poor egg quality, and preimplantation genetic diagnosis.

This information becomes useful in the evaluation of couples before undergoing IVF to optimize the chance for fertilization and embryo development. The most recent data from the Society for Assisted Reproductive Technology reveal an increase in male factor infertility with use of ICSI in IVF clinics across the country. Patients should be counseled appropriately about undergoing ICSI before attempting an IVF cycle. Studies suggest a small but significant increase in the risk of sex chromosomal abnormalities and congenital malformations in infants born to women who have undergone ICSI during ART procedures.

It is important to counsel patients that the use of ICSI in the treatment of male infertility caused by oligospermia or azoospermia (no sperm in the ejaculate) may result in new mutations or genetic transmission of chromosomal abnormalities in their offspring. Specific examples include Y microdeletions from DAZ (deleted in azoospermia) mutations in males with oligospermia, sex chromosomal abnormalities that may result from offspring of males with Klinefelter's syndrome (47, XXY), or the possibility of cystic fibrosis transmission in males with congenital bilateral absence of the vas deferens. These disorders have become more common presentations for fertility treatment in ART clinics. Thus, prenatal screening is justified in these couples until larger studies are completed.

Of the indications given, the low sperm count is the most appropriate indication for ICSI in this couple. Patients with normal semen parameters (eg, 50% motility) do not necessarily require ICSI with the associated risks described. Routine IVF is appropriate for these couples. Because sperm are processed in vitro before artificial insemination, a low semen volume with normal parameters does not indicate that ICSI should be needed. Despite normal semen parameters, the sperm morphology involves a close look at 200 sperm using strict criteria and may reveal a significantly lower percentage of normal forms. Recent data also show that abnormal strict morphology of spermatozoa (less than 5% normal forms) results in decreased fertilization rates resulting in lower ongoing pregnancy rates. Use of ICSI during an IVF cycle can overcome this decrease in fertilization and improve overall pregnancy rates. The choice indicated, 8% normal sperm, was above this recommended range for ICSI. Intracytoplasmic sperm injection may be an option for previously failed IVF but only after other more appropriate indications have been eliminated. This choice is not considered the most common indication for ICSI.

Although ICSI has become the mainstay of treatment for severe male factor, it does not prevent the possibility of passing on genetically abnormal sperm that may result in future infertility or aneuploidy in male offspring, even with highly specialized sperm function testing or sperm selection at the time of ICSI. Male factor patients must be evaluated and counseled appropriately because, even despite ICSI, the pregnancy rates are decreased with abnormal semen parameters including strict morphology. The unfortunate reality of male factor infertility is that other than the use of ICSI, medical therapy or urologic intervention do not significantly improve fertilization rates and overall pregnancy outcome, thus limiting the most successful options to ART with ICSI.

Assisted reproductive technology in the United States: 1999 results generated for the American Society for Reproductive Medicine/Society for Assisted Reproductive Technology Registry. American Society for Reproductive Medicine and Society for Assisted Reproductive Technology. Fertil Steril 2002;78:918–31.

Johnson MD. Genetic risks of intracytoplasmic sperm injection in the treatment of male infertility: recommendations for genetic counseling and screening. Fertil Steril 1998;70:397–411.

Palermo G, Joris H, Devroey P, Van Steirteghem AC. Pregnancies after intracytoplasmic injection of single spermatozoon into an oocyte. Lancet 1992;340:17–8.

Palermo GD, Neri QV, Hariprashad JJ, Davis OK, Veeck LL, Rosenwaks Z. ICSI and its outcome. Semin Reprod Med 2000;18:161–9.

105

Depot medroxyprogesterone and abnormal bleeding

A 25-year-old woman requests depot medroxyprogesterone acetate contraception. She is most interested in the convenience of this method because she lives close to a health center, which could provide the injections. She is concerned about rumors she has heard about bleeding problems associated with depot medroxyprogesterone acetate. The medical intervention that is likely to enhance continued use of this method is

      (A) intermittent estrogen
      (B) monthly depot medroxyprogesterone acetate injections
      (C) ibuprofen
*   (D) pretreatment counseling
      (E) raloxifene

Injectable contraception offers users convenient, safe, and reversible contraception that is more effective than sterilization. Depot medroxyprogesterone is provided in the United States in prefilled ampules or syringes containing 150 mg of aqueous microcrystalline suspension. Serum concentrations of medroxyprogesterone acetate are 1 ng/mL 3 months following injection of depot medroxyprogesterone acetate and are enough to prevent ovulation. Serum levels decrease to undetectable between 7–9 months, and when levels decrease to less than 0.1 ng/mL, ovulation returns.

Menstrual disturbances are the most common symptom and reason for depot medroxyprogesterone acetate discontinuation. In one study after 3 months of use, 46% of women reported amenorrhea, 46% reported irregular bleeding or spotting, and 26% reported longer menses. The rate of amenorrhea has been shown to increase over time, and at 1 year, it is nearly 70%. Among women who experience excessive bleeding, the bleeding decreases over time but remains at approximately 10% among users who continue depot medroxyprogesterone acetate after 1 year.

A World Health Organization study was completed on a large group of depot medroxyprogesterone acetate users who requested treatment for bleeding. Adding ethinyl estradiol (50 µg/day for 14 days) was compared with women who used estrone sulfate (2.5 mg/day for 14 days) and to women who took a placebo for bleeding episodes. Ethinyl estradiol successfully stopped the bleeding episode for which it was given in 93% of cases compared with 76% and 74% for estrone sulfate and placebo, respectively. The long-term bleeding reduction with a 2-week course of ethinyl estradiol was marginal, however, because bleeding became more unpredictable, and did not improve over the following weeks or months. User acceptability did not improve in any of the estrogen treatment groups.

Other progestin-only methods of contraception have similar problems with menstrual disturbances. Ibuprofen for 5 days has been investigated to help reduce the number of bleeding days with subdermal levonorgestrel implants (Norplant). A mild benefit was observed, but it was less than that seen with the addition of ethinyl estradiol. No published study to date has shown ibuprofen to improve continued use of depot medroxyprogesterone acetate. A pilot study using raloxifene with depot medroxyprogesterone acetate showed no decrease in number of bleeding days; therefore, it would not be the best option for this patient.

The effect of structured pretreatment contraceptive counseling has been studied with respect to depot medroxyprogesterone acetate. Subjects were informed of the expected hormonal effects and probable side effects of depot medroxyprogesterone acetate. Method discontinuation rates were significantly lower in the structured counseling group (11%) compared with the routine counseling group (42%). Side effects anticipated with depot medroxyprogesterone acetate are menstrual changes as described, with weight increases of 2.5 kg (5.5 lb) at 1 year, 3.6 kg (8 lb) at 2 years, and 6.35 kg (14 lb) at 4 years and mood changes (ie, depression reported at increased frequency at 3 months post injection) being the most common. Administration of depot medroxyprogesterone acetate will likely help alleviate dysmenorrhea, premenstrual symptoms, pain in women with endometriosis, and ovulatory pain.

Diaz S, Croxatto HB, Pavez M, Belhadj H, Stern J, Sivin I. Clinical assessment of treatments for prolonged bleeding in users of Norplant implants. Contraception 1990;42:97–109.

Kaunitz A. Injectable contraception. New and existing options. Obstet Gynecol Clin North Am 2000;27:741–80.

Lei ZW, Wu SC, Garceau RJ, Jiang S, Yang QZ, Wang WL, et al. Effect of pretreatment counseling on discontinuation rates in Chinese women given depo-medroxyprogesterone acetate for contraception. Contraception 1996;53:357–61.

Mishell DR Jr. Pharmacokinetics of depot medroxyprogesterone acetate contraception. J Reprod Med 1996;41(5 suppl):381–90.

Sangi-Haghpeykar H, Poindexter AN 3rd, Bateman L, Ditmore JR. Experiences of injectable contraceptive users in an urban setting. Obstet Gynecol 1996;88:227–33.

106

Insulin resistance in polycystic ovary syndrome

A 24-year-old woman with a longstanding history of oligomenorrhea, facial hirsutism, and acanthosis nigricans has recently received a diagnosis of insulin-resistant polycystic ovary syndrome (PCOS). Her oral glucose tolerance test (OGTT) revealed a glucose level of 156 mg/dL at 2 hours. The diagnosis was confirmed by a fasting plasma glucose level of 115 mg/dL and a serum insulin level of 30 µU/mL. The patient is confused about her diagnosis and wants to know why she is not considered to have diabetes at this point. You inform the patient that the criterion for a diagnosis of diabetes mellitus is

(A) a 2-hour plasma glucose level of at least 150 mg/dL
(B) a random plasma glucose level greater than or equal to 126 mg/dL
(C) an elevated fasting glucose to insulin ratio
* (D) a fasting plasma glucose level greater than or equal to 126 mg/dL
(E) an elevated 2-hour insulin level

Polycystic ovary syndrome affects approximately 5% of all women in the United States, approximately one half of whom demonstrate insulin resistance that leads to the development of hyperinsulinemia, even with normal pancreatic β-cell function. Several methods are used to identify insulin-resistant PCOS. Measuring glucose and insulin levels 2 hours postprandial or following a 75-g glucose intake will detect more than 80% of patients with PCOS who have insulin resistance and hyperinsulinemia. The American Diabetes Association recommends a fasting (not random) plasma glucose level of greater than or equal to 126 mg/dL be considered diagnostic for diabetes mellitus. If a patient has a fasting glucose level between 115 mg/dL and 140 mg/dL, an OGTT may help in the diagnosis of type 2 diabetes mellitus.

In patients with PCOS, excess insulin acts synergistically with luteinizing hormone on ovarian stroma, increasing androgen secretion. Insulin resistance predisposes these patients to the development of type 2 diabetes mellitus. A study that followed women for 22–31 years found that in women with PCOS, diabetes mellitus had been diagnosed in 15% of the women, compared with 2.3% of controls. Women with PCOS who have a family history of type 2 diabetes mellitus have a further increased risk of developing pancreatic β-cell dysfunction.

This patient does not meet the criteria for type 2 diabetes mellitus because her fasting glucose level does not exceed 125 mg/dL. However, insulin resistance often predisposes a woman to developing type 2 diabetes mellitus, especially if she is obese. In women younger than 50 years with PCOS, approximately 10% of nonobese women and 40–50% of obese women have insulin resistance or type 2 diabetes mellitus. One of the clinical signs associated with insulin resistance is acanthosis nigricans, observed in this patient, which also places her at greater risk for cardiovascular disease. Her ongoing care should include follow-up for possible development of diabetes mellitus, which is easily accomplished by measuring fasting glucose levels (Table 106-1) every 1–3 years. A fasting plasma glucose level of 126 mg/dL or greater confirmed by repeat testing is diagnostic of diabetes mellitus. Values between 110 mg/dL and 125 mg/dL imply impaired glucose tolerance and warrant follow-up.

Type 2 diabetes mellitus places patients at risk for retinopathy, nephropathy, neuropathy, and atherosclerotic coronary and peripheral vascular disease. In addition, the resulting hyperinsulinemia may lead to abdominal obesity, hypertension, hyperlipidemia, and coronary artery disease (ie, insulin resistance syndrome). Therefore, in overweight patients with type 2 diabetes mellitus, diet and exercise to reduce weight should be the most important considerations. If hyperglycemia is not improved by diet, a trial with an oral insulin-sensitizing agent, such as metformin, is indicated. Metformin may promote weight loss and reduces lipid levels by decreasing hepatic glucose production and may improve insulin sensitivity in those who lose weight.

TABLE 106-1. Testing for Diabetes

	Test		
Stage	**Fasting Plasma Glucose***	**Casual Plasma Glucose**	**Oral Glucose Tolerance Test**
Diabetes	Fasting plasma glucose[†] ≥126 mg/dL (7 mmol/L)	Casual[‡] plasma glucose ≥200 mg/dL (11.1 mmol/L) plus symptoms	2-h plasma glucose[§] 200 mg/dL
Impaired glucose homeostasis	Impaired fasting glucose = fasting plasma glucose ≥110 and <126 mg/dL		Impaired glucose tolerance = 2-h plasma glucose ≥140 and <200 mg/dL
Normal	Fasting plasma glucose <110 mg/dL		2-h plasma glucose <140 mg/dL

*The fasting plasma glucose is the preferred test for diagnosis, but any one of the three tests listed is acceptable. In the absence of unequivocal hyperglycemia with acute metabolic decompensation, one of these three tests should be used on a different day to confirm diagnosis.

[†]Fasting is defined as no caloric intake for at least 8 h.

[‡]Casual = any time of day without regard to time since the last meal; symptoms are the classic ones of polyuria, polydipsia, and unexplained weight loss.

[§]The oral glucose tolerance test should be performed using a glucose load containing the equivalent of 75 g anhydrous glucose dissolved in water. This test is not recommended for routine clinical use.

Rayburn WF. Diagnosis and classification of diabetes mellitus: highlights from the American Diabetes Association. J Reprod Med 1997;42:586

Dahlgren E, Johansson S, Lindstedt G, Knutsson F, Odén A, Janson PO, et al. Women with polycystic ovary syndrome wedge resected in 1956 to 1965: a long-term follow-up focusing on natural history and circulating hormones. Fertil Steril 1992;57:505–13.

Ehrmann DA, Sturis J, Byrne MM, Karrison T, Rosenfield RL, Polonsky KS. Insulin secretory defects in polycystic ovary syndrome. Relationship to insulin sensitivity and family history of non-insulin-dependent diabetes mellitus. J Clin Invest 1995;96:520–7.

Knochenhauer ES, Key TJ, Kahsar-Miller M, Waggoner W, Boots LR, Azziz R. Prevalence of the polycystic ovarian syndrome in unselected black and white women of the southeastern United States: a prospective study. J Clin Endocrinol Metab 1998;83:3078–82.

Legro RS, Kunselman AR, Dodson WC, Dunair A. Prevalence and predictors of risk for type 2 diabetes mellitus and impaired glucose tolerance in polycystic ovary syndrome: a prospective, controlled study in 254 affected women. J Clin Endocrinol Metab 1999;84:165–9.

107

Hydrosalpinges and success of in vitro fertilization

A 28-year-old nulligravid woman undergoes laparoscopy for persistent infertility and pelvic pain. Two years ago she had a bilateral neosalpingostomy. Based on the intraoperative findings (Figs. 107-1 and 107-2; see color plates), you perform a bilateral salpingectomy in preparation for future in vitro fertilization (IVF). The effect that the presence of hydrosalpinges during IVF would have is to

   (A) significantly increase the risk of pelvic infection after oocyte retrieval
   (B) decrease oocyte recruitment
* (C) decrease the rate of embryo implantation
   (D) retard in vitro embryonic cleavage rates

Tubal disease is one of the major causes of female infertility. Distal fallopian tube obstruction results in a hydrosalpinx. In vitro fertilization-embryo transfer (IVF-ET) was initially introduced to circumvent tubal disease as a cause of infertility. A hydrosalpinx can be diagnosed by hysterosalpingography or laparoscopy and occasionally by transvaginal ultrasonography. Normal fallopian tubes are difficult to discern via transvaginal ultrasonography unless pelvic fluid is present. In contrast, transvaginal ultrasonography may detect a hydrosalpinx by its adjacent location to the ovary and iliac vessels and its tubular appearance often with intraluminal longitudinal folds. The hydrosalpinx may increase in size during exogenous gonadotropin stimulation of the ovary during IVF-ET.

The presence of a hydrosalpinx adversely affects the success of IVF-ET. The number of oocytes harvested, the fertilization, and cleavage rates in women with hydrosalpinges who undergo IVF-ET are comparable with those of couples with male infertility or idiopathic causes of infertility. It is, therefore, hypothesized that retrograde flow of hydrosalpinx contents into the endometrial cavity adversely affects implantation rates. Hydrosalpinx contents may be directly toxic to embryos. In vitro murine embryo development is retarded when cultured in hydrosalpinx fluid.

The exact mechanism by which hydrosalpinx fluid may alter endometrial receptivity remains unclear. Endometrial glandular and stromal integrins are adhesion molecules that participate in cell-to-cell attachment and their presence may be crucial to implantation. Abnormal endometrial β-integrin expression has been described in women with hydrosalpinges. Integrin status has improved after salpingectomy.

Removal of the fallopian tubes has increased pregnancy rates in women with hydrosalpinges who subsequently undergo IVF-ET. It is unclear whether salpingectomy may adversely affect ovarian nerve and blood supply and, thus, have an impact on folliculogenesis and hormone production, but studies show no detrimental effect of salpingectomy on these parameters. One study concluded that laparoscopic salpingectomy should be considered for all women with hydrosalpinges who are scheduled to undergo IVF. Further research is required to assess the effectiveness of other pre-IVF surgical interventions, such as needle aspiration of hydrosalpinx fluid, which is associated with an extremely low incidence of pelvic infection, laparoscopic proximal tubal occlusion, or laparoscopic salpingostomy.

Eytan O, Azem F, Gull I, Wolman I, Elad D, Jaffa AJ. The mechanism of hydrosalpinx in embryo implantation. Hum Reprod 2001;16:2662–7.

Johnson NP, Mak W, Sowter MC. Laparoscopic salpingectomy for women with hydrosalpinges enhances the success of IVF: a Cochrane review. Hum Reprod 2002;17:543–8.

Meyer WR, Castelbaum AJ, Somkuti S, Sagoskin AW, Doyle M, Harris JE, et al. Hydrosalpinges adversely affect markers of endometrial receptivity. Hum Reprod 1997;12:1393–8.

108
Hormonal contraception and weight gain

A 17-year-old adolescent requests advice on different contraceptive methods. She currently uses an oral contraceptive (OC) with 20 µg ethinyl estradiol. She is unhappy with her current method because of a 4.5 kg (10 lb) weight gain. She desires reliable contraception. The most appropriate recommendation for contraception in this patient is to

* (A) continue use of current OC and begin counseling about diet and exercise
* (B) change to depot medroxyprogesterone acetate
* (C) change to a progestin-releasing intrauterine device (IUD)
* (D) change to a progestin-only OC
* (E) change to partner's use of latex condoms

Choices of contraceptive methods for the sexually active adolescent range from barrier techniques to hormonal contraception. The most commonly used contraceptive technique in this age group is the combination OC. In perfect use, OCs have a failure rate such that 0.1% of women experience an unintended pregnancy during the first year of use. Side effects of excessive weight gain have not been substantiated in controlled trials. In one study of 128 women over 4 cycles of OC use, 52% of women remained within 0.9 kg (2 lb) of their starting weight and 72% had either no weight change or a loss. Women who gain weight while using OCs should be counseled to increase their aerobic exercise per week and observe a diet plan.

Depot medroxyprogesterone acetate is an injectable progestin preparation administered intramuscularly every 3 months. Because the medication is given parenterally, compliance is optimal and the preparation is ideal for patients with contraindications to an estrogen-containing preparation. One prominent side effect noted by patients has been weight gain during depot medroxyprogesterone acetate use. In one study of 53 adolescent females who used depot medroxyprogesterone acetate, the average weight gain was 6 kg (13.2 lb) at 11 months and 9 kg (19.8 lb) at 17 months of use. In the first year of typical use, depot medroxyprogesterone acetate has a failure rate of 3%. Although it has a lower failure rate than OCs, the weight gain is greater with depot medroxyprogesterone acetate, a point that frequently is cited as a reason for discontinuation of its use. Therefore, depot medroxyprogesterone acetate would not be the treatment of choice for this patient who wishes to avoid weight gain.

Although the IUD has a low failure rate of 0.1% in its first year of use, the use of an IUD in the adolescent is not recommended because of the potential exposure to multiple sexual partners. The risk of developing pelvic inflammatory disease is unknown in this adolescent, but IUD use is best in a stable mutually monogamous relationship. Progestin-only OCs do not consistently inhibit ovulation, and, therefore, this method may not provide reliable contraception for this adolescent. The perfect use failure rate in the first year is 0.5%. Although latex condoms would provide the best protection from human immunodeficiency virus (HIV) and other sexually transmitted diseases (STDs), the failure rate in typical use is 15%. Natural membrane condoms may not provide adequate protection from STDs. For this adolescent, exclusive use of condoms by her partner may not give her the most reliable form of contraception she desires. If she does choose to rely exclusively on condom use, a prescription for emergency contraceptive pills (eg, Plan B or Preven) is advised. A condom break or slippage occurs in approximately 3–5% of acts of intercourse. The most common failure of the condom, however, is the male partner not using the condom during coitus. Condoms should be used in addition to other methods of contraception, such as OCs, to decrease the transmission of the HIV virus and other STDs. The use of these 2 "dual methods" would provide superior contraceptive protection than either method alone.

American College of Obstetricians and Gynecologists. Hyperprolactinemia and other pituitary disorders. In: Precis: an update in obstetrics and gynecology. Reproductive endocrinology. 2nd ed. Washington, DC: ACOG; 2002. p. 79–83.

Hatcher RA, Nelson AL, Zieman M, Darney PD, Creinin MD, Stosur HR, et al. A pocket guide to managing contraception. Tiger (GA): Bridging the Gap Foundation; 2003. p. 36–9, 51–4, 80–2, 117–8.

Rosenberg M. Weight change with oral contraceptive use and during the menstrual cycle. Results of daily measurements. Contraception 1998; 58:345–9.

Sangi-Haghpeykar H, Poindexter AN 3rd, Bateman L, Ditmore JR. Experience of injectable contraceptive users in an urban setting. Obstet Gynecol 1996;88:227–33.

109

Normal bone physiology

A 15-year-old adolescent presents with primary amenorrhea. There is no family history for developmental anomalies or delayed puberty. On physical examination, she is 1.73 m (5 ft 8 in.) tall, her arm span is 1.78 m (5 ft 10 in.), and she weighs 56.9 kg (127 lb). Her breasts are at Tanner stage I development, there is fine axillary hair, she has Tanner stage II pubic hair and a virginal introitus with small cervix, and the uterus is not palpable. Laboratory studies show normal thyroid-stimulating hormone and prolactin levels while follicle-stimulating hormone (FSH) and estradiol levels are low. She appears to have a normal sense of smell. The best next step in management is to obtain

(A) a pituitary stimulation test
(B) insulinlike growth factor (IGF)-1 level
(C) growth hormone (GH) level
* (D) an X-ray of her wrist
(E) karyotype

The delay in pubertal development and failure to achieve menstrual cycles are key features in patients with hypogonadotropic hypogonadism. This disorder is characterized by a deficiency in endogenous gonadotropin-releasing hormone (GnRH) secretion. This underlying defect could be caused by failure of the precursor GnRH neurons to migrate from the olfactory placode region to the mediobasal hypothalamus. Because the olfactory placode also may be affected, some patients with hypogonadotropic hypogonadism also will have defects in their sense of smell.

As a consequence of GnRH deficiency, both luteinizing hormone (LH) and FSH secretion are low and there is failure to appropriately stimulate ovarian follicular development and estradiol production. The other pituitary hormones remain unaffected. These hormones, which are responsible for adrenarche and pubarche (ie, adrenocorticotropic hormone) and skeletal growth (GH and IGF-I), will increase appropriately at puberty. The resultant phenotype is an individual with deficient estrogen and the lack of development or appropriate development in the estrogen target tissues, namely breast, uterus, endometrium, adipose tissue, and bone. Normal secretion of other pubertal hormones will lead to development of pubic and axillary hair and further skeletal growth. In the absence of estrogen, the bony epiphyses will undergo a delay in closure, allowing further disproportionate growth of long bones, which will lead to the arm span being greater than the overall height and a delay in bone age. Thus, bone age in these individuals will be less than chronologic age.

Recently, a male lacking functional estrogen receptor α was shown to have osteoporosis, reduced fertility, and failure of fusion of his long bones. This accident of nature serves to illustrate that estrogen plays a major role in bone mineralization in males and females as well as closure of the bony epiphyses.

Bone age can be estimated by an X-ray of the wrist using the Greulich and Pyle atlas and the adult height predicted using Bayley and Pinneau tables. In this patient, a delay in starting estrogen therapy will allow a longer growth period for the long bones before epiphyseal closure. Institution of estrogen therapy in this patient will result in an initial acceleration in growth followed by a closure of the epiphyses and attainment of her final adult height. In addition, estrogen will drive other estrogen-responsive target tissues resulting in further breast development, increase in hip fat deposition, as well as menses.

Pituitary stimulation testing will be normal for the thyroid, adrenal, and GH axes. Most commonly, there will be a lack of LH and FSH response to GnRH because the pituitary has not been adequately exposed to endogenous GnRH. This diagnostic approach will reaffirm that the patient has hypogonadotropic hypogonadism, but the tests will not affect her future management. Both GH and IGF-I levels will be in the normal range for her age because this neuroendocrine axis is unaffected by hypogonadotropic hypogonadism. Because the patient has demonstrated a growth pattern at the expected time, it is unlikely that there is abnormal secretion of GH and IGF-I. Individuals with hypogonadotropic hypogonadism do not have karyotypic abnormalities and ovarian reserve is normal.

de Waal WJ, Greyn-Fokker MH, Stijnen T, van Gurp EA, Toolens AM, de Munick Keizer-Schrama SM, et al. Accuracy of final height prediction and effect of growth-reductive therapy in 362 constitutionally tall children. J Clin Endocrinol Metab 1996;81:1206–16.

Gruber CJ, Tschugguel W, Schneeberger C, Huber JC. Production and actions of estrogens. N Engl J Med 2002;346:340–52.

Smith EP, Boyd J, Frank GR, Takahashi H, Cohen RM, Specker B, et al. Estrogen resistance caused by a mutation in the estrogen-receptor gene in a man. N Engl J Med 1994;331:1056–61.

Turner RT, Riggs BL, Spelsberg TC. Skeletal effects of estrogen. Endocr Rev 1994;15:275–300.

110

Transdermal patch versus vaginal ring

A 23-year-old nulligravid student requests a new contraceptive method. She wants something that has more predictable bleeding than an oral contraceptive because she is sometimes troubled by breakthrough bleeding. Her schedule is hectic, and she occasionally forgets to take her oral contraceptive but cannot always explain why she has spotting or delayed menses. She has contact dermatitis and a prior history of positive gonorrhea and chlamydia cultures. The contraceptive that you recommend is

    (A) copper intrauterine device (IUD)
* (B) vaginal contraceptive ring (NuvaRing)
    (C) transdermal contraceptive patch (Ortho Evra)
    (D) levonorgestrel intrauterine system

The NuvaRing is a novel contraceptive method approved by the U.S. Food and Drug Administration. It is inserted into the vagina and releases 15 µg of ethinyl estradiol and 120 µg of etonogestrel (active ingredient desogestrel), common ingredients in oral contraceptives. The Nuva-Ring completely inhibits ovulation during proper and extended use. Serum follicle-stimulating hormone is suppressed and no luteinizing hormone surge is detected in users. Progesterone levels are low, which means ovulation does not occur. Following discontinuation, there is rapid return to ovulation, much as with oral contraceptives. The ring is a transparent ethylene vinyl acetate copolymer that measures 54 mm (2.1 in.) in diameter and is 4 mm (0.16 in.) thick. It is inserted into the vagina for a 3-week period, then discarded. After 1 week (during which menses reliably occurs), a new ring is inserted. Timers are available to remind users to insert the ring after 7 days.

Breakthrough bleeding rates are less than 1% from the first month of use, and spotting occurs in approximately 4% of patients. In comparison studies, oral contraceptive users versus NuvaRing users show much higher breakthrough bleeding rates in the early months of use. Withdrawal bleeding occurred in 98.8% of all cycles in a study of 1,145 European women.

NuvaRing has been shown to have a neutral effect on body weight; 2% of users had a clinically significant (7% change) weight decrease, and 1.9% had a clinically significant weight increase. By contrast, among oral contraceptives users, 2% had a weight decrease but 7.6% experienced a significant weight increase. This difference could be related to decreased hepatic metabolism or lower estrogen levels with the ring. Over 3 menstrual cycles, 81% of users find the ring preferable to oral contraceptives, although 66% preferred oral contraceptives before trying the ring. Accordingly, with proper counseling, many women will find this method more satisfactory than their current approach. A small minority of partners (less than 5%) find the ring bothersome during intercourse, and the ring can be removed for 3 hours without any loss of efficacy. If left out for more than 3 hours, a back-up method is recommended during the next week because efficacy may decrease. Only 2.6% of women report ring expulsion.

The transdermal contraceptive patch (Ortho Evra) also is very well tolerated and has high user compliance. The patch delivers 20 µg of ethinyl estradiol and 150 µg of norelgestromin (17-deacetylnorgestimate) per day at a constant rate over 7 days. Menstrual cycle control is similar to oral contraceptive use. A major advantage over oral contraceptives is the 90% perfect adherence to the dosing schedule across all age groups. Partial or total detachment of the patch occurs at a rate of 3.8%, but the patch adheres well despite humid climates, vigorous exercise, or exposure to saunas and water baths. There is a transient increase in breast sensitivity and nipple tenderness in the first month that decreases thereafter. Effectiveness may be decreased in users who weigh more than 90 kg (198 lb). The transdermal patch may not be the preferred method in this patient with contact dermatitis.

The levonorgestrel intrauterine system (Mirena) releases levonorgestrel at a relatively constant rate over 5 years. Contraceptive effectiveness is similar to sterilization. A high rate of amenorrhea is observed after 3 months of use, but a substantial frequency of spotting occurs before that time. Reduction of menstrual flow is nearly 90%, comparable with endometrial ablation, and user satisfaction is high. Any IUD may not be the best choice for a woman with a history of sexually transmitted diseases. Such women should certainly be counselled about the use of condoms.

Bjarnadottir RI, Tuppurainen M, Killick SR. Comparison of cycle control with a combined contraceptive vaginal ring and oral levonorgestrel/ethinyl estradiol. Am J Obstet Gynecol 2002;186: 389–95.

Creasy GW, Abrams LS, Fisher AC. Transdermal contraception. Semin Reprod Med 2001;19:373–80.

Dieben TO, Roumen FJ, Apter D. Efficacy, cycle control, and user acceptability of a novel combined contraceptive vaginal ring. Obstet Gynecol 2002;100:585–93.

Mulders TM, Dieben TO, Bennink HJ. Ovarian function with a novel combined contraceptive vaginal ring. Hum Reprod 2002;17:2594–9.

Roumen F. Contraceptive efficacy and tolerability with a novel combined contraceptive vaginal ring, NuvaRing. Eur J Contracept Reprod Health Care 2002;7(suppl 2):19–24; discussion 37–9.

Zieman M, Guillebaud J, Weisberg E, Shangold GA, Fisher AC, Creasy GW. Contraceptive efficacy and cycle control with the Ortho Evra/Evra transdermal system: the analysis of pooled data. Fertil Steril 2002;77(2 suppl 2):S13–8.

111

Choice of agent in ovulation induction

A 28-year-old woman presents with a history of infrequent menstrual periods. Her last period was 4 months ago. Physical examination reveals a body mass index (BMI) of 26 kg/m^2 and galactorrhea bilaterally. Laboratory results show a negative β-hCG level, a normal thyroid-stimulating hormone (TSH) level, a dehydroepiandrosterone sulfate (DHEAS) level of 180 μg/dL, and a fasting prolactin level of 75 ng/mL. A repeat prolactin test confirms the prior elevated level. A magnetic resonance imaging (MRI) study of her pituitary gland is normal. The most appropriate next step in management is

     (A) clomiphene citrate (Clomid, Serophene)
     (B) dexamethasone (Decadron)
     (C) weight reduction
     (D) metformin (Glucophage)
*   (E) bromocriptine mesylate (Parlodel)

Chronic anovulation may result from a number of etiologies, including hyperprolactinemia, thyroid disorders, insulin resistance, or inappropriate gonadotropin secretion. In the evaluation of a patient with chronic anovulation with underlying hyperprolactinemia, the elevated prolactin level should be corrected before instituting any other therapy. Because an elevated level of thyroid-releasing hormone can lead to hyperprolactinemia, TSH should be measured to rule out primary hypothyroidism. Prolactin levels also may be elevated after meals, sleep, exercise, or breast stimulation or examination. To minimize falsely elevated levels, prolactin should be measured in a fasting state, a few hours after awakening. Although a pituitary microadenoma is not visualized in the anterior pituitary gland, a small focus of active prolactin-secreting adenoma cells (lactotropes) usually are present, which are below the detectable limit of the MRI study. Lactotrope cells make up 40–50% of the total pituitary cell population. They are located in the lateral wings of the anterior pituitary. If an adenoma increases in size leading to a visual disturbance, because of the position of the lactotropes, bitemporal hemianopsia results. Prolactin secretion is regulated by dopamine, which functions as a prolactin inhibiting factor. Use of a dopamine agonist, such as bromocriptine mesylate (Parlodel), is the mainstay of therapy.

Bromocriptine usually is started at a low dose at bedtime to prevent initial postural hypotension. Some patients will respond to 1.25 mg (one half a tablet) or 2.5 mg (1 tablet) of bromocriptine with a resumption of their menstrual cycles. Bromocriptine can be increased as often as weekly by measuring serum prolactin levels until they are in the normal range. If additional doses of bromocriptine are necessary, a morning dose of 2.5 mg can be added. The therapeutic dosage usually is 5–7.5 mg per day, up to a maximum of 10–15 mg per day, given in 2 or 3 divided doses. At higher doses, side effects are more frequent. Some gastrointestinal side effects (ie, nausea, vomiting) can be minimized by inserting the bromocriptine tablet in the vagina, where vaginal absorption in serum bromocriptine levels is comparable with oral administration. If side effects persist, some patients may demonstrate fewer symptoms with another dopamine agonist, cabergoline (Dostinex), which is given less frequently. Cabergoline is available as a 0.5 mg tablet. The initial dose is 0.25 mg (one half a tablet) twice weekly, which may be increased to a maximum of 1 mg twice weekly. Because of the increased cost of cabergoline, bromocriptine usually is instituted as first-line therapy. If prolactin levels return to normal and the patient is still anovulatory, clomiphene citrate can be added to the bromocriptine medication.

In this patient, who has no evidence of hyperandrogenism and a normal DHEAS level, the addition of dexamethasone (Decadron) to decrease the adrenal androgen level is not indicated. In an obese patient with a BMI greater than 28 kg/m², dietary counseling and daily exercise may be effective in development of spontaneous ovulatory cycles. If insulin resistance is present, correction with metformin (Glucophage) alone may result in ovulatory cycles. In a randomized, double-blind, placebo-controlled trial, metformin increased the ovulatory and pregnancy rates more than did clomiphene citrate in patients with polycystic ovary syndrome who were resistant to clomiphene citrate.

American College of Obstetricians and Gynecologists. Hyperprolactinemia and other pituitary disorders. In: Precis: an update in obstetrics and gynecology. Reproductive endocrinology. 2nd ed. Washington, DC: ACOG; 2002. p. 79–83.

Hoeger K. Obesity and weight loss in polycystic ovarian syndrome. Obstet Gynecol Clin North Am 2001;28:85–97, vi–vii.

Speroff L, Glass RH, Kase NG, eds. Clinical gynecologic endocrinology and infertility. 6th ed. Baltimore (MD): Lippincott Williams & Wilkins; 1999. p. 450–8.

Vandermolen DT, Ratts VS, Evans WS, Stovall DW, Kauma SW, Nestler JE. Metformin increases the ovulatory rate and pregnancy rate from clomiphene citrate in patients with polycystic ovary syndrome who are resistant to clomiphene citrate alone. Fertil Steril 2001;75:310–5.

112

Blastocysts and twinning

A couple with tubal factor infertility undergoes a treatment cycle with in vitro fertilization and transfer of one embryo on day 5 at the blastocyst stage. The transfer results in a twin pregnancy. The most likely explanation for this pregnancy outcome is

(A) embryology laboratory error
(B) spontaneous conception
(C) dizygotic twinning
* (D) monozygotic twinning

Multiple gestations are commonly associated with contemporary treatments for infertility that use assisted reproductive technology (ART). To increase the chance for pregnancy, more embryos are transferred into the uterus, resulting in a higher rate of multiple pregnancies. In recent years, embryo transfer at the blastocyst stage, 5 days after fertilization to decrease multiple gestations although improving implantation, has been associated with an increase in monozygotic twinning. In addition, some embryos that are left in culture until the blastocyst stage may not survive, thus limiting the number of embryos available for embryo transfer.

Monozygotic twinning occurs when an embryo splits before implantation during the first week after fertilization. Multiple fetuses may share one placenta or develop within the same gestational sac, depending on when the duplication occurs. The general incidence of monozygotic twinning is 0.42%. With blastocyst transfer, however, this increases to 1–9%, a 10-fold increase higher than the rate in the general population.

The mechanism of why there is an increase in monozygotic twinning with blastocyst transfer is unclear. One theory is that there is duplication of the embryo after splitting of the inner cell mass, which forms the embryo and placenta. Some studies reveal an increase in monozygotic twinning with micromanipulation where there is an opening made through the zona pellucida, the outer layer that surrounds the developing embryo. Micromanipulation involves procedures such as intracytoplasmic sperm injection to improve fertilization, assisted hatching to increase chance of implantation, and preimplantation genetic diagnosis, which can diagnose genetic defects in the developing embryo. Other studies that have made observations that are contrary to this theory have found that monozygotic twinning occurs at an increased rate despite micromanipulation after blastocyst transfer. In addition, the time of implantation, the use of ART, and the type of media used also have been linked to monozygotic twinning with blastocyst transfer. In comparison, the rate of monozygotic twinning is much lower after a more common day 3 or cleavage-stage embryo transfer than a day 5 blastocyst transfer.

Because only one embryo was transferred in this case, the possibility of dizygotic twins is eliminated. Compared with dizygotic twins, which develop within 2 different gestational sacs using 2 separate placentas, monozygotic twins are at increased risk for poor obstetric outcomes, including twin-to-twin transfusion, congenital malformations, as well as delivery and neonatal complications. Monozygotic twinning poses a risk to these pregnancies that is 3 times higher than dizygotic twins.

Overall, the literature supports a significant relationship between monozygotic twinning and the transfer of embryos at the blastocyst stage. In this case scenario, a laboratory error at the time of transfer or a spontaneous conception most likely would not be responsible for the monozygotic twinning. The clinical presentation represents an example of monozygotic twinning that occurred after a day 5 embryo transfer.

There is a significant increase in preterm birth rate in the United States because of the increase in multiple gestation directly related to the advent of ART. This recognized complication of ART can only be decreased by limiting the number of embryos that are transferred back into the uterus. Although blastocyst stage embryo transfer may decrease high-order multiple gestations, the iatrogenic risk of monozygotic twinning continues to exist and should be discussed with all couples that undergo this procedure.

Blickstein I, Verhoeven HC, Keith LG. Zygotic splitting after assisted reproduction. N Engl J Med 1999;340:738–9.

Milki AA, Jun SH, Hinckley MD, Behr B, Giudice LC, Westphal LM. Incidence of monozygotic twinning with blastocyst transfer compared to cleavage-stage transfer. Fertil Steril 2003;79:503–6.

Schachter M, Raziel A, Friedler S, Strassburger D, Bern O, Ron-El R. Monozygotic twinning after assisted reproductive techniques: a phenomenon independent of micromanipulation. Hum Reprod 2001;16:1264–9.

Tarlatzis BC, Qublan HS, Sanopoulou T, Zepiridis L, Grimbizis G, Bontis J. Increase in the monozygotic twinning rate after intracytoplasmic sperm injection and blastocyst stage embryo transfer. Fertil Steril 2002;77:196–8.

113

Achieving fertility with premature ovarian failure

A 29-year-old woman with type 1 diabetes mellitus has developed secondary amenorrhea as a result of premature ovarian failure. She is considering using an oocyte donor for in vitro fertilization. The donor who is most suitable for this patient is a

   (A) 17-year-old nulligravid sister with irregular menses
   (B) 24-year-old nulligravid half-sister with irregular menses
 * (C) 27-year-old, gravida 1, para 1, unrelated woman with regular menses
   (D) 22-year-old nulligravid unrelated woman with regular menses after chemotherapy
   (E) 33-year-old, gravida 3, para 3, unrelated woman with regular menses after tubal ligation

Oocyte donation to women with premature ovarian failure is associated with a high degree of success usually exceeding the cycle fecundability rate for spontaneously ovulatory women of the same age. The success of this process is dependent on multiple factors, including the choice of the oocyte donor. Some oocyte donors may be more preferable than others depending on their age, relationship to the donor, prior pregnancy history, and other risk factors.

With respect to age of the oocyte donor, the American Society for Reproductive Medicine recommends that donors be aged between 21 and 34 years. Donors younger than 30 years are preferable because they have a higher cycle fecundity rate than women older than 30 years. Although the sister of the woman with premature ovarian failure may be desirable for a genetic link, sisters of a woman with premature ovarian failure associated with an autoimmune disorder appear to be suboptimal in comparison with unrelated oocyte donors. In a study of 79 oocyte recipients, 66 recipients used unrelated anonymous donors whereas 13 used a sister as their oocyte donor. The cycle cancellations in the sisters group were 5-fold higher because of a poor response to gonadotropin stimulation. The mean baseline cycle day 3 follicle-stimulating hormone level in the sisters also was significantly higher than in the unrelated donors ($P < .05$), and sisters as a group used more gonadotropin ($P < .05$). In this study, if the cycle of stimulation was not cancelled, recipients using oocytes from a sister had a similar pregnancy rate as from an unrelated donor.

Oocyte donors with regular menstrual periods are preferable to donors with irregular menses. Although uncommon, any patient with irregular menses could have reduced ovarian reserve. In a study that examined the menstrual history of 48 women who developed spontaneous premature ovarian failure with a normal karyotype, menstrual irregularity was the most common initial symptom in 92% of the affected group. Women with a prior history of chemotherapy for Hodgkin's disease are at risk for the development of premature ovarian failure. In a study of 34 women with a history of regular menstrual cycles prior to chemotherapy, 76% became amenorrheic following treatment. In 10 women, their menses returned at a median age of 25 years (range 21–34 years), and there were 2 pregnancies in this group. In the remaining 16 women, amenorrhea persisted, and they became menopausal. In the original group of 34, 53% benefited from hormone therapy for chemotherapy-induced ovarian failure.

The optimal donor for this 29-year-old woman with type 1 diabetes and premature ovarian failure would be an unrelated woman, preferably younger than 30 years, with regular menses and no prior history of chemotherapy. The 17-year-old woman could donate, but donors younger than 21 years without children may regret their decision if they should subsequently become infertile. For the reasons listed previously, the 24-year-old nulligravid half-sister, with irregular menses would be less optimal because her cycles may be anovulatory or signify a predisposition to premature ovarian failure. In this clinical scenario, the 27-year-old unrelated woman, gravida 1, para 1, with regular menses would be the most suitable oocyte donor.

Alzubaidi NH, Chapin HL, Vanderhoof VH, Calis KA, Nelson LM. Meeting the needs of young women with secondary amenorrhea and spontaneous premature ovarian failure. Obstet Gynecol 2002;99:720–5.

Clark ST, Radford JA, Crowther D, Swindell R, Shalet SM. Gonadal function following chemotherapy for Hodgkin's disease: a comparative study of MVPP and a seven-drug hybrid regimen. J Clin Oncol 1995;13:134–9.

Guidelines for oocyte donation. American Society for Reproductive Medicine. Fertil Steril 2002;77(suppl 5):S6–8.

Remohi J, Gartner B, Gallardo E, Yalil S, Simon C, Pellicer A. Pregnancy and birth rates after oocyte donation. Fertil Steril 1997;67:717–23.

Sung L, Bustillo M, Mukherjee T, Booth G, Karstaedt A, Copperman AB. Sisters of women with premature ovarian failure may not be ideal ovum donors. Fertil Steril 1997;67:912–6.

114

Surgical therapy for septate uterus

A 28-year-old woman with history of recurrent abortion undergoes a diagnostic laparoscopy and subsequent operative hysteroscopy to incise a small uterine septum that occupies less than 50% of the uterine cavity. The procedure is uncomplicated, and there is no evidence of uterine perforation or damage to the surrounding endometrium. The most important next step in the clinical management of this patient in the postoperative period is

    (A) an intrauterine device (IUD)
    (B) oral estrogen for 2 weeks postoperatively
    (C) oral contraceptives
*   (D) hysterosalpingography (HSG)

Müllerian anomalies of the uterus constitute some of the most common types of malformations in the female reproductive tract, affecting 5% of this population. These congenital abnormalities are associated with recurrent pregnancy loss; infertility; and complicated obstetric outcomes, including preterm labor and abnormal fetal presentation. The most common of the uterine anomalies associated with the poorest reproductive outcome is the septate uterus. However, this particular type of congenital aberration is easily amenable to treatment by hysteroscopy. The uterine septum results after the müllerian ducts fuse but fail to resorb. The septum may be incomplete or extend into the cervix.

Diagnosis can be made by HSG, ultrasonography, or magnetic resonance imaging. However, all these imaging modalities have their limitations, and the diagnosis is commonly confirmed by the use of laparoscopy and hysteroscopy. Diagnostic evaluation at surgery may permit close evaluation of the uterine fundus and differentiate the septate uterus from the bicornuate.

Hysteroscopy has become the standard for surgical treatment of the septate uterus. Avoidance of laparotomy decreases the risks of intrauterine adhesions, uterine scarring from serosal incisions, decreases in uterine volume, and also negates the need for prolonged hospital stay and longer postoperative recovery.

Surgery for the septate uterus usually is performed in the proliferative phase of the menstrual cycle after menses have ceased. Preoperative preparation to thin the endometrium for best visualization can be done with hormonal manipulation using oral contraceptives, danazol (Danocrine), progestins, or gonadotropin-releasing hormone analogs.

Operative technique involves performing an incision on the septum to the level of the uterine fundus. This can be accomplished with the use of scissors, electrocautery, or laser. Because the septum is avascular, an incision through the septum between the anterior or posterior myometrial walls should result in minimal bleeding. The dissection is complete when both cornua can be visualized, and the operator can move easily from between the tubal ostia. Often, the second operator can visualize a uniform uterine "glow" through the laparoscope after the septum has been completed resected. The laparoscope also aids in monitoring the hysteroscopic portion of the surgery and may help enter a narrow cervix and prevent perforation.

After hysteroscopic lysis of the septum is performed, the patient can be managed in a variety of ways. However, there exists a lack of uniform consensus in the literature. The intrauterine device or balloon has not been proved to be effective in reducing adhesions. Use of antibiotics after surgery also has not been proved to be of benefit. In addition, a randomized study confirmed estrogen or hormonal therapy to promote epithelialization has no apparent role after resection of an avascular septum. Rather, this therapy might be useful after lysis of intrauterine adhesions to prevent recurrence within a damaged endometrial cavity.

Follow-up examination of the uterine cavity is uniformly recommended 1–2 months after hysteroscopic surgery. This can be accomplished with HSG, ultrasonography, or office hysteroscopy to ensure that resection of the septum is complete. An incomplete septum can be treated with a second procedure if this is deemed necessary. Residual septa less than 1 cm usually can be left alone and will not interfere with future fertility.

The uterine septum in this scenario is a likely cause for the recurrent pregnancy loss. After lysis of the septum, hormonal therapy with estrogen or oral contraceptives is not necessary nor is there the need for a uterine device, such as an IUD or pediatric Foley catheter. An HSG, ultrasonography, or hysteroscopy can be performed in the next menstrual cycle to ensure complete resolution of the septum. This allows pregnancy attempts to start no later than 2 cycles. The physician should be aware that on rare occasions a septum may still be evident on HSG even after it has been incised.

Hysteroscopic metroplasty has become a standard of treatment for the septate uterus to reduce poor reproductive outcomes. It is considered simple, safe, and effective when appropriate evaluation and skill are used.

Fedele L, Bianchi S. Hysteroscopic metroplasty for septate uterus. Obstet Gynecol Clin North Am 1995;22:473–89.

Grimbizis G, Camus M, Clasen K, Tournaye H, De Munck L, Devroey P. Hysteroscopic septum resection in patients with recurrent abortions or infertility. Hum Reprod 1998;13:1188–93.

Homer HA, Li TC, Cooke ID. The septate uterus: a review of management and reproductive outcome. Fertil Steril 2000;73:1–14.

Valle RF. Hysteroscopic treatment of partial and complete uterine septum. Int J Fertil Menopausal Stud 1996;41:310–5.

115

Markers for osteoporosis

A 43-year-old nulligravid woman requests a second opinion regarding treatment for osteoporosis. Osteoporosis has been diagnosed by dual-energy X-ray absorptiometry (DXA), and she has begun to take alendronate at her physician's recommendation. She takes calcium supplements, 1,500 mg per day, with vitamin D, 400 IU per day. She runs approximately 16 km (10 mile) per week and bikes 80.5 km (50 mile) every weekend. On physical examination, she is 1.7 m (5 ft 8 in.) tall, she weighs 57.2 kg (126 lb), her blood pressure level is 96/60 mm Hg, and pulse rate is 64 beats per minute. The remainder of her examination is unremarkable. Laboratory studies, including thyroid-stimulating hormone, estradiol, follicle-stimulating hormone, and serum prolactin levels, are normal. In addition, her electrolyte, human parathyroid hormone, serum calcium, and 24-hour urinary free calcium levels obtained while she is off calcium supplementation also are normal. To monitor her response to alendronate, the most appropriate next step in her management is

(A) repeat DXA scan
* (B) urinary N-telopeptide level
(C) lateral X-ray of spine
(D) urinary calcium excretion rate
(E) ultrasonography of calcaneus

During puberty, activation of the pituitary–ovarian axis, increased adrenal androgen secretion, and activation of the growth hormone axis result in growth of long bones and increased deposition of calcium into the bony matrix. Bone turnover during puberty and adolescence favors bone formation over bone resorption.

The finding of osteoporosis in reproductive-aged women is unusual. In these individuals, there may be a failure to achieve peak bone mass because of eating disorders or long periods of hypoestrogenism caused by hypothalamic amenorrhea and exercise-associated amenorrhea, such as seen in this patient. In other patients, hypoestrogenism can result from treatment with gonadotropin-releasing hormone agonists for endometriosis or hypogonadism secondary to other disorders. Other endocrine dysfunctions that can affect bone turnover, such as hyperthyroidism and hyperparathyroidism, must be considered. To determine if urinary calcium loss is excessive, it is prudent to screen for disorders of calcium metabolism and to measure serum calcium, parathyroid hormone, and 24-hour calcium excretion. This determination should be performed without additional calcium supplementation.

The criterion standard for assessment of fracture risk is a DXA scan. Bone mineral density testing of this patient indicates osteoporosis at the lumbar spine and at the femoral neck (T-score less than −2.5 at both sites). These are physical measurements of the calcium content in bone relative to a surface area. Another approach is measurement of biochemical breakdown products of bone formation or bone resorption in the serum and urine. The currently available bone turnover markers are listed in Appendix B. Most of the bone biomarkers for bone resorption are based on urinary measurements and must be indexed to creatinine. For this reason, there is a large variance in the day-to-day values for urinary N-terminal type I collagen telopeptides and C-terminal type I collagen telopeptides. Many of the bone formation biomarkers, such as osteocalcin and procollagen type I C-terminal propeptide, also have circadian rhythms and, therefore, timing of the blood sampling is important.

There are several theoretical uses of bone biochemical markers:

- Prediction of bone mass
- Prediction of fracture risk
- Prediction of bone loss
- Monitoring effectiveness of therapy

Unfortunately, the clinical data to support most of these indications are poor, in part because of the variability in the day-to-day values. The best established clinical use of bone markers is to monitor the effectiveness of therapy. Generally, after initiation of antiresorptive therapy, such as alendronate, there is a significant decrease in markers of bone resorption (ie, N-terminal type I collagen telopeptides and C-terminal type I collagen telopeptides) within 6 weeks. Markers of bone formation also will be decreased within 8–12 weeks.

In this patient, a urinary N-telopeptide determination would provide an early indication of clinical efficacy and would be expected to decrease from menopausal levels to low premenopausal levels. A repeat DXA scan in this patient would not be indicated for at least 1–2 years because of the variance in DXA measurements and the ability of the instrument to detect relatively modest changes in bone density. A lateral X-ray of the spine can be useful in assessment of subclinical spine fractures but is not helpful in assessing efficacy. A urinary calcium excretion can be a useful index of overall calcium intake and loss but has not been clinically correlated to efficacy of treatment. Ultrasonographic measurement of the calcaneus is a useful screening tool for osteoporosis but is not currently indicated as a technique for sequential monitoring of bone mass for treatment purposes.

Garnero P, Shih WJ, Gineyts E, Karpf DB, Delmas PD. Comparison of new biochemical markers of bone turnover in late postmenopausal osteoporotic women in response to alendronate treatment. J Clin Endocrinol Metab 1994;79:1693–700.

Khosla S, Kleerekoper M. Biochemical markers of bone turnover. In: Favus MJ, ed. Primer on the metabolic bone diseases and disorders of mineral metabolism. 4th ed. Philadelphia (PA): Lippincott Williams and Wilkins; 1999. p. 128–34.

Prestwood KM, Pilbeam CC, Burleson JA, Woodiel FN, Delmas PC, Deftos LJ, et al. The short-term effects of conjugated estrogen on bone turnover in older women. J Clin Endocrinol Metab 1994;79:366–71.

Tannenbaum C, Clark J, Schwartzman K, Wallenstein S, Lapinski, R, Meier D, et al. Yield of laboratory testing to identify secondary contributors to osteoporosis in otherwise healthy women. J Clin Endocrinol Metab 2002;87:4431–7.

116
Bilateral tubal ligation and future fertility

A 38-year-old woman, gravida 3, para 3, in a new relationship with a 32-year-old man, comes in for a fertility evaluation after a failed tubal ligation reversal that was done 18 months ago. The patient had a day 3 follicle-stimulating hormone (FSH) level of 5 mIU/mL. She has a normal hysterosalpingogram. Her partner has a semen analysis with normal parameters. The patient is interested in the in vitro fertilization (IVF) success rate in her particular case with a history of tubal factor infertility. The factor most likely to predict IVF success is

* (A) age of patient
   (B) failed tubal anastomosis
   (C) age of spouse
   (D) FSH level

Tubal sterilization remains the most common method of permanent contraception used by couples in the United States today. Among women who have undergone the procedure, 3–5% have been shown to express regret and to request a tubal ligation reversal. The increased rate of divorce in the United States with development of new relationships creates a need for reproductive technology to overcome iatrogenic secondary infertility. The most common reasons cited for regret and sterilization reversal include age younger than 30 years, sterilization at the time of cesarean delivery, and marital discord at the time of the procedure.

In vitro fertilization with embryo transfer offers an alternative to treatment for patients who are not candidates for surgery. The procedure overcomes tubal factor infertility by bypassing the fallopian tubes and allowing fertilization to be accomplished in the laboratory. Embryos created are then transferred back into the uterus with progesterone administration to support embryo implantation. With the ongoing advances in assisted reproductive technology, pregnancy rates with IVF have increased dramatically and surpass the normal cycle fecundity in many centers.

The age of the woman has been shown consistently to have the most dramatic effect on pregnancy success after sterilization reversal as well as IVF. As women delay childbearing and become older, the chance for pregnancy success decreases. Other factors that must be considered are semen parameters, status of the uterine cavity, ovarian reserve, and previous medical history. These factors also may play a significant role in IVF success.

Although IVF is considered a good alternative to sterilization reversal, the expense of a single cycle with decreased success should be carefully considered along with the chance for conception after multiple cycles following tubal reconstruction. The cumulative pregnancy rate of tubal reversal can reach 70%, whereas natural conception has been reported in up to 45% in women older than 40 years. With advancing age older than 37 years, IVF pregnancy rates decrease to less than 25% whereas live births in women older than 40 years decrease to 15% or less.

Couples who undergo IVF or tubal reversal should consider the risks of both procedures. Complications from IVF include ovarian hyperstimulation, infection or bleeding at the time of egg retrieval, multiple gestations, and ectopic pregnancy. Surgical risks associated with tubal anastomosis are those risks associated with laparotomy, laparoscopy, and anesthesia. Tubal anastomosis usually is accomplished through an outpatient surgical procedure with a short overnight stay if necessary.

This couple presents after a failed tubal reversal and is considering IVF. The most important risk factor for the couple is advanced maternal age because the uterine cavity is normal as are the semen parameters. Despite a normal day 3 FSH value and, thus, a normal ovarian reserve, the chance for success is lower than it is for patients younger than 35 years. The history of failed tubal reversal and age of the spouse should not significantly decrease the chance for success because the initial evaluation was normal.

Use of operative microsurgery and IVF over the past 2 decades have improved success for tubal factor infertility. In vitro fertilization has been deemed to be a reasonable alternative to tubal reversal but no data are presently available to confirm this finding. Careful evaluation and counseling should be undertaken for all couples who come in for evaluation after a tubal ligation.

Centers for Disease Control and Prevention, Department of Health and Human Services. 2001 Assisted reproductive technology success rates. National summary and fertility clinic reports. Atlanta (GA): Centers for Disease Control and Prevention; 2003.

Dubuisson JB, Chapron C, Nos C, Morice P, Aubriot FX, Garnier P. Sterilization reversal: fertility results. Hum Reprod 1995;10:1145–51.

Sitko D, Commenges-Ducos M, Roland P, Papaxanthos-Roche A, Horovitz J, Dallay D. IVF following impossible or failed surgical reversal of tubal sterilization. Hum Reprod 2001;16:683–5.

Templeton A, Morris JK, Parslow W. Factors that affect outcome of in-vitro fertilization treatment. Lancet 1996;348:1402–6.

Trimbos-Kemper TC. Reversal of sterilization in women over 40 years of age: a multicenter survey in The Netherlands. Fertil Steril 1990;53:575–7.

117
Primary amenorrhea

A 16-year-old adolescent comes in for evaluation of primary amenorrhea and lack of breast development. She denies being sexually active and has no history of vaginal bleeding. Her height is 134.6 cm (53 in.). She has Tanner stage I breast development and Tanner stage I pubic hair (Appendix D). She has a normal vaginal length, visible cervix, small palpable uterus, and no palpable ovaries. Initial laboratory evaluation reveals a negative serum pregnancy test result and normal levels of prolactin and thyroid-stimulating hormone (TSH). The serum measurement that would provide the most information to make the diagnosis is

* (A) follicle-stimulating hormone (FSH)
* (B) estradiol
* (C) testosterone
* (D) dehydroepiandrosterone sulfate (DHEAS)
* (E) 17-hydroxyprogesterone

Amenorrhea can be a transient, intermittent, or permanent condition resulting from dysfunction of the hypothalamus, pituitary gland, ovaries, uterus, or vagina. It often is classified as either primary (absence of menarche by age 16 years) or secondary (absence of menses for more than 3 cycles or 6 months in women who were previously menstruating). Menarche occurs at mean age 12.8 years, and 95% of girls begin to menstruate by age 16 years. The menstrual cycle is susceptible to outside influences; thus, missing a single menstrual period is rarely important. In contrast, prolonged amenorrhea may be the earliest sign of a reduction in general health or signal an underlying condition, such as a pituitary tumor.

Primary amenorrhea often is the result of a genetic or anatomic abnormality. All causes of secondary amenorrhea may be associated with primary amenorrhea. A logical approach to the woman with either primary or secondary amenorrhea is to consider disorders based on the level of control of the menstrual cycle: hypothalamus, pituitary, ovary, uterus, and vagina. For women with primary amenorrhea, outflow tract disorders should be excluded, which usually can be done by pelvic examination before studies to identify endocrine disorders are undertaken.

Congenital abnormalities of the female reproductive tract account for approximately 20% of cases of primary amenorrhea. Menses cannot occur without an intact uterus, endometrium, cervix, and vagina. Pelvic or lower abdominal pain is a common symptom in girls with primary amenorrhea and an obstructed reproductive tract.

The diagnostic approach to a woman with primary amenorrhea consists of a series of sequential steps. The physical examination in a female with primary amenorrhea should begin with an evaluation of pubertal development, including current height, weight, and arm span (normal arm span for adults is within 5 cm of height), and an evaluation of the woman's growth chart.

The laboratory evaluation of a woman with primary amenorrhea depends on the physical examination findings, in particular, whether müllerian structures are present or absent. The single most important step in the evaluation is to determine by physical examination or ultrasonography whether there are any anatomic abnormalities of the vagina, cervix, or uterus. For patients with normal müllerian structures and no evidence of an imperforate hymen, vaginal septum, or congenital absence of the vagina, an endocrine evaluation should be performed. This includes measurement of serum β-hCG levels to exclude pregnancy and serum FSH levels. Serum prolactin and TSH levels should be measured, especially if galactorrhea is present. If pelvic ultrasonography demonstrates an absent uterus and ovaries are identified, the probable diagnosis is müllerian agenesis.

A high serum FSH concentration is indicative of ovarian failure (hypergonadotropic hypogonadism). These patients usually have minimal breast development because of a lack of estrogen production from the ovaries; however, pubic hair development may be normal or absent as in this patient. A karyotype is then required and may demonstrate complete or partial deletion of the X chromosome (Turner's syndrome), a 46,XX karyotype (Fig. 117-1; see color plate), or the presence of Y chromatin. Patients with mixed gonadal dysgenesis (45,X, 46,XY) and those with 46,XY gonadal dysgenesis (Swyer syndrome) have a 20–30% risk of tumor formation, most commonly gonadoblastoma and dysgerminoma, and warrant surgical removal of the gonads.

A low serum FSH concentration represents a defect in gonadotropin release (hypogonadotopic hypogonadism), the cause for which could be either hypothalamic or pituitary in origin. A low FSH level necessitates an evaluation with computed tomography or magnetic resonance imaging to search for a central lesion and an endocrine evaluation consisting of prolactin, TSH, and renal function tests.

An estradiol level would not be useful in this patient. The lack of breast development is indicative of a low estrogen milieu. In this instance, the patient is her own physiologic bioassay.

A testosterone level would be useful in a patient with suspected androgen insensitivity syndrome, where the FSH concentration would be normal for an adult. However, the findings of a normal müllerian system (cervix and uterus) do not support the possibility of androgen insensitivity syndrome in this patient.

If there are signs or symptoms of hyperandrogenism (hirsutism, acne, or virilization), the patient's serum testosterone, DHEAS, and 17-hydroxyprogesterone levels or nonclassical 21-hydroxase deficiency should be measured to assess for an androgen-secreting tumor. Because this patient does not exhibit any signs or symptoms of hyperandrogenism, the measurement of these hormones is not warranted.

Edmonds DK. Congenital malformations of the genital tract. Obstet Gynecol Clin North Am 2000;27:49–62.

Pletcher JR, Slap GB. Menstrual disorders. Amenorrhea. Pediatr Clin North Am 1999;46:505–18.

Slap GB. Menstrual disorders in adolescence. Best Pract Res Clin Obstet Gynaecol 2003;17:75–92.

118
Recurrent pregnancy loss

A 27-year-old woman, gravida 4, para 0, is referred to you with a history of recurrent first-trimester pregnancy loss and a normal hysterosalpingogram. Her records from 2 months ago indicate normal endocrine parameters, positive anticardiolipin immunoglobulin (Ig) G, and normal parental karyotypes. A repeat anticardiolipin IgG is elevated. The most effective therapy is

    (A) clomiphene citrate (Clomid, Serophene)
    (B) progesterone
*   (C) heparin and low-dose aspirin
    (D) initiation of intravenous immune globulin

Recurrent first-trimester pregnancy loss occurs in approximately 1% of reproductive-aged women. A definitive cause for such losses can be established in approximately 50% of these couples. A generally accepted definition of recurrent pregnancy loss is 2 or more consecutive miscarriages.

Antiphospholipid syndrome is an autoimmune disorder that is accepted as a cause of recurrent first-trimester pregnancy loss. The disorder is characterized by the presence of significantly elevated levels of at least 1 of the antiphospholipid antibodies (IgM, IgG, and lupus anticoagulant) on 2 occasions separated by at least 6 weeks and at least 1 of the following clinical scenarios: recurrent pregnancy loss, thrombosis, or stillbirth. When the diagnosis is established, the current recommendations are for the use of unfractionated heparin (5,000 units subcutaneously twice daily) and low-dose aspirin (81 mg per day) during pregnancy. Research suggests that low molecular weight heparin is as effective as unfractionated heparin with fewer complications.

A deficiency in the luteal phase production of progesterone has long been thought to play a role in infertility and specifically in spontaneous abortion but remains unproved. A variety of medications have been proposed to correct this deficiency. Two of the more commonly referenced medications include clomiphene citrate and various formulations of progesterone. It is important to understand that making the diagnosis of luteal phase deficiency is extremely problematic, and treatment of this entity is not clear. As such, the American Society for Reproductive Medicine does not recommend evaluation of women for luteal phase deficiency.

Clomiphene citrate is a selective estrogen receptor modulator that acts as a weak estrogen antagonist. Use of this oral agent will lead to increased production of follicle-stimulating hormone and luteinizing hormone by the hypothalamic–pituitary axis. This increase in gonadotropin levels has the potential to improve folliculogenesis leading to potentially improved progesterone production in the luteal phase of the menstrual cycle. In this patient with identified antiphospholipid antibodies, the use of clomiphene citrate would not be helpful.

Progesterone, either in the form of vaginal suppositories, intramuscular injections, or oral formulations, has been promoted as another method to correct luteal phase deficiency and decrease the chance for early pregnancy loss. The evidence for establishing the diagnosis of luteal phase deficiency and the use of progesterone for therapeutic benefit remains controversial. The use of progesterone would not be appropriate in this patient with a clearly defined diagnosis of antiphospholipid syndrome.

Some investigators have proposed alloimmune mechanisms as a reason for recurrent first-trimester pregnancy losses. Alloimmunity implies that immunologic differences between partners are the source for these miscarriages. A variety of specific mechanisms have been proposed, including an increased percentage of natural killer cells in the maternal circulation, embryotoxic factors similar to interferon gamma, and excessive levels of tumor necrosis factor α. Although such factors may play a role, it has been difficult for laboratories to standardize this type of testing and for other investigators to reproduce their findings. Furthermore, researchers who claim that abnormalities in these factors are primarily responsible for recurrent first-trimester pregnancy losses have yet to consistently demonstrate a reliable treatment modality. Many advocate the use of intravenous Ig. Several clinical trials have produced conflicting results and recent meta-analyses of the data do not support the use of intravenous immunoglobulin as a treatment modality. In this patient with antiphospholipid syndrome, use of intravenous immune globulin would not be appropriate.

American College of Obstetricians and Gynecologists. Management of recurrent pregnancy early pregnancy loss. ACOG Practice Bulletin 24. Washington, DC: ACOG; 2001.

Empson M, Lassere M, Craig JC, Scott JR. Recurrent pregnancy loss with antiphospholipid antibody: a systematic review of therapeutic trials. Obstet Gynecol 2002;99:135–44.

Ogasawara M, Kajiura S, Katano K, Aoyama T, Aoki K. Are serum progesterone levels predictive of recurrent miscarriage in future pregnancies? Fertil Steril 1997;68:806–9.

119

Complications of intrauterine insemination

A 29-year-old woman comes in for intrauterine insemination (IUI) with her husband's washed semen sample. The couple has unexplained infertility, and they have just completed their fourth IUI with the co-administration of clomiphene citrate (Clomid, Serophene). Before her initial procedure, her cervical cultures were negative for gonorrhea and chlamydia. The most common side effect associated with an IUI is

    (A) acute salpingitis
    (B) anaphylactoid reaction to components in the media used to prepare the semen
    (C) formation of antisperm antibodies
* (D) uterine contractions
    (E) transmission of viruses into the uterine cavity

Intrauterine insemination (IUI) of washed sperm following ovarian hyperstimulation with clomiphene citrate often is the first treatment for a woman with unexplained infertility. Side effects following an IUI procedure are rare, with uterine cramping or contractions cited as the most common. Uterine contractions are minimized by separating the sperm from fluids that contain prostaglandins. Previous attempts at inseminating semen directly into the uterus without prior washing of the semen were associated with marked uterine contractions and a higher rate of infection after insemination. The rate of infection after semen washing is approximately 1 in 500 inseminations. After IUI with sperm, there are isolated case reports of anaphylactoid reactions to components in the media and added antibiotics (eg, severe reactions to bovine serum albumin, streptomycin, and penicillin in the media). Patients with a history of marked atopy should be considered for screening before performing an IUI. Formation of new antisperm antibody (ASA) has not been documented to occur after IUI of washed sperm samples. Semen samples with ASA attached to the sperm often are washed and inseminated into the uterine cavity for the treatment of ASA.

Sperm washing techniques have been effective in reducing the transmission of viruses into the uterine cavity. This is especially important in the infertility treatment of human immunodeficiency virus (HIV)-negative women who want to conceive using sperm from their HIV-positive partner. Semen preparation protocols have been developed to reduce the transmission of the HIV virus to undetectable levels at a few specialized infertility centers.

Chrystie IL, Mullen JE, Braude PR, Rowell P, Williams E, Elkington N, et al. Assisted conception in HIV discordant couples: evaluation of semen processing techniques in reducing HIV viral load. J Reprod Immunol 1998;41:301–6.

Ombelet W, Vandeput H, Janssen M, Cox A, Vossen C, Pollet H, et al. Treatment of male infertility due to sperm surface antibodies: IUI or IVF? Hum Reprod 1997;12:1165–70.

Orta M, Ordoqui E, Aranzabal A, Fernandez C, Bartolome B, Sanz ML. Anaphylactic reaction after artificial insemination. Ann Allergy Asthma Immunol 2003;90:446–51.

Speroff L, Glass RH, Kase NG. Clinical gynecologic endocrinology and infertility. 6th ed. Baltimore (MD): Lippincott Williams & Wilkins; 1999. p. 1088–90.

120
Add-back therapy with analogs

A 23-year-old nulligravid woman recently received a diagnosis of midline pelvic pain secondary to endometriosis. A laparoscopy performed 8 months ago demonstrated stage I disease with endometriosis implants localized to the cul-de-sac and bilateral ovarian fossae. Her implants were ablated. Postoperatively, she was managed with continuous oral contraceptives for 4 months, but they were discontinued because of irregular bleeding and recurrent pelvic pain. She was subsequently placed on leuprolide acetate (Lupron) at a dose of 3.75 mg per month. On this new regimen, her pain has improved, but she reports dyspareunia and severe vasomotor symptoms. In addition to prescribing a gonadotropin-releasing hormone (GnRH) agonist, the most appropriate daily management will be

(A) norethindrone acetate, 10 mg
(B) combination oral contraceptives
(C) 0.625 mg of conjugated estrogens
* (D) 0.625 mg of conjugated estrogens and 5 mg of norethindrone acetate
(E) 10 mg of medroxyprogesterone acetate

Long-term medical suppression of the pituitary–ovarian axis with GnRH agonists has become the most common choice for conservative treatment of young patients with endometriosis accompanied by pelvic pain that is unresponsive to oral contraceptives. This approach is very effective in reducing circulating estradiol levels into the castrate range, but it also is accompanied by hot flushes, vaginal dryness, and loss in bone mineral density. A variety of "add-back" hormonal strategies have been proposed to reduce hot flushes and bone loss, to maintain pain relief, and to reduce the frequency of surgical intervention.

One approach is to provide low doses of estrogen–progestin therapy similar to that administered to postmenopausal women. In principle, this approach would provide sufficient estrogen to minimize hot flushes, reduce dyspareunia, and maintain bone density, but it would still remain less than the threshold needed to stimulate endometrial or endometriosis growth and development. In longer trials, this approach has demonstrated clinical efficacy. Thus, use of 0.625 mg of conjugated estrogens and 5 mg of norethindrone acetate is appropriate in this patient.

A second approach is to use pharmacologic doses of progestins, such as norethindrone acetate, 2.5–5 mg daily, to maintain bone mineral density. Currently, norethindrone acetate, 5 mg daily, is the only U.S. Food and Drug Administration-approved steroid for add-back therapy. These progestins have the ability to relieve hot flushes and can induce or maintain a decidual reaction in endometrium or endometriosis. In some individuals, the GnRH agonist can be discontinued and the patient maintained on long-term progestin therapy at a reduced cost.

The combination of a GnRH agonist with progestin add-back can be effective for treatment of pelvic pain. However, this patient reports occasional uterine bleeding coinciding with return of her pelvic pain. Because the GnRH agonist has essentially suppressed the pituitary–ovarian axis, the uterine bleeding should reflect progestin action on the endometrial target tissue. Clinically this phenomenon can occur during transient endometrial breakdown from prolonged progestin activity on the endometrium and may be similar to progestin breakthrough bleeding. The addition of low doses of estrogen may be sufficient to stimulate limited endometrial development and regenerate estrogen receptors in these tissues. The addition of higher doses of progestin (such as norethindrone acetate, 5 mg, or medroxyprogesterone acetate, 10 mg) could exacerbate this situation. Interestingly, in limited trials, antiprogesterone compounds, such as mifepristone, have been shown to be effective in reducing pelvic pain associated with endometriosis. These compounds may act centrally to reduce GnRH release, inhibit gonadotropin secretion, inhibit ovulation, and may have direct effects on endometrial tissue.

Suppression of pituitary gonadotropin output also can be successfully achieved with GnRH antagonists. These newer peptides compete directly with native GnRH for the pituitary GnRH receptors and shut down follicle-stimulating hormone and luteinizing hormone release within hours of administration without the flare response. However, long-acting depot preparations of GnRH antagonists currently are not available.

Edmonds DK, Howell R. Can hormone replacement therapy be used during medical therapy of endometriosis? Br J Obstet Gynaecol 1994;101(suppl 10):24–6.

Hornstein MD, Surrey ES, Weisberg GW, Casino LA. Leuprolide acetate depot and hormonal add-back in endometriosis: a 12-month study. Lupron Add-Back Study Group. Obstet Gynecol 1998;91: 16–24.

Kettel LM, Murphy AA, Mortola JF, Liu JH, Ulmann A, Yen SS. Endocrine responses to long-term administration of the anti-progesterone RU486 in patients with pelvic endometriosis. Fertil Steril 1991; 56:402–7.

Kiilholma P, Tuimala R, Kivinen S, Korhonen M, Hagman E. Comparison of the gonadotropin-releasing hormone agonist goserelin acetate alone versus goserelin combined with estrogen-progestogen add-back therapy in the treatment of endometriosis. Fertil Steril 1995; 64:903–8.

Surrey ES, Hornstein MD. Prolonged GnRH agonist and add-back therapy for symptomatic endometriosis: long-term follow-up. Obstet Gynecol 2002;99:709–19.

Surrey ES, Voigt B, Fournet N, Judd HL. Prolonged gonadotropin-releasing hormone agonist treatment of symptomatic endometriosis: the role of cyclic sodium etidronate and low-dose norethindrone "add-back" therapy. Fertil Steril 1995;53:747–55.

121

Migraines and hormonal contraception

A 23-year-old woman comes in for contraception and management of her migraines. She is in a monogamous relationship. She currently takes a β-blocker, which has reduced the number and severity of her migraines. She denies a history of neurologic prodromes associated with her migraines and states that her headaches are worse during her menses. She inquires whether hormonal contraception will further ameliorate her migraines. She does not smoke and does not have a history of sexually transmitted diseases or abnormal Pap test results. Physical examination and vital signs are normal. The most appropriate contraceptive for this patient is

* (A) continuous low-dose monophasic oral contraceptives (OCs)
* (B) triphasic low-dose OCs
* (C) progestin-only OCs
* (D) progestin-containing intrauterine device (IUD)
* (E) copper-containing IUD

Many women report increased frequency of migraines in association with menstruation. The term menstrual migraine often is used despite the lack of an agreed definition. The International Headache Society has classified most headaches but not menstrual migraines. A proposed definition is based on the finding that the prevalence of the migraine headache increases within 2 days of menses onset. Headaches that occur at this time of the menstrual cycle typically are without aura.

Effective acute therapy is the mainstay of management for menstrual and nonmenstrual attacks. There is some evidence that attacks linked to menstruation are less responsive to treatment compared with migraines at other times of the cycle. If several attacks occur throughout the menstrual cycle, standard prophylactic agents should be used. Women with exclusive menstrual migraines may benefit from perimenstrual prophylaxis, but this should only be instituted once the association between the migraine and menstruation has been confirmed with prospective records kept for a minimum of 3 menstrual cycles. Nonsteroidal antiinflammatory drugs are the treatment of choice in reducing migraines associated with menorrhagia or dysmenorrhea.

Menstrual migraines are a treatment challenge for both the patient and the physician. Some women with menstrual migraines may respond to acute and preventive therapies for nonmenstrual migraines; however, others continue to experience refractory menstrual migraines. These women may respond to hormonal interventions, which may reduce the frequency of menstrual migraines, thereby reducing the need for abortive migraine therapies, decreasing migraine-related disability, and improving quality of life. Menstrual migraines appear to have a distinct pathophysiology. Published studies have shed light on the effectiveness of a variety of hormonal interventions, including OCs, estrogen therapy, selective estrogen receptor modifiers, danazol (Danocrine), and leuprolide acetate (Lupron).

Studies indicate that menstrual migraine headaches are caused by the decrease in estradiol levels that occurs in the late luteal phase. Continuous administration of estrogen in any of several forms, including in combination monophasic low-dose OCs, often is effective in reducing or eliminating menstrual migraines. Newer OCs, which allow for withdrawal bleeding every 3 months, may be effective in the reduction of migraine attacks. However, no data are available in regard to these newer OCs and menstrual migraines.

The data regarding stroke and migraine headaches make it difficult to decide whether to give OCs to women with migraines. The incidence of stroke in women with migraines generally is increased approximately 3-fold and appears to be increased even more among cigarette smokers with migraine. Migraine with aura may increase the risk approximately 6-fold. The incidence of stroke in women with migraines also may be increased among users of combination OC agents: one study reported no increase in the incidence of stroke, while another noted a 4-fold increase in stroke. One investigation noted a 34-fold increase in the risk of stroke in women who smoke and use OCs. It is difficult to estimate these relationships with precision because the incidence of stroke is low in young women, whether they smoke, have migraine headaches, or use OCs.

The International Headache Society Task Force has concluded that there is no contraindication to the use of OCs in women with migraine in the absence of migraine aura or other risk factors. Thus, it would seem reasonable to offer low-dose combination OCs in women with menstrual migraine who require contraception and whose migraine headaches are not entirely relieved by β-blockers, calcium channel blockers, and antidepressants. Given the information about strokes and migraine, it would seem reasonable to limit OC use to women without focal neurologic components to their headaches.

The frequency of menstrual migraine headache can be reduced by decreasing the frequency of withdrawal episodes when using OCs. Thus, Seasonale is one alternative. To reduce the severity of the withdrawal headaches, the episodes of withdrawal can be decreased in length to less than 7 days. For women who do not spot or bleed irregularly, continuous OCs can be used.

Triphasic OCs should not be used in this setting because the variation in steroid levels may cause breakthrough bleeding and precipitate a headache. Currently, there are no data to demonstrate the efficacy of the patch or vaginal ring in reducing menstrual headaches. Theoretically, continuous use should be efficacious because steady-states hormonal levels are achieved.

If OCs are contraindicated, depot medroxyprogesterone acetate may be an alternative, because it also inhibits ovulation and may improve migraines, provided amenorrhea is achieved. However, no data document efficacy at this time. Oral progestin-only contraception has little place in the management of menstrual migraines, because it does not inhibit ovulation and often is associated with a disrupted menstrual cycle. Likewise, there is no evidence to suggest that the progestin-containing IUD, copper-containing IUD, vaginal spermicide, or the diaphragm will reduced the frequency or severity of menstrual-associated migraines.

Chavanu KJ, O'Donnell DC. Hormonal interventions for menstrual migraines. Pharmacotherapy 2002;22:1442–57.

Lidegaard O. Oral contraceptives, pregnancy and the risk of cerebral thromboembolism: the influence of diabetes, hypertension, migraine and previous thrombotic disease. Br J Obstet Gynaecol 1995;102:153–9.

MacGregor A. Migraine associated with menstruation. Funct Neurol 2000;15(suppl 3):143–53.

Silberstein SD. Headache and female hormones: what you need to know. Curr Opin Neurol 2001;14:323–33.

Stewart WF, Lipton RB, Chee E, Sawyer J, Silberstein SD. Menstrual cycle and headache in a population sample of migraineurs. Neurology 2000;55:1517–23.

Sulak PJ, Cressman BE, Waldrop E, Holleman S, Kuehl TJ. Extending the duration of active oral contraceptive pills to manage hormone withdrawal symptoms. Obstet Gynecol 1997;89:179–83.

122

Medical management of metabolic syndrome

A 68-year-old woman comes in for her annual examination with no specific symptoms. She is 1.6 m (5 ft 4 in.) tall, weighs 82 kg (181 lb), has a body mass index (BMI) of 31 kg/m², and a waist circumference of 99 cm (39 in.). She has a blood pressure reading of 129/83 mm Hg. She walks 30 minutes per day, 3 times per week. She smoked one half a pack of cigarettes per day until 4 years ago. She takes no medications. Two sisters are overweight and one has taken metformin hydrochloride (Glucophage) for 2 years for type 2 diabetes mellitus. Her mother died from a heart attack at age 69 years. Her fasting laboratory results are as follows: glucose level of 121 mg/dL, total cholesterol level of 230 mg/dL, triglyceride level of 240 mg/dL, high-density lipoprotein (HDL) cholesterol level of 38 mg/dL, and low-density lipoprotein (LDL) cholesterol level of 134 mg/dL. You make a diagnosis of metabolic syndrome and recommend that she make therapeutic lifestyle changes with regard to diet, weight loss, and increased exercise. In addition to an increased risk of type 2 diabetes mellitus, this patient has an increased risk of

* (A) hypertension
  (B) hyperthyroidism
  (C) pancreatic cancer
  (D) hepatic failure
  (E) renal disease

Metabolic syndrome or insulin resistance syndrome is characterized by abdominal obesity (ie, waist circumference in women in excess of 88.9 cm [35 in.]), low HDL cholesterol level less than 50 mg/dL, increased triglyceride levels greater than 150 mg/dL, and impaired glucose tolerance (ie, fasting glucose level between 110–125 mg/dL). Increased coagulation factors and hyperuricemia can be associated with metabolic syndrome. Low HDL cholesterol and high triglyceride levels are more common than high LDL cholesterol levels in this syndrome. In contrast, women with hypothyroidism, renal insufficiency, steroid use, and obstructive liver disease tend to present with much higher LDL cholesterol levels. Given evidence-based literature, this patient is at an increased risk for hypertension and type 2 diabetes mellitus.

Triglyceride levels greater than 150 mg/dL are one of the criteria for metabolic syndrome according to the report of the National Cholesterol Education Program Adult Treatment Panel III. This report recommended that non-HDL cholesterol be considered a secondary target of therapy in patients with metabolic syndrome. Because non-HDL cholesterol contains all known and potentially atherogenic lipid particles, it is a reliable predictor for coronary heart disease (CHD). Non-HDL cholesterol is calculated as total cholesterol minus HDL cholesterol. The therapeutic goal is set at 30 mg/dL higher than the therapeutic value for LDL cholesterol. Target therapeutic levels of LDL cholesterol are based on CHD risk factors (Table 122-1).

Insulin resistance links hypertension and dyslipidemia. A relationship between serum lipids and blood pressure

TABLE 122-1. National Cholesterol Education Program (NCEP) Adult Treatment Panel III (ATP III) Risk Categories and Lipid Goals

Risk Category	Lipid Goal (mg/dL)	Low-density Lipoprotein Level To Initiate Total Life Changes (mg/dL)	Low-density Lipoprotein Level To Consider Drug Therapy (mg/dL)
Coronary heart disease or CHD risk equivalents (10-year risk >20%)	LDL level <100; non-HDL level <130	>100	>130 (100–129: LDL lowering drug optional)
>2 Risk factors (10-year risk <20%)	LDL level <130; non-HDL level <160	>130	10-year risk 10–20%: >130 10-year risk <10%: >160
<1 Risk factor	LDL level <160; non-HDL level <190	>160	>190 (160–189: LDL lowering drug optional)

Abbreviations: CHD, coronary heart disease; HDL, high-density lipoprotein cholesterol; LDL, low-density lipoprotein cholesterol.

Expert Panel on Detection, Evaluation, and Treatment of High Blood Cholesterol in Adults. JAMA 2001;285:2486–97. Copyright © 2001, American Medical Association. All rights reserved.

can be found after adjustment for age and BMI. Hyperinsulinemia may result in hypertension because insulin increases the sympathetic drive, promotes sodium retention, and stimulates vascular hypertrophy.

Hypertriglyceridemia (ie, level greater than 500 mg/dL) is occasionally associated with pancreatitis but not with pancreatic cancer. Metabolic syndrome may have associated hyperuricemia. Hyperthyroidism, renal disease, and hepatic failure are not sequelae associated with metabolic syndrome.

Executive Summary of the Third Report of the National Cholesterol Education Program (NCEP) Expert Panel on Detection, Evaluation and Treatment of High Blood Cholesterol in Adults (Adult Treatment Panel III). Expert Panel on Detection, Evaluation and Treatment of High Blood Cholesterol in Adults. JAMA 2001;285:2486–97.

Han TS, Williams K, Sattar N, Hunt KJ, Lean ME, Haffner SM. Analysis of obesity and hyperinsulinemia in the development of metabolic syndrome: San Antonio Heart Study. Obes Res 2002;10: 923–31.

Reaven G. Metabolic syndrome: pathophysiology and implications for management of cardiovascular disease. Circulation 2002;106: 286–8.

Schrott HG, Bittner V, Vittinghoff E, Herrington DM, Hulley S. Adherence to National Cholesterol Education Program Treatment goals in postmenopausal women with heart disease. The Heart and Estrogen/Progestin Replacement Study (HERS). The HERS Research Study Group. JAMA 1997;277:1281–6.

123

Cost-effective use of antiandrogens

A 29-year-old woman requests alternatives to oral contraceptives to treat her long-standing abnormal facial hair growth. She has used oral contraceptives for control of acne and facial hair growth for the past 9 years but is not satisfied with the results. You recommend for treatment of her hirsutism

    (A) gonadotropin-releasing hormone agonist (Lupron)
    (B) flutamide
    (C) ketoconazole (Nizoral)
*   (D) spironolactone

Hirsutism is defined as the presence of unwanted terminal hair on the face, breasts, abdomen, and lower extremities. Dihydrotestosterone, which is formed by enzymatic conversion from testosterone in hair follicles, is the androgen primarily responsible for hair growth and hirsutism. Approximately 25% of testosterone production in women originates from the ovary, an additional 25% comes from the adrenal gland, and the remainder is produced by peripheral conversion. The ovary produces more androgen in the presence of enhanced luteinizing hormone or insulinlike growth factor I secretion. Thus, women with disorders such as polycystic ovarian syndrome produce more androgen and are more apt to be hirsute.

Therapies for hirsutism are directed at reducing the androgen production from either ovarian or adrenal sources or reducing peripheral conversion from testosterone to dihydrotestosterone. A reduction in androgen production or hair follicle receptivity will change the existing dark and thickened terminal hair to a thinner and lighter vellus type of hair and reduce or eliminate new hair growth.

Gonadotropin-releasing hormone (GnRH) agonists ultimately produce pituitary suppression, which leads to a hypogonadotropic and hypoestrogenic state, reducing the luteinizing hormone effect on the ovary and leading to a direct reduction in ovarian androgen production. It is this mechanism of action that will promote a reduction in hirsutism scores. However, the long-term use of GnRH agonists is limited by their side effects related to hypoestrogenism and costs. Thus, they would not offer a long-term solution for this patient.

Flutamide is a potent androgen-receptor antagonist used in the treatment of prostate cancer. It has been shown to be effective in the management of hirsutism. However, the potential for significant liver toxicity has limited its use and makes this a poor choice for long-term use in this patient. Additionally, the potential for feminization of a male fetus requires the use of reliable contraception in women at risk of pregnancy.

Ketoconazole (Nizoral) also has been shown to be effective in cases of hirsutism. Its mechanism of action is inhibition of the cytochrome P450 pathway responsible for steroid synthesis. The use of this medication is limited by the side effects of potential hepatotoxicity, and the possible potentiation of warfarin, making this a poor choice for long-term use in this patient.

Spironolactone is an aldosterone antagonist structurally related to progestins. Spironolactone will inhibit steroidogenesis, act as an androgen antagonist, and inhibit 5α-reductase activity. It is effective in the management of hirsutism associated with chronic anovulation or idiopathic hirsutism. In patients with normal renal function, hyperkalemia is a rare complication. Hypotension is another potential side effect that usually is more common in older patients. Spironolactone offers the best long-term solution for this patient. Because of the antiandrogen activity of this medication, spironolactone should be used in conjunction with reliable contraception to avoid the potential for failure of masculinization of male genitalia. The combination of oral contraceptives and spironolactone seems to be more effective for the management of hirsutism than spironolactone alone.

Acien P, Mauri M, Gutierrez M. Clinical and hormonal effects of the combination gonadotropin-releasing hormone agonist plus oral contraceptive pills containing ethinyl-oestradiol (EE) and cyproterone acetate (CPA) versus the EE-CPA pill alone on polycystic ovarian disease-related hyperandrogenisms. Hum Reprod 1997;12:423–9.

Azziz R, Carmina E, Sawaya ME. Idiopathic hirsutism. Endocr Rev 2000;21:347–62.

De Leo V, Fulghesu AM, la Marca A, Morgante G, Pasqui L, Talluri B, et al. Hormonal and clinical effects of GnRH agonist alone, or in combination with a combined oral contraceptive or flutamide in women with severe hirsutism. Gynecol Endocrin 2000;14:411–6.

Fruzzetti F, Bersi C, Parrini D, Ricci C, Genazzani AR. Treatment of hirsutism: comparisons between different antiandrogens with central and peripheral effects. Fertil Steril 1999;71:445–51.

Serafini P, Lobo RA. Increased 5 alpha-reductase activity in idiopathic hirsutism. Fertil Steril 1985;43:74–8.

124

Use of androgen–estrogen for increasing bone mineral density

A 32-year-old woman underwent bilateral oophorectomy with uterine preservation 5 years ago for severe endometriosis. Since then she has experienced decreased libido. Vasomotor symptoms persist despite an increase in the daily dose of conjugated estrogens and medroxyprogesterone acetate. Results of dual-energy X-ray absorptiometry are consistent with osteoporosis. Secondary causes of osteoporosis have been excluded. Her lipid profile is normal. The medication most likely to manage her symptoms and address her bone mineral density (BMD) is

* (A) methyltestosterone
 (B) venlafaxine hydrochloride (Effexor)
 (C) clonidine (Catapres-TTS)
 (D) black cohosh (*Cimicifuga racemosa*) (Remifemin)
 (E) yohimbine

Testosterone levels do not decrease appreciably with menopause. Possibly because of elevated levels of luteinizing hormone, the postmenopausal ovary secretes more testosterone than the premenopausal ovary. In contrast, levels of testosterone decrease markedly after bilateral oophorectomy. Hence, the quality of life in surgically castrated women may be enhanced by the addition of oral methyltestosterone to standard hormone therapy. Significantly improved sexual sensation and desire have been observed in some studies within 4 weeks of oral estrogen–androgen treatment when compared with estrogen alone or placebo. However, most studies have used pharmacologic doses of testosterone. Sex hormone-binding globulin levels increase with estrogen but decrease with estrogen–androgen therapy. Increased availability of endogenous and exogenous free androgens caused by decreased sex hormone-binding globulin levels may improve the libido and BMD of patients. It would seem prudent to use an estrogen–androgen preparation in an attempt to improve her libido and BMD before using a nonhormonal antiresorptive treatment for osteoporosis.

When used in addition to estrogen therapy, methyltestosterone (Estratest) over a 2-year period was more effective than estrogen alone in increasing BMD of both the spine and hip. High-density lipoprotein cholesterol and triglyceride levels decreased significantly in the estrogen–androgen group. Side effects of androgen therapy may include acne, increased facial hair, and weight gain.

The selective serotonin uptake inhibitor, venlafaxine hydrochloride (Effexor), blocks uptake of both serotonin and norepinephrine. Venlafaxine may prove effective in alleviating vasomotor symptoms, but it would not improve BMD in this patient.

Clonidine (Catapres-TTS) blocks presynaptic uptake of norepinephrine. It may reduce hot flushes by 45%, compared with 25% in placebo. Side effects of clonidine include hypotension, fatigue, constipation, dry mouth, and drowsiness, but it has no apparent effect on BMD. Black cohosh has been found in some but not all placebo-controlled trials to ameliorate vasomotor symptoms but likewise does not appear to affect BMD.

Yohimbine is derived from the bark of an African tree and the South American herb quebracho. It has traditionally been marketed as a stimulant and aphrodisiac. Yohimbine is a competitive blocker of presynaptic α-2-adreno-receptors that cause an increase in the release of norepinephrine, which may increase the risk of hot flushes, hypertension, anxiety, and tachycardia. There is no evidence that yohimbine is effective in preventing or improving BMD.

Jacobson JS, Troxel AB, Evans J, Klaus L, Vahdat L, Kinne D, et al. Randomized trial of black cohosh for the treatment of hot flashes among women with a history of breast cancer. J Clin Oncol 2001;19: 2739–45.

Sarrel P, Dobay B, Wiita B. Estrogen and estrogen-androgen replacement in postmenopausal women dissatisfied with estrogen-only therapy. Sexual behavior and neuroendocrine responses. J Reprod Med 1998; 43:847–56.

Sloan JA, Loprinzi CL, Novotny PJ, Barton DL, Lavasseur BI, Windschitl H. Methodologic lessons learned from hot flash studies. J Clin Oncol 2001;19:4280–90.

Watts NB, Notelovitz M, Timmons MC, Addison WA, Wiita B, Downey LJ. Comparison of oral estrogens and estrogens plus androgen on bone mineral density, menopausal symptoms, and lipid-lipoprotein profiles in surgical menopause. Obstet Gynecol 1995;85: 529–37.

125
Hyperthyroidism

A 35-year-old woman, gravida 1, para 1, presents with occasional palpitations and fatigue. She is 2 months postpartum after an uncomplicated vaginal delivery. She is breastfeeding exclusively. Her medical history and antenatal history are unremarkable. Vital signs reveal a resting pulse rate of 102 beats per minute and a blood pressure reading of 110/72 mm Hg. The physical examination is normal with the exception of a mildly enlarged thyroid gland. She has a normal complete blood count and free thyroxine (T_4) level of 2.1 ng/dL. Her thyroid-stimulating hormone (TSH) level is 0.15 µU/mL. The most appropriate immediate management for this patient is

(A) levothyroxine
(B) methimazole
(C) radioactive iodine
(D) thyroidectomy
* (E) β-blocker

Postpartum thyroiditis is a common but relatively benign condition that develops in 5–10% of parturients within 6 months of delivery and is characterized by a diffusely enlarged, firm, painless thyroid gland and only chemical or mildly symptomatic hyperthyroidism. It is much more common in women with diabetes mellitus. One half of these patients become euthyroid within 1 year, whereas the other half develop a mild transient hypothyroidism that in most cases will resolve spontaneously. Treatment with antithyroid medications may be required, although most patients are not sufficiently symptomatic to require treatment during the hyperthyroid phase.

Postpartum thyroiditis is likely to recur after each subsequent pregnancy, and permanent hypothyroidism ultimately develops in 20–30% of patients. The classic pattern consists of a thyrotoxic phase, which develops in the first 3 months postpartum and lasts 1–2 months; followed by a hypothyroid phase, which develops 4–8 months postpartum and lasts 4–6 months; and finally spontaneous restoration to euthyroidism. However, the disease also can manifest as either transient thyrotoxicosis alone or hypothyroidism alone.

Postpartum thyroiditis also can occur after spontaneous or induced abortion. Postpartum thyroiditis, like subacute lymphocytic thyroiditis, is considered a variant form of chronic autoimmune thyroiditis (Hashimoto's thyroiditis). Most women with postpartum thyroiditis have high serum concentrations of antithyroid microsomal (thyroid peroxidase) antibodies, and many eventually develop hypothyroidism or a goiter.

The symptoms and signs of hyperthyroidism, when present, are typically mild and consist mainly of anxiety, weakness, irritability, palpitations, tachycardia, and tremor. Similarly, hypothyroidism usually is mild, leading to lack of energy, sluggishness, and dry skin. The biochemical findings are very similar to those of painless thyroiditis: high or high–normal serum free T_4 and T_3 concentrations, low serum TSH concentrations, and low thyroid radioiodine uptake values during the hyperthyroid phase, which may be overt or subclinical. During the hypothyroid phase, serum T_4 concentrations are low or low normal and serum TSH concentrations are high (ie, either overt or subclinical hypothyroidism).

Most women with postpartum thyroiditis need no treatment during either the hyperthyroid or the hypothyroid phases of their illness. Beta-blockers are given to alleviate palpitations, irritability, and nervousness. Patients who have bothersome symptoms of hyperthyroidism should be treated with a β-blocker daily. Any woman who has had postpartum thyroiditis should be told that she is at substantial risk for the later development of hypothyroidism or goiter and informed of these symptoms. It is recommended that a diagnosis of postpartum thyroiditis be considered for any thyroid gland abnormality that occurs within 1 year after delivery or miscarriage.

Treatment of postpartum thyroiditis is indicated in only the more severe cases. Thyrotoxic symptoms are alleviated by β-blockers and hypothyroid symptoms by levothyroxine. Levothyroxine should be discontinued after several months and thyroid function re-evaluated 6 weeks thereafter. Antithyroid drugs (propylthiouracil and methimazole) are the preferred initial therapy for thyrotoxicosis. Radioactive iodine therapy frequently is used to treat hyperthyroidism. Treatment by means of radioactive iodine therapy is contraindicated during pregnancy because the fetal thyroid gland can accumulate iodine at 10–12 weeks of gestation.

Surgical removal of a large part of the thyroid (subtotal thyroidectomy) is indicated in patients with large obstructing glands or glands that contain nodules identified as malignant or equivocal on fine-needle aspiration. Pregnant women with severe hyperthyroidism, which is difficult to control with antithyroid drugs, can be treated with thyroidectomy during the second trimester. In addition, young patients with hyperthyroidism that is difficult to control with antithyroid drugs, patients with toxic reactions to antithyroid drugs, and patients who are not candidates for antithyroid drugs and refuse radioactive iodine are treated by surgery.

Hall R, Richards CJ, Lazarus JH. The thyroid and pregnancy. Br J Obstet Gynaecol 1993;100:512–5.

Seely BL, Burrow GN. Thyroid disease and pregnancy. In: Creasy RK, Resnik R, eds. Maternal-fetal medicine. 4th ed. Philadelphia (PA): WB Saunders; 1999. p. 996–1014.

Stuckey BG, Kent GN, Allen JR. The biochemical and clinical course of postpartum thyroid dysfunction: the treatment decision. Clin Endocrinol (Oxf) 2001;54:377–83.

Thyroid disease in pregnancy. ACOG Practice Bulletin No. 37. American College of Obstetricians and Gynecologists. Obstet Gynecol 2002;100:387–96.

126

Hormonal contraceptive methods choices

The method of hormonal contraception associated with the lowest failure rate at 1 year of use is

(A) combined oral contraceptives
(B) transdermal patch
(C) vaginal ring
* (D) levonorgestrel intrauterine system
(E) progestin-only pill

A higher percentage of young women in the United States become pregnant than do their counterparts in other Western countries. The adolescent pregnancy rate of northern European countries ranges from 13% to 53% of the U.S. rate. The difference almost disappears after age 25 years, due in large part to the use of surgical sterilization in the United States. As more contraceptive choices become available to U.S. women, obstetrician–gynecologists must understand all forms of reversible contraception, their benefits and risks, as well as their failure rates to assist women to make informed contraceptive choices.

Table 126-1 shows the typical pregnancy rates for different birth control methods after 1 year of use. The levonorgestrel intrauterine system has the lowest pregnancy rates, is effective immediately, and does not require any type of user compliance other than verification 1 month after placement that the system has not been extruded from the uterine cavity. Therefore, user dependency is eliminated. The levonorgestrel intrauterine system contains 52 mg of levonorgestrel, released at a rate of 15 µg per day. The levonorgestrel intrauterine system lasts up to 10 years and reduces menstrual blood loss and dysmen-

TABLE 126-1. Percent of Women Experiencing Unintended Pregnancy by Various Birth Control Methods (For 1 Year of Use)

Method	Rate of Pregnancy With Typical Use (%)
Male sterilization	0.15
Female sterilization	0.5
Medroxyprogesterone acetate	0.3
Combined pill (estrogen/progestin)	5
Mini-pill (progestin-only)	5
Copper-T	0.8
Levonorgestrel intrauterine system	0.1
Male latex condom	14
Spermicide (gel, foam, suppository, film)	26
Withdrawal	19
Contraceptive transdermal patch	1
Contraceptive vaginal ring	1–2
No method	85

Data from Hatcher RA, Trussell J, Stewart F, Cates W, Stewart GK, Guest F, et al. Contraceptive technology. 17th ed. New York (NY): Irvington Publishers, 1998, and Speroff L, Darney P. A clinical guide for contraception. 2nd ed. Baltimore (MD): Williams and Wilkins; 1996. p. 5.

orrhea with a significant reduction in ectopic pregnancy rates. It currently is being marketed in the United States for up to 5 years of use. Because it is a progestin-only release system, it can be used safely in patients who have relative contraindications, such as hypertension, smoking, and glucose intolerance, to combined hormonal oral contraceptives.

Each of the other methods of reversible contraception may be useful with particular patients. It should be recognized that those methods are user dependent and, therefore, have high typical failure rates.

Arias RD. Compelling reasons for recommending IUDs to any woman of reproductive age. Int J Fertil Womens Med 2002;47:87–95.

Burkman RT. The transdermal contraceptive patch: a new approach to hormonal contraception. Int J Fertil Womens Med 2002;47:69–76.

French RS, Cowan FM, Mansour D, Higgins JP, Robinson A, Procter T, et al. Levonorgestrel-releasing (20 microgram/day) intrauterine systems (Mirena) compared with other methods of reversible contraceptives. BJOG 2000;107:1218–25.

Peterson HB, Xia Z, Hughes JM, Wilcox LS, Tylor LR, Trussell J. The risk of pregnancy after tubal sterilization: findings from the U.S. Collaborative Review of Sterilization. Am J Obstet Gynecol 1996; 174:1161–8; discussion 1168–70.

127

Male infertility: retrograde ejaculation

A 39-year-old man with a 10-year history of type 1 diabetes mellitus is referred for evaluation of an abnormal semen analysis. He and his wife have a 3-year history of infertility. The referring physician has completed an infertility workup on the couple. The wife's evaluation and history are unremarkable. The man has had 3 semen analyses in the past year, each after 48–72 hours of abstinence, which demonstrated a volume of 0.1–0.3 mL, sperm concentration of 1–2 million per mL, normal motility, and normal morphology. He denies a history of dysuria, urethral discharge, radiation, or testicular trauma. You explain to the couple that the next step in his evaluation is

    (A) repeat semen analysis after a longer period of abstinence
*   (B) collect a postejaculate urine sample
    (C) testicular ultrasonography
    (D) testicular biopsy
    (E) gonadotropin-releasing hormone (GnRH) stimulation test

Basic semen analysis measures volume, pH, liquefaction, round cells, sperm density, motility, and morphology (Appendix E). Before obtaining the semen specimen, the patient is instructed to abstain from ejaculation for a minimum of 48 hours and no longer than 7 days. The optimal period of abstinence has not been determined. However, a longer period of abstinence does not produce significantly improved results and most likely will result in a decreased motility as the fructose is used.

Retrograde ejaculation often is associated with diabetic neuropathy. Any process that interferes with the peristaltic function of the vas deferens and closure of the bladder neck may result in either failure of emission or retrograde ejaculation. Retrograde ejaculation should be suspected in any patient with low-volume (less than 1 mL) or absent ejaculate and should be distinguished from anorgasmia. Retrograde ejaculation is diagnosed by examining the postejaculate urine for sperm. The diagnosis is suggested by low semen volume and is confirmed by a high number of sperm in the urine after ejaculation. Although exact criteria have not been established for a positive postejaculate urinalysis, the finding of greater than 10–15 sperm per high-power field confirms the presence of retrograde ejaculation.

The causes of ejaculatory dysfunction can be divided into anatomic and functional. Patients with retrograde ejaculation from anatomic causes, including bladder neck surgery and transurethral resection of the prostate, do not respond to medical therapies. In contrast, patients with ejaculatory dysfunction from neurologic abnormalities, such as diabetes mellitus, multiple sclerosis, and retroperitoneal surgery, may respond to medical intervention.

The treatment for retrograde ejaculation is to collect and process sperm from a urine specimen immediately after ejaculation for intrauterine insemination or assisted reproduction. The urine pH and osmolarity are optimized for sperm survival in the urine by adjusting the patient's fluid intake and by the administration of sodium bicarbonate or baking soda (2 tablespoons the night before and 2 hours before ejaculation). Sperm are recovered from the urine by centrifugation and then washed in an appropriate insemination media. Deposition of pH-adjusted media into the bladder before ejaculation will reduce the toxic effect of urine and may be used as an adjunct to protect the sperm if the other methods are not successful.

Congenital absence of the vas deferens can be diagnosed by the absence of fructose in the semen and confirmed by testicular ultrasonography. Treatment options for men with obstructive abnormalities include microsurgical vasovasostomy or a testicular biopsy and sperm harvest procedure combined with assisted reproduction and intracytoplasmic sperm injection. Sperm harvest procedures include open and percutaneous epididymal aspiration and sperm extraction from testicular biopsy specimens.

The GnRH stimulation test result may be abnormal in men with suboptimal semen quality, demonstrating an exaggerated pituitary response. An abnormal GnRH test result does not alter treatment. Therefore, routine GnRH stimulation testing is not advocated.

Kamischke A, Nieschlag E. Treatment of retrograde ejaculation and anejaculation. Hum Reprod Update 1999;5:448–74.

Schuster TG, Ohl DA. Diagnosis and treatment of ejaculatory dysfunction. Urol Clin North Am 2002;29:939–48.

Shangold GA, Cantor B, Schreiber JR. Treatment of infertility due to retrograde ejaculation: a simple, cost-effective method. Fertil Steril 1990;54:175–7.

World Health Organization. WHO laboratory manual for the examination of human semen and sperm-cervical mucus interaction. Cambridge, England: Cambridge University Press; 1999.

128
Diethylstilbestrol exposure

A 69-year-old woman used diethylstilbestrol (DES) during 2 pregnancies. She has never smoked cigarettes or consumed alcohol. Based on current information, compared with women of a similar age, this patient is at increased risk for cancer of the

    (A) endometrium
    (B) cervix
    (C) lung
*   (D) breast
    (E) colon

Diethylstilbestrol is a synthetic nonsteroidal estrogen that was prescribed for the prevention of miscarriages or premature deliveries between 1948 and 1971. The use of DES in pregnant women was discontinued when research linked its administration to the development of clear cell adenocarcinoma of the vagina and cervix in the daughters of women exposed to DES. It is estimated that 5–10 million women and their offspring were exposed to DES. Because of the high doses used and the variable duration of DES exposure, there have been concerns that estrogen-sensitive sites like the breast and endometrium may be at increased risk for the development of future neoplasms.

Two studies from the same group of investigators have demonstrated that women who used DES had an increased risk for breast cancer compared with women who did not use DES. The initial study examined the incidence of breast cancer in 3,033 women exposed to DES during 1940–1960 and a comparable group of women who did not use DES. No data suggest that the daughters of women who used DES have an increased risk of breast cancer. The women exposed to DES had a relative risk of 1.4 (95% confidence interval, 1.1–1.9) for breast cancer. The actual risk for breast cancer per 100,000 women-years was 134 cases in the exposed group versus 93 in the unexposed group. These findings represent an overall increase of 41 cases of breast cancer per 100,000 women-years. This study was extended with a follow-up report, which demonstrated a persistent increased relative risk of 1.35 (95% confidence interval, 1.05–1.74) for breast cancer. This second report indicated that the relative risk does not appear to increase over time.

In another study, which examined breast cancer mortality, there was a modest positive associated risk with DES use with a relative risk of 1.34 (95% confidence interval, 1.06–1.69). Women who used DES in pregnancy are advised to follow the usual breast cancer screening guidelines of a monthly self-examination and an annual mammography and breast examination by a health care provider.

In case–control studies, women exposed to DES are not at increased risk of developing endometrial cancer. Similarly, these women are not at greater risk of developing cervical cancer. Only the daughters of women exposed to DES appear to be at increased risk of developing clear cell adenocarcinoma of the cervix during their reproductive years. Because daughters exposed to DES are aging, they will need to be observed for a possible increased incidence of clear cell adenocarcinoma of the cervix, which normally occurs in women at ages 50–80 years. In women exposed to DES who have a negative tobacco smoking history, there does not appear to be a greater risk for the development of lung cancer. Although the incidence of colon cancer increases with age, women who used DES do not appear to be at greater risk compared with nonusers.

Goldberg JM, Falcone T. Effect of diethylstilbestrol on reproductive function. Fertil Steril 1999;72:1–7.

Herbst AL. Behavior of estrogen-associated female genital tract cancer and its relation to neoplasia following intrauterine exposure to diethylstilbestrol (DES). Gynecol Oncol 2000;76:147–56.

Mitka M. CDC resource focuses on DES exposure [news]. JAMA 2003; 289:1624.

129
Sperm physiology

A couple is referred to your office for evaluation of primary infertility. The 34-year-old woman has a normal history, workup, and examination. The 36-year-old man has a history of testicular cancer and recently completed alkylating chemotherapy. His semen analysis demonstrates a volume of 3.2 mL, sperm concentration of 3.7 million sperm per mL, sperm motility of 25%, and normal sperm morphology of 35%. The cell type most affected by the chemotherapy in this patient is the

* (A) spermatogonium
(B) primary spermatocyte
(C) secondary spermatocyte
(D) spermatid
(E) spermatozoa

Each germ cell (spermatogonium) that undergoes differentiation after puberty gives rise to 16 primary spermatocytes, each of which then enters meiosis and gives rise to 4 spermatids and finally 4 spermatozoa (Fig. 129-1; see color plate). Therefore, each of the 3 million spermatogonia that begin the process of differentiation each day gives rise to 64 spermatozoa. One half of potential sperm are lost during this process leaving approximately 100 million sperm produced each day. Sperm formation takes approximately 70 days from the spermatocyte stage. The transport of sperm through the epididymis to the ejaculatory ducts requires approximately 14 days. Some maturation of sperm occurs during passage through the epididymis, as evidenced by enhancement of motility, but the final maturation (or capacitation) of sperm takes place in the female urogenital tract after ejaculation.

Drugs and medications may impair male fertility through 4 basic mechanisms:

1. Direct gonadotoxic effects
2. Alteration of the hypothalamic–pituitary–gonadal axis
3. Impairments in ejaculation and erectile function
4. Adverse effects on libido

Gonadotoxins affect spermatogenesis most directly by damaging spermatogonia in the testis or by inhibiting the function of the supporting Sertoli cells. These agents are less likely to affect later stages in sperm development including primary and secondary spermatocytes, spermatids, and spermatozoa. Adverse effects on spermatogenesis may be permanent in nature.

The severity of the gonadotoxic effects depends on the agents used, individual doses, and the time interval over which treatment is administered. The germinal epithelium with its rapid cell division is the target of these drugs. The sensitivity of dividing germ cells to chemotherapeutic agents has been recognized from the onset of their use. Total destruction of spermatogenic stem cells in the testes leads to permanent sterility; however, with some forms of combination therapy, the toxicity of individual agents can be reduced by combining agents in lower doses, limiting damage to stem cells, and increasing the possibility of eventual restoration of fertility.

The chemotherapeutic agents that are most gonadotoxic are shown in Box 129-1. Treatment of testicular cancer with cisplatin and carboplatin regimens leads to temporary azoospermia and oligozoospermia in most men, with a recovery to normospermia in 80% of men by 5 years. The use of lower doses of alkylating agents for decreased numbers of cycles also can reduce gonadotoxicity. It is not always possible to regain sperm production following chemotherapy; therefore, it is essential to offer patients the option of sperm cryopreservation before the initiation of chemotherapy.

The issue of retrieving and preserving sperm from the adult male patient who is about to undergo ablative or destructive therapies poses no ethical obstacles. The male ejaculate is easily obtainable, and the cryopreservation techniques are readily available in sperm banks. The useful life of such stored specimens may be indefinite. The stored sperm may be used for artificial insemination, intrauterine insemination, or in vitro fertilization techniques.

BOX 129-1

Chemotherapeutic Agents That Are Most Gonadotoxic

Alkylating agents
- Cyclophosphamide (Cytoxan)
- Chlorambucil (Leukeran)
- Melphalan (Alkeran)
- Carmustine (BiCNU, Gliadel)
- Lomustine (CCNU, CeeNU)

Antimetabolites
- Cytarabine

Vinca alkaloids
- Vinblastine

Others
- Procarbazine hydrochloride (Matulane)
- Cisplatin (Platinol)
- Nitrogen mustard (Mustargen)
- Carboplatin

Howell SJ, Shalet SM. Testicular function following chemotherapy. Hum Reprod Update 2001;7:363–9.

Meirow D, Schenker JG. Cancer and male infertility. Hum Reprod 1995;10:2017–22.

Thompson ST. Prevention of male infertility: an update. Urol Clin North Am 1994;21:365–76.

130
Bone density studies

A 59-year-old woman with severe osteoarthritis and recent multiple lumbar vertebral fractures comes in for a bone mineral density (BMD) study. The patient is a smoker, and her mother has severe osteoporosis. Four years ago, a dual-energy X-ray absorptiometry (DXA) scan showed a spine T-score of -2. She has taken a bisphosphonate for 4 years. Based on her history, the best next step in evaluation is a

- (A) ultrasonography of the calcaneus
- (B) lateral spine X-ray
- (C) peripheral DXA of the wrist
- (D) central DXA of the spine
- * (E) quantitative computed tomography scan

The most commonly used diagnostic test for determining BMD is central DXA, which measures BMD at various anatomic sites. Although central DXA scan was initially used to make the diagnosis of osteopenia in this patient, the intervening variables (ie, fracture and severe osteoarthritis) may make quantitative computed tomography the optimal and most precise mode of monitoring this women's response to bisphosphonates.

A newer method of assessing BMD is quantitative ultrasonography of the heel (calcaneus), which has the advantages of portability, low cost, and ease of operation. This method, however, has several disadvantages: it may underestimate the "true" incidence of osteoporosis as determined by central monitoring; it should not be used to monitor the progress of therapy used in treating osteopenia or osteoporosis; and it does not monitor sites where fractures predominate (ie, spine and hip).

A lateral spine X-ray may be useful for detecting an asymptomatic crush vertebral fracture, but it is an insensitive tool if used to monitor response to treatment for osteoporosis. Usually, asymptomatic lumbar vertebral fractures are detected serendipitously at the time of a lateral chest X-ray obtained to rule out pulmonary disease.

Studies have demonstrated that peripheral BMD testing correlates with a woman's global fracture risk. However, in most cases, a central measurement at the site at risk for fracture (eg, spine or hip) is a much better predictor of future fracture at that particular site than measurement at a different site. The lack of correlation between peripheral BMD measurements and central DXA is the main reason these devices should not be used to monitor response to treatment.

Central DXA is considered to be the criterion standard for the noninvasive prefracture diagnosis of osteoporosis. It provides an estimate of BMD based on area. The recommended skeletal site for monitoring is the posteroanterior lumbar spine at vertebrae lumbar 1–4 and the total hip. The lateral spine, Ward's region of the hip, or peripheral skeletal sites (other than the forearm) should not be used. As in the current case, previous compression fractures and osteoarthritis may falsely elevate BMD measurements of the spine with DXA. Additionally, body weight changes and curvature of the spine may alter BMD measurements when central DXA is used.

Hamdy RC, Petak SM, Lenchik L. Which central dual x-ray absorptiometry skeletal sites and regions of interest should be used to determine the diagnosis of osteoporosis? International Society for Clinical Densitometry Position Development Panel and Scientific Advisory Committee. J Clin Densitom 2002;5(suppl):S11–8.

Lenchik L, Leib ES, Hamdy RC, Binkley NC, Miller PD, Watts NB. Executive summary International Society for Clinical Densitometry position development conference Denver, Colorado July 20–22, 2001. International Society for Clinical Densitometry Position Development Panel and Scientific Advisory Committee. J Clin Densitom 2002; 5(suppl):S1–3.

Miller PD, Njeh CF, Jankowski LG, Lenchik L. What are the standards by which bone mass measurement at peripheral skeletal sites should be used in the diagnosis of osteoporosis? International Society for Clinical Densitometry Position Development Panel and Scientific Advisory Committee. J Clin Densitom 2002;5(suppl):S39–45.

131
Occlusion of the fallopian tubes

A 30-year-old woman with primary infertility of 1-year duration undergoes hysterosalpingography (HSG), which reveals a normal uterine cavity but bilateral proximal tubal occlusion at the uterotubal junction. The patient has no history of previous abdominal surgery, sexually transmitted diseases, pelvic pain, or dysmenorrhea. She would prefer not to undergo surgery or anesthesia at this time. An appropriate next step for examination of the fallopian tubes is

   (A) 3-dimensional ultrasonography
* (B) repeat HSG
   (C) sonohysterography
   (D) office hysteroscopy

Proximal tubal occlusion is a common finding on HSG, and it occurs in up to 15% of patients. The occlusion is seen at the uterotubal junction, wherein radiographic contrast fails to enter into the isthmic fallopian tube. This occlusion can be secondary to a number of pathologic conditions (eg, acute or chronic salpingitis, salpingitis isthmica nodosa, cornual fibroids, pelvic adhesive disease, endometritis, prior ectopic pregnancy, and adenomyosis). However, in a large proportion of cases, the proximal occlusion may indeed be functional. The interstitial portion of the fallopian tube is a complex region anatomically. It is in this area of the fallopian tube that the myometrium of the uterus transitions into the 3 layers of muscle that make up the fallopian tube. In addition, there is parasympathetic and sympathetic innervation to the fallopian tube, which aids in the peristaltic movements necessary for gamete transport. Instrumentation of the uterus during the HSG procedure may indeed lead to tubal spasm and nonfilling of the fallopian tube with contrast.

A number of techniques have been described over the past decade to overcome uterotubal junction occlusion: selective salpingography, transcervical tubal cannulation (by fluoroscopy or by simultaneous hysteroscopy and laparoscopy), transcervical balloon tuboplasty, falloposcopy, and more recently sonohysterography. All of these methods have utility but most require some anesthesia to perform, which is undesirable in this case. These procedures may be performed if repeat HSG reveals bilateral tubal occlusion. If repeat HSG reveals one fallopian tube is patent, further diagnostic testing is not necessary.

Sonohysterography detects the accumulation of fluid in the pelvis by ultrasound as evidence of tubal patency. It is known to make false-positive diagnosis of tubal occlusion at a rate that may exceed that of HSG.

The simplest way to confirm the presence of proximal tubal occlusion is to repeat the HSG in 1 month, and this should be the next step for this patient. A recent study of 40 patients with proximal tubal occlusion showed that repeat HSG revealed that the affected tubes were actually patent in 60% of cases. Hysterosalpingography requires no anesthesia, requires minimal lost time from work, and, thus, would be the best next step for examination of the fallopian tubes in this case. In some settings, it is possible to schedule a repeat HSG with concomitant selective salpingography (tubal cannulation). If this is successful, the patient will potentially avoid a surgical approach that would require anesthesia.

Office hysteroscopy provides little ability to visualize the proximal tube and is not appropriate here. Three-dimensional ultrasonography alone does help detect the presence of fibroids, but otherwise is not specific for the evaluation of tubal patency.

Dessole S, Meloni GB, Capobianco G, Manzoni MA, Ambrosini G, Canalis GC. A second hysterosalpingography reduces the use of selective technique for treatment of a proximal tubal obstruction. Fertil Steril 2000;73:1037–9.

Flood JT, Grow DR. Transcervical tubal cannulation: a review. Obstet Gynecol Surv 1993;48:768–76.

Sankpal RS, Confino E, Matzel A, Cohen LS. Investigation of the uterine cavity and fallopian tubes using three-dimensional saline sonohysterosalpingography. Int J Gynaecol Obstet 2001;73:125–9.

132–135

Hysterosalpingography versus sonohysterogram

For each of the following clinical scenarios (132–135), match the most appropriate diagnostic tools (A–D).

(A) Hysterosalpingography (HSG)
(B) Sonohysterography
(C) Hysteroscopy
(D) Transvaginal ultrasonography

A 132. A 32-year-old woman comes in for follow-up 6 months after a tubal ligation reversal.

B 133. A 30-year-old woman presents with continuous vaginal bleeding refractory to medical therapy for 4 months. Her pelvic examination in the office is normal.

A 134. A 25-year-old woman presents with a history of pelvic inflammatory disease and infertility.

D 135. A 33-year-old woman presents with a positive pregnancy test result and pelvic pain.

Imaging modalities used to evaluate pelvic anatomy have advanced rapidly over the past 2 decades. Hysterosalpingography, sonohysterography, hysteroscopy, and transvaginal ultrasonography are invaluable diagnostic tools that aid providers in evaluation and treatment. Important indications for use include preoperative assessment of the uterus and adnexa, infertility evaluation, pregnancy monitoring, and screening for gynecologic pathology. It is essential to understand the proper indications, contraindications, potential benefits, and be aware of any important complications before using these procedures in a clinical setting.

Hysterosalpingography, the best diagnostic tool for patients 132 and 134, is a radiologic procedure that involves injection of contrast dye through the reproductive tract under fluoroscopy in a radiology outpatient setting. It is used to evaluate the internal anatomy of the cervix, uterine cavity, and fallopian tubes and to document tubal patency. Indications for use include evaluation of infertility and gynecologic disorders (such as abnormal uterine bleeding), evaluation of recurrent miscarriage, and location of a lost intrauterine device (IUD). Hysterosalpingography is contraindicated in pregnancy, during active pelvic infection, during menstrual bleeding, or in a case with a documented history of iodine allergy. The most common side effect is uterine cramping.

Hysterosalpingography can be used to evaluate for tubal patency after a sterilization reversal. In fact, of the choices listed, HSG is the only imaging modality that can visualize the fallopian tubes and document patency. Injecting fluid with sonohysterography can visualize fluid in the cul de sac to document at least 1 patent fallopian tube, but it cannot image the fallopian tubes directly. If a patient has a hydrosalpinx, there is an increased risk of postprocedure infection, and antibiotics are recommended. In patients with these risk factors, the risk of severe infection approaches 3%.

Sonohysterography, the best diagnostic step for patient 133, is a simple procedure that enhances the use of vaginal ultrasonography to evaluate the uterine cavity for abnormalities. A small catheter is introduced into the cervix to instill fluid to distend the uterine cavity. Transvaginal ultrasonography is used to scan the fluid-filled cavity to enhance endometrial polyps, submucous myomas, intrauterine adhesions, müllerian anomalies, and abnormal uterine bleeding. The procedure is simple and without significant risk. Most patients who undergo the procedure experience little discomfort. It is easily used in the office setting and training is minimal. The only contraindications are active infection or pregnancy.

Hysteroscopy involves direct visualization of the uterine cavity and is considered the criterion standard to diagnose and treat uterine pathology. It can be used in an office or operating room setting. In the office, the patient is commonly given a paracervical block along with an oral analgesic before introducing a small hysteroscope into the uterine cavity through the cervix. Usually, there is no need for cervical dilation. Indications and contraindications are similar to those for sonohysterography. Use in the operating room usually involves treatment of more complicated pathology, such as resection of submucous myomas, polyps, or a uterine septum, with an operating hysteroscope that is larger than one used in the office setting. The patient with abnormal uterine bleeding with large submucous myomas would be best treated with a hysteroscopic procedure. Patients treated with advanced hysteroscopic procedures are at higher risk for electrolyte abnormalities from fluid use, uterine perforation, and cervical laceration.

Of all the imaging tools available to the gynecologist, transvaginal ultrasonography is used most frequently in the office and provides an accurate evaluation of the uterus and adnexa. Ultrasound probes are used transabdominally or transvaginally to visualize the pelvis with high intensity sound waves. Transvaginal ultrasonography cannot clearly define uterine cavity anatomy or pelvic pathology with certainty. Other forms of imaging are necessary to further evaluate abnormalities noted. Ultrasonography is very helpful to monitor the ongoing pregnancy as well as ovulation induction and embryo transfer, visualize lost IUDs, and diagnose ovarian cysts and uterine fibroids. Color flow Doppler ultrasonography combined with transvaginal ultrasonography can enable a closer look at uterine and adnexal structures and their vascularity.

The patient who is pregnant with pelvic pain, as in the case of patient 135, is a good candidate for transvaginal ultrasonography in the clinic. Routine use of transvaginal ultrasonography in the office can quickly correlate presenting symptoms with pelvic pathology, including the presence of an ectopic pregnancy, ovarian cysts, or uterine fibroids. Any of these conditions may be found in the clinical scenario presented.

Heard MJ, Carson SA. Hysterosalpingography: a clinical update. Female Pat 2001;26(4):29–31, 35, 39–40.

Prevedourakis C, Loutradis D, Kalianidis C, Makris N, Aravantinos D. Hysterosalpingography and hysteroscopy in female infertility. Hum Reprod 1994;9:2353–5.

Snowden EU, Jarrett JC 2nd, Dawood MY. Comparison of diagnostic accuracy of laparoscopy, hysteroscopy, and hysterosalpingography in evaluation of female infertility. Fertil Steril 1984;41:709–13.

Soares SR, Barbosa dos Reis MM, Camargos AF. Diagnostic accuracy of sonohysterography, transvaginal sonography, and hysterosalpingography in patients with uterine cavity diseases. Fertil Steril 2000;73: 406–11.

136–138

Evaluation of bleeding with hormone therapy

For each postmenopausal woman taking hormone therapy (HT) referred for evaluation of uterine bleeding (136–138), select the most appropriate management (A–D).

(A) Sonohysterography
(B) Endometrial biopsy
(C) Dilation and curettage
(D) Observation

D **136.** A 52-year-old symptomatic woman, gravida 3, para 3, started taking combination HT 6 weeks ago. She has experienced episodic daily spotting for the past 2 weeks, requiring sanitary protection. Her gynecologic medical history is unremarkable.

B **137.** A 37-year old nulliparous woman began taking combination HT after a bilateral oophorectomy 3 years ago for endometriomas. She experienced no bleeding for the first 2 years of HT but has bled for 3–4 days on 4 occasions in the past 8 months.

A **138.** A 62-year-old nulliparous woman has undergone multiple dilation and curettage procedures for uterine polyps before menopause. She has been taking HT for more than 10 years and has had 2 recent 1-day episodes of bleeding.

Distinguishing between a normal perimenopausal pattern and abnormal uterine bleeding can be difficult. Typical patterns indicative of abnormal uterine bleeding include heavy bleeding resulting in anemia or bleeding with clots; uterine bleeding lasting more than 7 days or 2 more days longer than normal; intervals shorter than 21 days between uterine bleeding episodes; and uterine bleeding after intercourse. These patterns are different from those usually seen after initiating HT, which in itself is associated with bleeding.

Postmenopausal women with an intact uterus who receive HT generally are prescribed estrogen plus progestin to reduce the risk of endometrial hyperplasia. For many patients, unscheduled bleeding with HT usually is a reason for discontinuation of therapy; however, when HT is initiated early in the perimenopause, such unscheduled bleeding is not uncommon. In the first 6 months of therapy, episodes of irregular bleeding will occur in more than one third of women taking cyclic or continuous combined therapy. After the first year of treatment, amenorrhea will occur in approximately 70–80% of patients taking continuous combined HT. Therefore, the best step in managing patients in that period would be observation, and this is the appropriate management of patient 136.

Continued observation of a patient who has had no bleeding for the first 2 years on HT followed by repeated episodes of bleeding over the past 8 months would be contraindicated in patient 137, who should be further evaluated for a pathologic etiology for her abnormal bleeding. Several modalities may be used to evaluate the endometrial cavity. An appropriate first step would be an endometrial biopsy to rule out abnormal endometrial histology.

Endometrial thickness evaluated by transvaginal ultrasound also has been promoted to screen for asymptomatic disease before or during HT, and it has been used as a less invasive adjunct to biopsy for endometrial hyperplasia. Although it is useful to rule out other pelvic pathology, data do not support its use as the sole evaluation of postmenopausal women.

In postmenopausal women, an endometrial lining that exceeds a thickness of 5 mm generally warrants evaluation to rule out endometrial hyperplasia or carcinoma. The Postmenopausal Estrogen/Progestin Intervention (PEPI) study, a large multicenter randomized trial, called into question the practice of using ultrasonography to monitor the endometrium. In a largely asymptomatic cohort of postmenopausal women, the PEPI study compared 2 methods, ultrasonography and endometrial biopsy. After the first year, the investigators were able to determine concordance of ultrasonography with endometrial thickness directly via histopathology of endometrial biopsy specimens. Endometrial thickness was greater in women who received estrogen alone than in women who received cyclic or continuous estrogen–progesterone or placebo for 3 years; although associated with detection of endometrial hyperplasia, it was not associated with detection of more serious diagnoses. The PEPI study concluded that the high false-positive rate rendered ultrasonography an impractical screening procedure in asymptomatic women regardless of whether they were receiving HT.

Performance of a hysteroscopy with dilation and curettage is not indicated at this point. At a minimum, endometrial biopsy should be performed to rule out endometrial hyperplasia. Sonohysterography and an endometrial biopsy would strengthen the detection for endometrial pathology.

Patient 138 should undergo sonohysterography, which is more sensitive than ultrasonography, and an office endometrial biopsy to determine the cause of her recent episodes of bleeding, which are most likely a recurrence of her uterine polyps. Sonohysterography also is useful to detect the exact location of any polyps and, thus, will help to plan the surgical approach. Given the recent findings from the Women's Health Initiative study, this patient's history also should be reassessed to determine what risks she faces if she were to continue taking HT. Current U.S. Food and Drug Administration recommendations for the use of any systemic estrogen-containing treatment regimen are that it should be used in symptomatic women for the shortest amount of time.

Langer RD, Pierce JJ, O'Hanlan KA, Johnson SR, Espeland MA, Trabal JF, et al. Transvaginal ultrasonography compared with endometrial biopsy for the detection of endometrial disease. Postmenopausal Estrogen/Progestin Interventions Trial. N Engl J Med 1997;337; 1792–8.

Rossouw JE, Anderson GL, Prentice RL, LaCroix AZ, Kooperberg C, Stefanick ML, et al. Risks and benefits of estrogen plus progestin in healthy postmenopausal women: principal results from the Women's Health Initiative randomized controlled trial. Writing Group for the Women's Health Initiative Investigators. JAMA 2002;288:321–33.

Turner RT, Berman AM, Topel HC. Improved demonstration of endometrial polyps and submucous myomas using saline-enhanced vaginal sonohysterography. J Am Assoc Gynecol Laparosc 1995;2: 421–5.

The Writing Group for the PEPI Trial. Effects of hormone replacement therapy on endometrial histology in postmenopausal women: the Postmenopausal Estrogen/Progestin Interventions (PEPI) Trial. JAMA 1996;275:370–5.

139–141
Uterine and associated anomalies

Match the following clinical scenarios (139–141) with the most appropriate uterine anomaly (A–D).

(A) Unicornuate uterus
(B) Obstructed hemivagina
(C) Rudimentary uterine horn
(D) Uterine septum

A **139.** A 31-year-old woman with history of preterm delivery has an irregular shaped uterus and one fallopian tube seen at cesarean delivery.

B **140.** A 13-year-old adolescent with pelvic pain has irregular menstrual cycles, an absent right kidney, and a right pelvic mass.

D **141.** 25-year-old woman with secondary infertility and recurrent miscarriage has an abnormal hysterosalpingogram and normal uterine fundus noted on laparoscopy.

Congenital anomalies of the müllerian system (Fig. 139–141-1) are common and are reported in 1 in every 200–600 women of childbearing age. Both multifactorial and familial modes of inheritance have been reported. Some anomalies are asymptomatic while others produce symptoms during puberty. Up to 25% of women with these abnormalities have difficulty conceiving and many pregnancies are complicated with spontaneous abortion, preterm delivery, and abnormal fetal lie. In addition, müllerian anomalies are associated with renal, muscular, and skeletal abnormalities that could be clinically significant and should be routinely investigated.

The development of the müllerian system involves fusion of the müllerian ducts, which create the fallopian tube, uterus, and upper two thirds of the vagina. This fuses with the lower vagina to form the complete reproductive tract. Defects along this developmental pathway can cause uterine abnormalities, but their true etiology is unknown. Congenital uterine anomalies are the results of lack of fusion, underdevelopment, and defective resorption or canalization of müllerian ducts.

A fusion defect is responsible for the formation of the bicornuate uterus. Abnormal fusion all along the ducts can result in partial or total duplication of the uterus. This ranges from a small indentation at the fundus termed the arcuate uterus to the uterine didelphys, which is complete duplication of the uterus. These anomalies often are asymptomatic unless outflow obstruction occurs in one horn or they are discovered on hysterosalpingogram during the evaluation for recurrent miscarriage or infertility. Delivery complications that can occur include preterm delivery, cervical incompetence, and dysfunctional labors. Unification of a bicornuate uterus is rarely recommended and only after recurrent pregnancy loss.

A developmental problem that involves one side of the müllerian ducts results in the unicornuate uterus or partial or lack of formation of one side. The anomaly often goes unrecognized unless there is obstruction and is associated with ipsilateral renal agenesis. Although preterm delivery is common, patients can go to term without complications. Patient 139, who had an irregular uterus discovered at cesarean delivery with only one tube, most likely has a unicornuate uterus. Her pelvis should be inspected for a rudimentary horn, and it also is essential that she be investigated for renal anomalies.

An obstructed hemivagina occurs where there is lack of resorption of the upper vaginal septum during development causing an outlet obstruction of one side. In virtually all cases of obstructed hemivagina, there is associated an absent ipsilateral kidney. Associated with other müllerian abnormalities, this uterine anomaly can lead to a backup of menstrual flow at menarche causing a hematocolpos, hematometra, and ultimately ovarian and pelvic endometriosis. Timely diagnosis and treatment with relief of the obstruction will treat pain as well as preserve future fertility. Patient 140, the adolescent with pelvic pain, irregular menses, and a pelvic mass is one example of an obstructed hemivagina. The pelvic mass most likely is a hematocolpos, hematometra, or possibly a hematosalpinx. Despite the history of irregular menstrual cycles, the patient had a thickened endometrial stripe which was present in the obstructed horn with backup of menstrual blood. Sometimes, damage to the adnexa from retrograde menstruation requires operative intervention to treat a hematosalpinx or ovarian endometrioma. The affected uterine horn may be left in situ, removed by hemihysterectomy if it is damaged, or unified with the open horn and allowed to function normally in the future.

CLASSIFICATION OF MÜLLERIAN ANOMALIES

Patient's name _____ Date _____ Chart # _____

Age _____ G _____ P _____ Sp Ab _____ VTP _____ Ectopic _____ Infertile Yes _____ No _____

Other significant history (eg, surgery, infection) _____
_____

HSG _____ Sonography _____ Photography _____ Laparoscopy _____ Laparotomy _____

Examples

I. Hypoplasis/Agenesis	II. Unicornuate	III. Didelphus
a. Vaginal* b. Cervical	a. Communicating b. Noncommunicating	IV. Bicornuate
c. Fundal d. Tubal e. Combined	c. No cavity d. No horn	a. Complete b. Partial
V. Septate	VI. Arcuate	VII. DES Drug Related
a. Complete† b. Partial		

*Uterus may be normal or take a variety of abnormal forms.
†May have two distinct cervices.

Type of anomaly

　　　Class I _____　　　Class V _____
　　　Class II _____　　　Class VI _____
　　　Class III _____　　　Class VII _____
　　　Class IV _____

Treatment (surgical procedures) _____
_____

Prognosis for conception and subsequent viable infant*

___ Excellent (>75%)　　___ Good (50–75%)
___ Fair (25–50%)　　　 ___ Poor (<25%)

• Based on physician's judgment.

Recommended follow-up treatments _____
_____

For additional supply contact:
American Society for Reproductive Medicine
1209 Montgomery Highway
Birmingham, AL 35216-2809
Tel: 205-978-5000 • Fax: 205-978-5018

Additional findings _____
_____
_____
Vagina _____
Cervix _____
Tubes: Right _____ Left _____
Kidneys: Right _____ Left _____

Drawing
L　　　　　　　　　　　　　　　　R

Property of
American Society for Reproductive Medicine

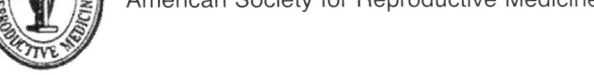

FIG. 139–141-1. American Fertility Society classification of mullerian anomalies. (Allen FS, Feste JR. Pelvic disease classifications. Fertil Steril 1989;51:199–201.)

Where formation of a müllerian horn is incomplete as in a fusion defect, a unicornuate uterus is present along with a rudimentary horn that lies away from the other horn and disconnected from the vagina. If functioning endometrium is present, an obstructed hematometra can result causing abdominal pain and a pelvic mass. The standard treatment for this finding is removal. Surgical caution should be taken not to misdiagnose structures like a pelvic kidney instead because renal anomalies may occur along with müllerian abnormalities.

The most common müllerian anomaly is the uterine septum. Its etiology results from failure of the fused müllerian ducts to resorb, creating a septum. This can be partial or complete, spanning the entire uterus down into the cervix and upper vagina. These abnormalities are nonobstructive and can be diagnosed with ultrasonography, sonohysterography, hysterosalpingography, or magnetic resonance imaging. The criterion standard for diagnosis has been to image a smooth fundus by laparoscopy with a septum noted by hysteroscopy. The risk of miscarriage is increased if the septum is not resected. It also can lead to malpresentation in pregnancy and complicate delivery. A uterine septum can easily be resected by performing a hysteroscopic lysis of the septum with the use of scissors, cautery, or laser. Patient 141, with secondary infertility and recurrent miscarriage with an abnormal hysterosalpingography and smooth fundus on laparoscopy, most likely has a clinically significant uterine septum that should be treated.

Congenital müllerian anomalies are common abnormalities that present during the infertility evaluation or as an obstetric problem. Aberrant embryologic development can result in several different malformations that have clinical importance. Complete evaluation should be undertaken before planning any surgical procedure. Preservation of fertility and good obstetric outcome are the ultimate goals.

Acien P. Reproductive performance of women with uterine malformations. Hum Reprod 1993;8:122–6.

Buttram VC Jr, Gibbons WE. Mullerian anomalies: a proposed classification (an analysis of 144 cases). Fertil Steril 1979;32:40–6.

Nahum GG. Uterine anomalies. How common are they, and what is their distribution among subtypes? J Reprod Med 1998;43:877–87.

Raga F, Bauset C, Remohi J, Bonilla-Musoles F, Simon C, Pellicer A. Reproductive impact of congenital Mullerian anomalies. Hum Reprod 1997;12:2277–81.

142–145

Laser characteristics and safety

For each of the following types of gynecologic surgery (142–145), select the laser (A–D) that has the most appropriate characteristics and safety history.

(A) Carbon-dioxide laser
(B) Argon laser
(C) KTP laser
(D) Neodymium:yttrium-aluminum-garnet (nd:YAG) laser

A 142. Standard glass lenses (eg, those commonly used in reading glasses) are sufficient to defuse laser energy and prevent eye injury.

D 143. When used in the noncontact mode, laser energy has a depth of tissue penetration of 3–7 mm.

A 144. The wavelength of energy produced is highly absorbed by the water within cells and, thus, has minimal tissue penetration.

C 145. The wavelength of the energy produced is altered during passage through a crystal before traveling to the surgical handpiece.

Laser, light amplification by stimulated emission, is a means for delivering energy to tissue. A number of lasers are now in common use in therapeutic medicine. Each laser, by virtue of its physical properties, has characteristic effects on human tissues, different capabilities, and quite different inherent safety issues. The effect of laser energy on tissue is one of reflection, transmission, scattering, and absorption. For the most part, the effect a given laser energy has on tissue is the consequence of absorption by the tissue and is determined by the wavelength of the laser energy and the physical properties of the tissue. When laser energy is absorbed by tissue, it is converted to heat energy that creates the effect.

Water and blood are present in significant amounts in the various tissues. Because water is a major component of cellular structure, its interaction with laser energy is predominant. Hemoglobin, also present in abundance in many tissues, interacts with laser energy but with characteristics different from water. When lasers are used therapeutically, it is important for the surgeon to understand the characteristics of the different laser modalities and how they interact with tissues, especially the hemoglobin and water components, to insure safe and effective use.

The lasers in common use today are confined to the visible, ultraviolet, and infrared portions of the spectrum. Table 142–145-1 presents a list of the therapeutic lasers and their respective wavelengths. For lasers with wavelengths that render them invisible, it is common to use a visible spotting guide so that the operator can see where the laser is being focused. Most often, the spotting beam is a helium-neon laser that provides a visible red beam.

Whether of visible or invisible wavelengths, laser energy has the potential for serious harm to patients and physicians.

Perhaps the most commonly used laser in gynecologic surgery is the carbon-dioxide laser. Because of its long wavelength (10,600 nm), carbon-dioxide laser energy is highly absorbed by water and, thus, has its greatest effect on tissues with relatively large water content. As the laser energy is absorbed by water, it is converted to thermal energy and heats the water. The water temperature increases almost instantaneously creating steam that explodes the cell. Because water absorbs nearly 90% of the laser energy within 100 μm of the tissue surface exposed, the initial depth of injury is stated to be 0.1–0.2 mm. However, carbon-dioxide laser energy is poorly absorbed by hemoglobin and, thus, fails to effectively initiate

TABLE 142–145-1. Characteristics of Lasers Used in Gynecology

Type of Laser	Color	Wavelength (nm)
Carbon-dioxide	Mid-far infrared	10,600
Nd:YAG 1.06	Near infrared	1,064
Nd:YAG 1.32	Near infrared	1,218
Excimer	Ultraviolet	200–400
Visible wavelengths		
Helium-neon	Red	630
Dye laser	Yellow/green	577
KTP	Green	532
Argon	Blue	488

Abbreviation: Nd:YAG, neodymium:yittrium-aluminum-garnet.

hemostasis. For these reasons, most clinicians choose to use the carbon-dioxide laser for the treatment of epithelial lesions. If bleeding is encountered during treatment of an epithelial lesion with a carbon-dioxide laser, the operator can defocus the laser beam by pulling the surgical handpiece away from the tissue. This increases the diameter of the laser spot and reduces the power density (ie, the amount of laser energy per centimeter of surface area). The result is diffusion of energy and slower heat generation sufficient to stimulate coagulation.

Safety issues involved with the use of carbon-dioxide lasers, as with all lasers, are based on the physical properties of the laser energy. Because carbon-dioxide laser energy is highly absorbed by water, there is a danger of corneal injury if the beam is directed at the eyes or if it is reflected toward the eyes. In addition, because the carbon-dioxide laser beam is invisible, safety goggles or glasses are mandatory. Because of the relatively long wavelength, virtually any type of glass lens is sufficient to defuse the beam and protect the corneas.

Although carbon-dioxide laser energy is minimally scattered, the beam can be reflected off shiny surfaces. Therefore, surgical instruments used during laser procedures should be sand blasted or subjected to other treatment to roughen the surface and reduce reflectiveness. This is especially true of flat instruments, such as vaginal speculums, as well as rounded instruments that may reflect in multiple directions. Simply blackening or anodizing instruments is insufficient to prevent reflection of the invisible laser beam. Proper alignment of mirrors in the laser instrument will ensure accurate delivery of the laser beam. Because carbon-dioxide laser energy is effectively absorbed by water, an additional safety measure is frequent irrigation and the isolation of the tissue site of interest with moistened laparotomy sponges. A fire hazard also exists with the use of carbon-dioxide lasers and all drapes should be fire retardant and moistened or covered with moistened towels.

The nd:YAG laser is another laser in common use in gynecologic surgical procedures. Similar to the carbon-dioxide laser, the nd:YAG laser has a wavelength in the invisible portion of the spectrum. The nd:YAG laser has a wavelength of 1,064 nm and has characteristics and, thus, safety issues quite distinct from that of the carbon-dioxide laser. The wavelength of the nd:YAG laser is in the near infrared portion of the spectrum, but it is still invisible and, thus, requires a helium: neon-aiming beam. This wavelength of energy is transmissible through quartz fibers, so most devices use flexible fibers for transmission to handpieces and instruments adaptable to laparoscopes and hysteroscopes. The laser energy of the nd:YAG laser is poorly absorbed by water. Special eyeglasses of optical density greater than 5 at 1,064 nm are required. The nd:YAG laser is transmitted through the cornea and focused by the lens on the retina and can result in permanent retinal damage if protective lenses of sufficient optical density are not used. This wavelength of energy is less well absorbed by hemoglobin rich tissues than the argon or KTP lasers.

When used in the "free beam" mode, nd:YAG laser energy has a depth of penetration of 3–7 mm. The surgeon needs to be aware of this characteristic because dark tissues well beneath the visible surface may be damaged during application of the laser energy. Reflective surfaces on surgical instruments need to be treated for use with the nd:YAG laser in "free beam" mode just as with the carbon-dioxide laser. The advent of synthetic sapphire or quartz tips that can be attached to the end of the transmission fiber allows the nd:YAG laser to be turned into an energy conversion device. The synthetic tips are coated with an infrared absorbent material that converts the laser energy into thermal energy in the tip. The "hot" tip is then applied to tissues for the desired effect. With these tips, the depth of penetration is less than 0.5 mm.

The 2 lasers with wavelengths that are in the visible spectrum and that are used regularly in gynecologic surgery, the argon and KTP lasers, have characteristics that make them particularly useful for coagulation. The KTP laser has a wavelength that is created by passing the nd:YAG laser beam (with a wavelength of 1,064 nm) through a KTP crystal that halves the wavelength to 532 nm. Its depth of penetration is 0.5–2.5 mm, which is similar to that of the argon laser. Because of their high absorbance by hemoglobin, both the KTP and the argon laser are used in heme-rich tissues, such as retina and liver. The KTP and the argon lasers are poorly absorbed by water and are transmissible through quartz fibers. Thus, both laser wavelengths can be used in fluid media. To protect the patient, the operator, and assistants, special colored lenses or eye filters on various scopes are mandatory for use with argon and KTP lasers.

Frank F. Noncontact delivery systems and accessories for the application of nd:YAG laser in endoscopy and surgery. In: Joffe SN, Oguro Y, eds. Advances in Nd:YAG laser surgery. New York (NY): Springer-Verlag; 1988. p. 10–8.

Keckstein J. Tissue effects of different lasers and diathermy. In: Sutton C, Diamond MP, eds. Endoscopic surgery for gynecologists. New York (NY): WB Saunders; 1993. p. 60–70.

Sinai R. Laser physics and laser instrumentation. In: Donnez J, Nisolle M, eds. An atlas of laser operative laparoscopy and hysteroscopy. New York (NY): The Parthenon Publishing Group; 1994. p. 1–20.

146–149
Uterine anomalies

Select the most appropriate associated clinical scenario (146–149) based on current understanding of normal physiology of müllerian development (A–D).

(A) Absence of *bcl-2* protein
(B) Failure of bi-directional resorption
(C) Defects in pericentric region of chromosome 8
(D) X-linked laterality sequence

A 146. A normal female fetus at 18 weeks of gestation with normal uterus and no uterine septum.

C 147. A 16-year-old adolescent with a blind ending vagina, mild mental retardation, and facial asymmetry.

B 148. A 26-year-old woman with a single uterus, complete uterine septum, cervical duplication, and complete longitudinal vaginal septum.

D 149. A 38-year-old woman with uterine septum and hypertelorism has 2 daughters with uterine septa and hypertelorism.

The uterus, cervix, and fallopian tubes are derived embryologically from the paired müllerian ducts. Traditional theory indicates that the 2 ducts fuse medially and form a solid Y-shaped uterovaginal primordium that subsequently canalizes to create 2 adjacent lumina. Cellular proliferation in the upper portion of what will become the uterus leads to the formation of a wedgelike upper median septum. The septum then resorbs resulting in the formation of a single uterine cavity. Anatomic anomalies develop when these processes fail to occur in the normal sequence or when the different components of the process fail to go to completion.

An important mechanism in the regulation of normal müllerian development appears to be apoptosis, or programmed cell death. Through apoptosis, it is possible for unwanted cells to be eliminated. Apoptosis has been described in the adult female reproductive organs and is involved in follicular atresia as well as in the endometrial sloughing that occurs during menses. Apoptosis is regulated by many genes, but one, *bcl-2*, a protein that protects cells from apoptosis and promotes cell survival, appears to be specifically involved in normal human female development. This protein has been localized to certain portions of the myometrium and endometrium. In recent studies, it has been demonstrated that the embryonic expression of *bcl-2* is absent from the embryonal uterine septum while present in superior, inferior, and lateral myometrium as well as in the tubal epithelium and muscularis. Thus, in the case of a normal female fetus, as with patient 146, the absence of *bcl-2* allows for normal resorption of the septal tissue. It remains to be determined whether *bcl-2* is present in the septal tissue of adult women with septate uterus.

Conventional or unidirectional theory states that fusion of the paired müllerian ducts and subsequent recanalization commences caudally and proceeds cephalad. Thus, failure to fuse followed by normal canalization results in a completely duplicated system, ie, 2 vaginas, 2 cervices, and 2 uteri, each with one fallopian tube. Partial fusion would be expected to result in a single vagina, single cervix, and bicornuate uterus. Complete fusion but incomplete canalization would lead to the single vagina, single cervix, and septate uterus.

Recent reports, however, call into question the unidirectional theory. Different investigators have now reported the finding of a single uterus with complete septum, cervical duplication, and complete longitudinal vaginal septum. One author reported the finding of different degrees of uterine septa in 3 sisters. After these reports, the classic unidirectional theory has been challenged and a new bi-directional theory proposed. This theory suggests that fusion and resorption begin at the isthmus and proceed simultaneously in both cranial and caudal directions. According to this theory, a septate uterus could develop following failure of fusion of the most caudal müllerian ducts and may result in a normal uterine fundus with a complete uterine septum, cervical duplication, and longitudinal vaginal septum as described in patient 147.

Müllerian aplasia is defined as congenital absence of the uterus and upper vagina, with normal ovaries, normal breast development, and female patterns of sex hair, also known as Mayer-Rokitansky-Küster-Hauser syndrome. Importantly, in addition to müllerian aplasia, embryologically related somatic anomalies are not infrequent. Thus, among women with müllerian abnormalities, it is not uncommon to observe renal and lower vertebral anomalies as well. These conditions have been defined as the müllerian duct aplasia, renal agenesis/ectopia, cervical somite dysplasia association or the genital, renal, ear, skeletal syndrome. The cause or causes remain(s) unclear, but the consensus among investigators is that it is multifactorial. Most patients with these conditions have completely normal female karyotypes and only a few patients are found to have chromosomal abnormalities (eg, reciprocal translocations). A single patient report suggests that genes in the pericentric region of chromosome 8 may be involved in the regulation of müllerian development because partial trisomy 8 mosaicism has been identified in a woman with müllerian aplasia, renal and skeletal abnormalities, and minor dysmorphic signs. The features described for patient 148 are the result of such a defect.

Other genetic abnormalities have been suggested in the etiology of müllerian anomalies. Fetal lateralization defects usually consist of either situs inversus (reversal of the sides of normally midline organs) or bilateral left- or right-sidedness. An X-linked form of lateralization defect has been described in males, and recent reports suggest that there is a carrier state in females. Heterozygous manifestations of the X-linked laterality sequence in females may vary among family members because of variable inactivation of the X chromosomes. Among obligate carriers of this defect, females have been found to have uterine septa and hypertelorism, now regarded as carrier manifestations. Thus, it appears that the X chromosomes contain a gene or genes that have an effect on right–left asymmetry as described in patient 149. The incidence of the abnormality among women with uterine septa is not known.

Ergun A, Pabuccu R, Atay V, Kucuk T, Duru NK, Gangor S. Three sisters with septate uteri: another reference to bi-directional theory. Hum Reprod 1997;12:140–2.

Lee DM, Osathanondh R, Yeh J. Localization of Bcl-2 in the human fetal mullerian tract. Fertil Steril 1998;70:135–40.

Loeffler J, Soelder E, Erdel M, Utermann B, Janecke A, Duba HC, et al. Mullerian aplasia associated with ring chromosome 8p12q12 mosaicism. Am J Med Genet 2003;116A:290–4.

Mikkila SP, Janas M, Karikoski R, Tarkkila T, Simola KO. X-linked laterality sequence in a family with carrier manifestations. Am J Med Genet 1994;49:435–8.

150–151

Mechanism of action of oral contraceptives

Select the steroid hormone (150–151) found in the combination oral contraceptive that results in the mechanism of action (A–E).

(A) Increases free testosterone
(B) Increases follicle-stimulating hormone (FSH) secretion
(C) Increases luteinizing hormone (LH) secretion
(D) Inhibits LH secretion
(E) Increases sex hormone-binding globulin

E 150. Ethinyl estradiol

D 151. Norethindrone

In the combination oral contraceptive, the combined action of the estrogen and progestin steroids leads to the contraceptive and noncontraceptive benefits of this medication. In the area of contraception, the estrogen component (ethinyl estradiol) suppresses FSH release and inhibits folliculogenesis. The estrogen also potentiates the action of the progestin by increasing the intracellular progesterone receptor pool and further stabilizes the decidualized endometrium. The progestin component (norethindrone) inhibits LH secretion and prevents the release of the oocyte by inhibiting the LH surge. The estrogen component potentiates the effect of progestin in suppressing LH secretion. Although estrogen is contained within the oral contraceptive, the pill is primarily progestin-dominant which leads to eventual endometrial atrophy and thickened cervical mucus. The presence of these 2 additional contraceptive mechanisms is preserved even when the dose of ethinyl estradiol is decreased to 20 µg per day.

In the area of noncontraceptive benefits, oral contraceptives are used to decrease hirsutism and acne. The estrogen component, ethinyl estradiol, is responsible for increasing the level of sex hormone-binding globulin. Increased levels of sex hormone-binding globulin lead to more binding of testosterone and less circulating free testosterone to bind to the androgen receptors. In a study of a new oral contraceptive, sex hormone-binding globulin levels were increased 296% and free testosterone levels were decreased 64% from baseline levels. The progestin component decreases LH secretion resulting in less stimulation of ovarian testosterone production. Progestins further inhibit 5α-reductase activity in the skin, which is responsible for conversion of testosterone to dihydrotestosterone, the primary androgen that stimulates the pilosebaceous unit and hair follicles in the skin.

American College of Obstetricians and Gynecologists. Hormonal agents as contraceptives. Precis: an update in obstetrics and gynecology. Reproductive endocrinology. 2nd ed. Washington, DC: ACOG; 2002. p. 162–7.

Boyd RA, Zegarac EA, Posvar EL, Flack MR. Minimal androgenic activity of a new oral contraceptive containing norethindrone acetate and graduated doses of ethinyl estradiol. Contraception 2001;63:71–6.

Rossmanith WG, Steffens D, Schramm G. A comparative randomized trial on the impact of two low-dose oral contraceptives on ovarian activity, cervical permeability, and endometrial receptivity. Contraception 1997;56:23–30.

152–154

Screening before hormone therapy

For each woman (152–154) who presents with severe vasomotor symptoms, and who has had a recent normal mammogram, a normal lipid profile 2 years previously, and a last menstrual cycle at least 12 months ago, select the most appropriate test for screening before beginning hormone therapy (HT) (A–E).

(A) Dual-energy X-ray absorptiometry (DXA) bone density study
(B) Lipid profile
(C) Fasting glucose and insulin levels
(D) *BRCA1*
(E) Follicle-stimulating hormone (FSH) test

B 152. A 54-year-old Hispanic woman, gravida 3, para 3, with type 2 diabetes mellitus is mildly obese and smokes 1–2 packs of cigarettes daily.

D 153. A 48-year-old Caucasian nulliparous woman exercises regularly and has never smoked. Breast cancer was diagnosed in her mother and maternal aunt at age 45 years.

A 154. A 50-year-old African-American woman, gravida 2, para 2, has a history of asthma and requires periodic steroid treatment.

Assessment of each woman should begin with a thorough medical and social history, including family history and lifestyle characteristics, that may affect her risk–benefit ratio in deciding whether to start HT. The patient also should have a complete physical examination, including a pelvic, rectal, and breast examination; mammogram; and Pap test. Presence of vasomotor symptoms, especially hot flushes, may be documented using the Menopause-Specific Quality of Life (MENQOL) questionnaire (Appendix F) or the Greene Climacteric Scale questionnaire, both at baseline and after administration of therapy to demonstrate benefit of the use of HT.

The American College of Obstetricians and Gynecologists supports baseline screening mammography at age 40 years followed by mammography at the following intervals: women aged 40–49 years should have screening mammography every 1–2 years, and women aged 50 years and older should have annual screening mammography. Women should be encouraged to perform monthly breast self-examinations throughout their lives. All women should have a clinical breast examination as part of their annual physical examination.

The importance of cardiovascular risk factors, such as age, smoking, hypertension, family history, dyslipidemia, obesity, and type 2 diabetes mellitus, in predicting cardiovascular disease in women becomes more important after menopause. Studies indicate that postmenopausal women usually have increases in low-density lipoprotein (LDL) cholesterol levels and decreases in high-density lipoprotein (HDL) cholesterol levels compared with premenopausal women. Increases in total cholesterol and triglyceride levels also have been observed in postmenopausal women. Elevated levels of total cholesterol and LDL cholesterol have both been associated with an increased risk of cardiovascular disease in women aged 65 years and younger. In addition, triglyceride levels are an independent predictor of cardiovascular disease in older women. With the onset of menopause, changes occur in fat distribution, with the predominant change being an increase in central adiposity. Estrogen loss also alters carbohydrate metabolism, resulting in decreases in insulin sensitivity and secretion, increasing the risk for type 2 diabetes. Diabetes mellitus also is linked to elevated triglyceride levels and reduced HDL cholesterol levels, especially in women. The risk for myocardial infarction in women who have diabetes is twice that for women of the same age who do not have diabetes. Dietary and pharmacologic lipid-lowering strategies can improve lipid profiles in women. In women with diabetes, with or without cardiovascular disease, the target LDL cholesterol level is at or less than 100 mg/dL. Although HT has been demonstrated to have a beneficial effect on lipids, on the basis of randomized prospective trials, HT is not recommended for the primary or secondary prevention of heart disease. In patient 152, a lipid profile should be repeated because of her increased risk for cardiovascular disease.

Family history is a nonmodifiable risk factor for breast cancer that is not considered a contraindication for HT unless the woman is a carrier of mutations in the *BRCA1* tumor suppressor gene and, thus, predisposed to develop both breast and ovarian cancer. In a prospective cohort study of 41,837 women aged 55–69 years, the risk of breast cancer in HT users with a family history of breast cancer did not differ significantly from nonusers. For patient 153, the correct choice would be a test to determine if she carries a mutation in the *BRCA1* gene before initiation of HT.

Dual-energy X-ray absorptiometry is the diagnostic test of choice for measurement of bone mineral density. Nonmodifiable and potentially modifiable risk factors for osteoporosis are summarized in Appendix C. The World Health Organization (WHO) criteria for defining osteoporosis based on bone mineral density measured by DXA scanning is as follows: a *T*-score of greater than −1 is normal; −1 to −2.5 is osteopenia; and less than or equal to −2.5 is osteoporosis. Severe, or established, osteoporosis is defined as a *T*-score of less than or equal to −2.5 with a fracture.

Many physicians currently measure *T*-scores using peripheral devices (ie, scans of the heel, forearm, or finger). Although peripheral devices are useful to screen for decreased bone mineral density, as demonstrated in the National Osteoporosis Risk Assessment study, they should not be used with WHO criteria for diagnosis of osteopenia or osteoporosis or for monitoring. Because of the lack of precision of peripheral devices, a low *T*-score by a peripheral device should be confirmed by a central DXA scan. All skeletal sites yield similar predictions of overall fracture risk.

Patient 154 is at increased risk for osteoporosis secondary to her periodic steroid use for treatment of asthma and menopausal status. Osteoporosis in women increases significantly following menopause because women lose approximately 20% of the expected lifetime bone loss during the first 5–7 years after menopause. Long-term glucocorticoid therapy induces osteoporosis by impairing calcium intestinal absorption, suppressing osteoblastic formation, and stimulating osteoclastic activity. Although African-American women have a 25% reduced risk of hip fractures than white women, their prevalence of osteopenia may be as high as 32%.

A fasting blood glucose test is the appropriate diagnostic test to detect type 2 diabetes mellitus in women who are obese and have elevated cholesterol levels with or without a family history of diabetes or gestational diabetes. Although fasting insulin may be used in the future to assist in the diagnosis of the phenomenon referred to as the metabolic syndrome, its use clinically is only for research purposes at this time.

A diagnostic FSH test is not indicated in any of these patients. They are symptomatic and had their last menstrual periods at least 1 year ago.

American Heart Association. Silent epidemic: the truth about women and heart disease. Dallas (TX): American Heart Association; 1995.

Greene JG. Guide to the Greene Climacteric Scale. Glasgow, Scotland: University of Glasgow; 1991.

Lafage-Proust MH, Boudignon B, Thomas T. Glucocorticoid-induced osteoporosis: Pathophysiological data and recent treatments. Joint Bone Spine 2003;70:109–18.

National Osteoporosis Foundation. America's bone health: the state of osteoporosis and low bone mass in our nation. Washington, DC: NOF; 2002.

Rossouw JE, Anderson GL, Prentice RL, LaCroix AZ, Kooperberg C, Stefanick ML, et al. Risks and benefits of estrogen plus progestin in healthy postmenopausal women: principal results from the Women's Health Initiative randomized controlled trial. Writing Group for the Women's Health Initiative Investigators. JAMA 2002;288:321–33.

The Rotterdam ESHRE/ASRM-Sponsored PCOS Consensus Workshop Group. Revised 2003 consensus on diagnostic criteria and long-term health risks related to polycystic ovary syndrome. Fertil Steril 2004;81:19–25.

Siris ES, Miller PD, Barrett-Connor E, Faulkner KG, Wehren LE, Abbott TA, et al. Identification and fracture outcomes of undiagnosed low bone density in postmenopausal women: results from the National Osteoporosis Risk Assessment. JAMA 2001;286:2815–22.

155–158
In vitro fertilization versus surgery

For each of the following patients with infertility (155–158), select the most appropriate treatment option to help achieve pregnancy (A–E).

(A) In vitro fertilization (IVF) with intracytoplasmic sperm injection (ICSI)
(B) Bilateral salpingectomy followed by IVF
(C) IVF alone
(D) Bilateral neosalpingostomy
(E) Bilateral tubal reversal

B 155. A 34-year-old woman has bilateral hydrosalpinges greater than 3 cm confirmed on ultrasonography. Her husband has 44 million sperm per cc on multiple semen analysis.

C 156. A 35-year-old woman has a history of severe dysmenorrhea, stage III endometriosis, and severe pelvic adhesive disease. Her husband has 66 million sperm per cc.

A 157. A 29-year-old woman with a history of chlamydial salpingitis, has bilateral proximal tubal occlusion confirmed on hysterosalpingography. Her husband has 2 million sperm per cc.

E 158. A 27-year-old woman with Hulka clip tubal sterilization is newly married and desires 2 more children. Her husband has 34 million sperm per cc.

Tubal disease is one of the major causes of female infertility and includes a variety of disorders, including blockage at various places along the tubal length, peritubal adhesions, and hydrosalpinges. Inflammatory conditions, such as infection, salpingitis isthmica nodosa, endometriosis, previous surgery, and ectopic pregnancy can all lead to tubal disease. Often, fallopian tubes are blocked intentionally for the purpose of sterilization, but the long-range intentions of patients can change so that fertility after tubal sterilization sometimes can become an issue.

A hydrosalpinx implies distal occlusion of the fallopian tube. The mucosa lining the interior of the fallopian tube is secretory, and without a distal outlet for the secretions, there often is an accumulation of fluid that causes distension of the tube throughout its length. This fluid may drain into the uterus and impair or prevent embryonic implantation. Hydrosalpinx fluid has been demonstrated to be embryotoxic to developing embryos. Poor endometrial receptivity has been demonstrated in the presence of hydrosalpinges. The chance of pregnancy is approximately halved if a hydrosalpinx is in place and IVF is performed.

Diagnosis of a hydrosalpinx is made by a number of techniques. They are most commonly diagnosed on hysterosalpingography but also can be diagnosed by laparoscopy. On ultrasonography, hydrosalpinges are observed as elongated and irregular tubelike structures adjacent to the ovaries. In young patients with mild distortion of the fallopian tube (ie, few tubal adhesions and minimal dilation), repair of the tube with careful neosalpingostomy can lead to respectable pregnancy rates (Table 155–158-1). If the fallopian tubes are bound with adhesions, are dilated, or if the patient is past her mid-thirties, removal of the tube and IVF is the option with the highest pregnancy rate.

If both tubes are hydrosalpinges, both must be repaired or removed. Fallopian tubes that are repaired often close again. If pregnancy does not occur within 6–12 months, repeat imaging studies should be performed. The patient should be warned of the risk of repeat hydrosalpinx if repair is chosen. Removal of hydrosalpinges leads to improved IVF pregnancy rates, comparable with patients without hydrosalpinx. Salpingectomy is recommended for those patients with hydrosalpinx who will be undergoing IVF. For patient 155, these dilated and distally occluded fallopian tubes will perform poorly if repaired and, thus, should be removed and IVF pursued. Should the situation arise that the fallopian tube cannot be removed safely, proximal occlusion combined with fenestration of hydrosalpinx and drainage of the fluid leads to enhanced IVF rates.

Endometriosis may cause impairment of fertility. Patients with minimal and mild endometriosis seeking fertility have fertility rates of approximately 5% per month, whereas those with moderate or severe endometriosis (as in patient 156) have rates of less than 1% per month. In vitro fertilization often is successful in producing pregnancy in women with endometriosis in a way that is independent of the stage of the disease. A delivery rate of 40% per cycle is reported for patients with endometrio-

TABLE 155–158-1. Classification of Tubal Disease With Distal Fimbrial Obstruction

Extent of Disease	Observations
Mild	Absent or small hydrosalpinx ≤15 mm diameter
	Inverted fimbriae easily recognized when patency is achieved
	No significant peritubal or periovarian adhesions
	Rugal pattern on preoperative hysterogram
Moderate	Hydrosalpinx 15–30 mm diameter
	Fragments of fimbriae not readily recognized
	Periovarian or peritubular adhesions without fixation, few cul-de-sac adhesions
	Absence of rugal pattern on preoperative hysterogram
Severe	Large hydrosalpinx ≥30 mm diameter
	No fimbriae
	Dense pelvic or adnexal adhesions with fixation of the ovary and fallopian tube to broad ligament, pelvic sidewall, omentum, or bowel
	Obliteration of the cul-de-sac
	Frozen pelvis (adhesion formation so dense that limits of organs are difficult to define)

Modified from Rock JA, Katayama KP, Martin EJ, Woodruff JD, Jones HW Jr. Factors influencing the success of salpingostomy techniques for distal fimbrial obstruction. Obstet Gynecol 1978;52:591.

sis, a rate that is not different from that for age-matched patients with other causes of tubal factor infertility.

Male factor infertility is successfully treated with ICSI. The more abnormalities present on the semen analysis, the lower the IVF rate. When sperm concentration is less than 10 million total motile sperm on the semen analysis, IVF with ICSI may be the most cost-effective therapy, even if identifiable female infertility does not exist. In the case of severe male factor infertility presented in patient 157, IVF with ICSI is the most appropriate treatment.

Sterilization is the most common method of contraception in the United States for women older than 30 years. Factors that affect success after tubal reanastomosis include the type of sterilization procedure performed, the location of the anastomosis, the age of the patient, and the existence of other tubal pathology. Sterilization procedures causing the least tubal damage (ie, Silastic rings, Hulka clips) have the highest success rate following reversal, eg, a 83% term pregnancy rate in one series. The most successful site for tubal anastomosis is isthmic-isthmic and cornual-isthmic with 81% and 67% term delivery rates, respectively. Patient 158 will have the best chance of pregnancy with tubal reversal. For younger patients with good prognosis tubal disease, tubal reversal carries a high pregnancy rate and allows for multiple conceptions. For patients older than 40 years and those with poor prognosis tubes, tubal reversal is controversial. Neither tubal reversal nor IVF offer a high chance of pregnancy for women older than 40 years. Oocyte donation may be an option for this patient because of its high success rate.

Benadiva CA, Kligman I, Davis O, Rosenwaks Z. In vitro fertilization versus tubal surgery: is pelvic reconstructive surgery obsolete? Fertil Steril 1995;64:1051–61.

Henderson SR. The reversibility of female sterilization with the use of microsurgery: a report on 102 patients with more than one year of follow-up. Am J Obstet Gynecol 1984;149:57–65.

Nackley AC, Muasher SJ. The significance of hydrosalpinx in in vitro fertilization. Fertil Steril 1998;69:373–84.

Olivennes F, Feldberg D, Liu HC, Cohen J, Moy F, Rosenwaks Z. Endometriosis: a stage by stage analysis—the role of in vitro fertilization. Fertil Steril 1995;64:392–8.

Van Voorhis BJ, Barnett M, Sparks AE, Syrop CH, Rosenthal G, Dawson J. Effect of the total motile sperm count on the efficacy and cost-effectiveness of intrauterine insemination and in vitro fertilization. Fertil Steril 2001;75:661–8.

Reproductive Endocrinology and Infertility

159–162
Secondary amenorrhea

For each patient (159–162) who presents with a history of secondary amenorrhea, negative β-hCG level, and a partial evaluation at referral, select the most appropriate next test (A–G).

(A) Vaginal smear
(B) Karyotype
(C) Echocardiography
(D) Antithyroid antibodies
(E) Thyroid-stimulating hormone (TSH)
(F) Serum prolactin
(G) Imaging study of the head

A 159. An 18-year-old adolescent presents with amenorrhea of 8 months' duration. She experienced menarche at age 16 years followed by 3 menses at approximately 2-month intervals before the onset of amenorrhea.

B 160. A 32-year-old woman with a 10-year history of irregular menses and amenorrhea for the past 6 months was referred with a negative progestin challenge test result and a follicle-stimulating hormone (FSH) level of 110 mIU/mL.

C 161. A 15-year-old adolescent is referred with amenorrhea of 7 months' duration. Her first menses occurred at age 13 years and was followed by 1½ years of bleeding twice monthly. Evaluation by her primary care physician reveals an FSH level of 160 mIU/mL, TSH level of 1.5 µU/mL, normal intravenous pyelogram, and chromosome analysis of 45,X/47,XXX.

G 162. A 16-year-old adolescent is referred for evaluation of secondary amenorrhea of 18 months' duration. Menarche occurred at age 12½ years and was followed with monthly menses until the sudden cessation of bleeding reported to her primary care physician. Her vaginal mucosa was atrophic and cervical mucus was absent. Prior evaluation included FSH level of 3 mIU/mL, prolactin level of 5 ng/mL, and TSH level of 1.8 µU/mL.

Secondary amenorrhea has been defined classically as cessation of menstrual cycles for a period of 6 months duration or longer. This definition, however, should not imply that physicians should wait for 6 months to begin a complete evaluation in an individual who has been previously menstruating regularly. Depending on the menstrual history for a given woman, evaluation may be appropriate far sooner and in incremental steps. For example, abrupt cessation in a very regular patient would signal, at the least, pregnancy testing. A partial evaluation also is appropriate in patients who initially exhibit signs or symptoms of a particular disease process (eg, thyroid dysfunction, hyperprolactinemia, or polycystic ovary syndrome). In the absence of such clues or evidence of an identifiable inciting event (eg, life stressor), it would be appropriate for the clinician to initiate an evaluation after several missed menses.

The first step in the evaluation of a patient with secondary amenorrhea, who is not pregnant and who does not have signs or symptoms of other conditions (patient 161), is to assess the status of estrogen production. No perfect method for determining estrogen status is available. In addition, none of the findings of currently used methodologies has been correlated with changes in bone mineral density or the adverse endometrial finding of hyperplasia. The appearance of the vaginal mucosa or absence of cervical mucus are the best clinical markers but can be misleading because of subjectivity. Vaginal cytology is presently the most objective marker, but it is only helpful if it denotes a hypoestrogenic smear. Furthermore, it is most helpful if performed and interpreted in the office.

The progestin challenge test similarly is considered most helpful if the results are negative and suggests a hypoestrogenic state. For the positive test result, differences in amount of bleeding are difficult to quantitate or correlate with degrees of estrogen production. In addition, physicians have to wait 2 weeks to determine the outcome, and, for patients who do not bleed, questions of compliance, absorption, and appropriate dosage for the very obese always linger. For these reasons, the role of the progestin challenge test in clinical paradigms has recently been questioned and even eliminated. The use of ultrasonography to measure the endometrial stripe as a biologic marker of estrogen production may be the easiest and most reliable method but has not been studied. Unless it is performed in the office as a part of the patient examination, it is too expensive to justify its use.

For patient 159, visual evaluation of the vaginal mucosa and endocervical canal for mucus may be helpful in suggesting a hypoestrogenic state, if it exists. If available in the office, vaginal cytology may corroborate this assessment. Vaginal cytology is best obtained by lightly rolling a cotton-tipped applicator over the lateral vaginal wall and then rolling this onto a glass slide. The glass slide is then flooded with any laboratory stain for several minutes before it is washed off and examined under the microscope. Pap test and Gram or Sedi (for urologic sediment) stains or indigo ink can all be used. The presence of greater than 20% superficial cells usually denotes a vagina with enough estrogen. Less than 20% superficial cells, 100% intermediate cells, or any parabasal cells all suggest a patient with hypoestrogenemia (Fig. 159–162-1; see color plates). If done in the office and immediately examined, the vaginal smear can be a valuable tool for this first step of the evaluation.

Once the patient is considered to have hypoestrogenemia, an FSH level can be obtained to determine if the patient has ovarian failure (ie, hypergonadotropism) or a hypothalamic–pituitary etiology (ie, hypogonadotropism). Patient 160 was identified to have an FSH level of 110 mIU/mL. The next step for her is to obtain a karyotype to better understand the cause of her ovarian failure. Previously, it was common to obtain chromosome analysis in these patients only if they developed ovarian failure before age 30 years. This patient may not have previously been studied. However, today it is important to complete this study in patients who develop ovarian failure through age 40 years. Although patients with either 46,XY or 45,X/46,XY gonadal dysgenesis will never have regular menstrual cycles, 5% of patients with all other forms of Turner's syndrome may have cyclic menses even well into their 30s before developing germ cell depletion and amenorrhea. Patients with Turner's syndrome of any karyotype need to be studied for a number of associated abnormalities (eg, Hashimoto's thyroiditis, coarctation of the aorta, bicuspid aortic valve with or without regurgitation or stenosis, dilation of the ascending aorta, and horseshoe kidney). With time, they may develop dilation of the ascending aorta, a major risk factor for aortic dissection and rupture. In addition, more of these women now desire pregnancies with donor oocyte and at older ages. Pregnancy appears to be a major risk factor for dilation, dissection, and rupture of the ascending aorta. If patient 160 has Turner's syndrome, as does patient 161, the next most important study would be echocardiography. Patients identified with 46,XX ovarian failure may have fragile X syndrome autoimmune dysfunction.

Patient 162 is found to be hypoestrogenic by appearance of her vaginal mucosa and absence of cervical mucus. If these findings had not been as obvious, a vaginal smear may have helped to corroborate the hypoestrogenic state. Furthermore, she was found to be hypogonadotropic. These patients with hypogonadotropic hypogonadism may have hypothyroidism or hyperprolactinemia. Many of them have a form of hypothalamic suppression, the etiology being evident for some but not all of such patients. A careful history is extremely important in identifying etiologies such as eating disorders. Other stressors may be identified, such as situational stress or intense exercise regimens. In the absence of such obvious causes of hypothalamic suppression, an imaging study of the head is necessary to rule out a central nervous system lesion. Two thirds of pituitary gland tumors are secretory, and 30–50% of them are prolactinomas in both children and adults. The second most common endocrinologically functional tumor produces growth hormone and represents 8% of all pituitary tumors among children younger than 20 years. The craniopharyngioma is the most common nonfunctional tumor in adolescents.

Kunwar S, Wilson CB. Pediatric pituitary adenomas. J Clin Endocrinol Metab 1999;84:4385–9.

Lin AE, Lippe B, Rosenfeld RG. Further delineation of aortic dilation, dissection, and rupture in patients with Turner syndrome. Pediatrics 1998;102:e12.

Reindollar RH, Nowak M, Tho SP, McDonough PG. Adult-onset amenorrhea: a study of 262 patients. Am J Obstet Gynecol 1986;155: 531–43.

Teramoto A, Hirakawa K, Sanno N, Osamura RY. Incidental pituitary lesions in 1000 unselected autopsy specimens. Radiology 1994;193: 161–4.

163–166
Risks of endoscopic surgery

For each of the patients (163–166) who comes in for tubal ligation, select the potential complications (A–E) that must be considered during laparoscopy.

(A) Decreased cardiac output resulting in cardiovascular collapse
(B) Alveolar rupture resulting in permanent lung injury
(C) Atrioventricular dissociation resulting in severe hypotension
(D) Postoperative atelectasis resulting in severe hypoxemia
(E) Pulmonary hypertension leading to pulmonary edema

A **163.** A 29-year-old obese woman with a history of cardiomyopathy of pregnancy.

B **164.** A 37-year-old woman with a history of extensive pulmonary fibrosis secondary to asbestos exposure.

C **165.** A 33-year-old woman with a history of recurrent vasovagal reaction to the placement of an intrauterine device.

D **166.** A 42-year-old woman with a history of neck cancer treated surgically followed by irradiation, who has an elevated hemidiaphragm.

Laparoscopy, like most techniques for minimal access surgery, has the advantages of reduced length of stay, shorter recovery period, rapid return to normal activity, and reduced postoperative pain. As a result, more extensive laparoscopic procedures in older patients are now being performed. It is not uncommon for the public, and even the inexperienced surgeon, to think of laparoscopy as a minor procedure that is unlikely to be associated with significant complications. Serious complications, such as vascular, bowel, bladder, and ureteral injuries, can and do occur. The competent surgeon should have a firm grasp of the types of complications that may occur and the medical conditions that may predispose patients to them. It is wise to have an anesthesia or internal medicine consultation in these higher risk patients.

Laparoscopy is associated with several hemodynamic changes that can lead to serious complications if not recognized and anticipated. Under ordinary conditions, the induction of pneumoperitoneum and Trendelenburg's position are associated with increases in systemic vascular resistance and arterial blood pressure levels. Changes in cardiac filling pressure depend on intraabdominal pressure changes. Cardiac output does not change in healthy individuals but may decrease in women with significant preexisting cardiopulmonary disease or in women with limited cardiac reserve as in patient 163, who has a history of cardiomyopathy. In this latter case, the pneumoperitoneum should be induced with the patient in the horizontal position rather than Trendelenburg's position. The intraabdominal pressure should be monitored rigorously to minimize excessive insufflation.

Changes in pulmonary function that are observed during laparoscopy include reduced lung volume, increased peak airway pressure, and decreased pulmonary compliance because of increased intraabdominal pressure and Trendelenburg's position. In addition, the increase in minute ventilation required to maintain normocapnia leads to further increases in peak airway pressures and a tendency toward hypercapnia. The major pulmonary complications observed during laparoscopic surgery include significant hypoxemia and hypercapnia. Hypoxemia occurs because of ventilation perfusion mismatching and intrapulmonary shunting secondary to decreased functional residual capacity. In addition, with vigorous attempts to improve ventilation and the resulting increased alveolar pressures, alveolar rupture can occur and lead to permanent lung injury, particularly in patients with extensive, preexisting pulmonary disease.

It has been suggested that preoperative pulmonary function testing be considered in women who have significant pulmonary disease, as in patient 164. When laparoscopy is performed, arterial blood gases should be monitored. If refractory hypercapnia and hypoxemia develop, or if high airway pressures are noted, the pneumoperitoneum should be released. Reinsufflation can then follow with maintenance of lower intraabdominal pressures.

The incidence of dysrhythmias during laparoscopy has been reported to be approximately 14% of patients. Most commonly seen are bradyarrhythmias that include severe bradycardia, atrioventricular dissociation, nodal rhythm, and even asystole. Most of these conditions have been attributed to vagal stimulation that results from the insertion of the Veress needle or the trocar, peritoneal stretching induced by the establishment of pneumoperitoneum, or stimulation of the fallopian tube during tubal ligation as in patient 165. The most important aspects in the management of these conditions are immediate cessation of surgical stimulation and immediate release of the pneumoperitoneum, as well as administration of anticholinergic medications (eg, atropine or glycopyrrolate). Tachyarrhythmias have been reported less commonly and are likely the result of increased carbon dioxide concentrations and catecholamines released as part of the stress response.

Following the termination of surgery and abdominal deflation, it can take up to 45 minutes for carbon dioxide concentrations to return to preinsufflation levels. Patients with impaired ventilation, especially those with cardiopulmonary disease, may be significantly affected during the immediate postoperative period. Patients who have impaired diaphragmatic function (eg, with nerve trauma during radical neck surgery, as in patient 166) may be particularly prone to hypercarbia during the immediate postoperative period. Because of the positive pressure ventilation during the procedure, the upwardly displaced diaphragm can lead to severe pulmonary atelectasis that goes unnoticed. With the resumption in spontaneous respiration, hypoxemia ensues and may lead to respiratory failure.

Brantley JC III, Riley PM. Cardiovascular collapse during laparoscopy: a report of two cases. Am J Obstet Gynecol 1988;159:735–7.

Joshi GP. Complications of laparoscopy. Anesthesiol Clin North America 2001;19:89–105.

Sadovnikoff N, Maxwell LG. Respiratory failure after laparoscopic cholecystectomy in a patient with chronic hemidiaphragm paralysis. Anesthesiology 1997;87:996–8.

Sprung J, Abdelmalak B, Schoenwald PK. Recurrent complete heart block in a healthy patient during laparoscopic electrocauterization of the fallopian tube. Anesthesiology 1998;88:1401–3.

167–170

Hypogonadism as a cause of male infertility

For each man who presents with azoospermia (167–170), select the most likely differential diagnosis (A–G).

(A) Klinefelter's syndrome
(B) Laurence-Moon syndrome
(C) Idiopathic hypogonadotropic hypogonadism
(D) Kallmann syndrome
(E) Gonadotropin-releasing hormone (GnRH) receptor gene mutation
(F) *DAX-1* gene mutation
(G) Follicle-stimulating hormone (FSH) receptor gene mutation

F 167. A 29-year-old man diagnosed with adrenal insufficiency at age 2 years and with hypogonadism at age 15 years despite corticoid therapy.

C 168. An otherwise healthy 32-year-old man with complete pubertal development and FSH level of 4 mIU/mL, luteinizing hormone level of 2 mIU/mL, and testosterone level of 60 ng/dL.

A 169. A 28-year-old man who is taller than predicted mid-parental height with reduced lean body mass and scanty pubic hair. Laboratory evaluation included FSH level of 24 mIU/mL, testosterone level of 98 ng/dL, and fasting blood glucose level of 145 mg/dL.

G 170. A 32-year-old man of Scandinavian descent with a normal physical examination except for reduced testicular size. A sister received a diagnosis with ovarian failure at age 19 years and a brother was evaluated for infertility and found to have a low sperm count.

Although as many as 50% of men with a significant compromise of sperm production do not have an identifiable cause, etiologies are increasingly being identified for men with severe oligospermia or azoospermia. In particular, men identified with hypogonadism can be easily categorized and often diagnosed. Both hypogonadotropic and hypergonadotropic causes of azoospermia have been well delineated.

Most men with hypogonadotropic hypogonadism are identified during the adolescent years with delayed puberty, well before concerns for spermatogenesis arise. Although most present with completely absent testicular function, some heterogeneity exists and, for a few syndromes, men may present after pubertal development with only absent spermatogenesis. A number of genetic causes of hypogonadotropic hypogonadism exist, most of which prevent spontaneous pubertal development. Although mutations of the GnRH gene have not been identified in humans with seeming isolated gonadotropin deficiency, such mutations have been observed in the hypogonadal mouse. Mutations of the GnRH receptor gene have been identified in these men. The phenotype of hypogonadotropic hypogonadism associated with mutations within the GnRH receptor gene is variable depending on the specific mutations present. Variable degrees of pubertal underdevelopment may be present. However, all affected men demonstrate absent spermatogenesis.

Mutations of the X-linked *KAL* and *DAX-1* genes produce well-characterized hypogonadotropic hypogonadism syndromes. The first of these gene defects causes a form of Kallmann syndrome and the latter is associated with congenital adrenal hypoplasia. For Kallmann syndrome, patients may variably present with anosmia, midline facial defects, and unilateral renal agenesis in addition to hypogonadotropic hypogonadism and delayed puberty. The *KAL* gene produces anosmin, a cell adhesion protein particularly important during embryogenesis for migration and synapses of the GnRH and olfactory neurons from the olfactory placode to the hypothalamus. Although GnRH is produced in patients with Kallmann syndrome, it is unable to be transported from the arcuate nucleus to the median eminence for pituitary stimulation.

The *DAX-1* gene encodes a nuclear hormone receptor that is similarly important during embryogenesis and that plays a key role in the development of the permanent zone of the adrenal cortex and the hypothalamic–pituitary–gonadal circuit. As an X-linked disorder, many of the affected men present within the first 2 weeks of life with a salt-losing crisis and adrenal insufficiency. Others, such as patient 167, do not develop overt adrenal insufficiency until as late as age 2–3 years. In even milder cases, adrenal insufficiency has been reported to develop during the third decade of life. This condition was previously often misdiagnosed as 21-hydroxylase deficiency. Unlike congenital adrenal hyperplasia that is associated with elevations of precursor steroids and androgens, none of the adrenal steroids can be produced for patients with congenital adrenal hypoplasia. Previously, these males died in infancy and childhood because of the adrenal insufficiency and salt-wasting crises. For males correctly diagnosed and treated with adrenal steroids, a second component of the clinical phenotype becomes apparent during adolescence, hypogonadotropic hypogonadism manifested by delayed puberty. Evidence suggests that defects may be present within both the hypothalamus and pituitary to cause the hypogonadotropic hypogonadism. The pituitary dysfunction, however, is limited to the inability for gonadotropin production and secretion. Clinical heterogeneity has been reported for hypogonadotropic hypogonadism in these patients as well as for time onset of the adrenal insufficiency. For example, incomplete puberty and milder hypogonadotropic hypogonadism were reported in an individual who developed adrenal insufficiency at age 28 years.

In addition to hypogonadotropic hypogonadism associated with Kallmann syndrome and congenital adrenal hypoplasia, men with Prader-Willi and Laurence-Moon syndromes also develop hypogonadotropic hypogonadism at puberty in addition to the phenotypes of their separate genetic disorders. Rarely, infiltrative disorders of the hypothalamus or pituitary gland may secondarily cause hypogonadotropic hypogonadism. Included in this list are histiocytosis, hemochromatosis, lymphocytic hypophysitis, and sarcoidosis. Most males with hypogonadotropic hypogonadism, however, do not have an identifiable cause for their deficient gonadotropin secretion. Although all males with hypogonadotropic hypogonadism have previously been categorized as having idiopathic hypogonadotropic hypogonadism, only those without an identifiable cause, such as patient 168, now meet this definition. For most, puberty will not spontaneously develop. However, for some males similar to patient 168, puberty may incompletely or completely develop with the laboratory findings of low gonadotropin and testosterone levels and azoospermia. There appears to be an adult onset form of this syndrome, not unlike hypothalamic amenorrhea in women.

Klinefelter's syndrome is the most common cause of hypergonadotropic hypogonadism in men and accounts for nearly 15% of all cases of azoospermia. Ninety percent of these men have a 47,XXY karyotype. Mosaicism, usually 46,XY/47,XXY, is found in the remainder of patients. The gonadal process associated with the extra X chromosome begins as early as the childhood years and progresses with time. It involves hyalinization and fibrosis of the seminiferous tubules with near total loss of germ cells in 99% of men. The same process appears to similarly affect Leydig cell function. As the testes become more hyalinized and fibrotic, androgen production decreases. Although most males with Klinefelter's syndrome initiate the pubertal process, levels of testosterone are rarely much higher than the lower limit for normal adults. Puberty, therefore, usually is incomplete.

Males with Klinefelter's syndrome (patient 169) have small genitalia; decreased pubic, axillary, facial, and body hair; increased adiposity in a feminine distribution often accompanied by gynecomastia; and decreased muscle mass. They are taller than predicted by parental height because of the extra X chromosome and delayed epiphyseal closure secondary to hypogonadal androgen production and subsequent conversion to estrogen. Laboratory studies demonstrate elevated gonadotropin levels, reduced androgen levels, and, in virtually all patients, azoospermia. Rarely, men who are genetically mosaic will have a few spermatozoa in the ejaculate; some nonmosaic and mosaic men will have a few immature spermatozoa in the testes to allow for successful in vitro fertilization with intracytoplasmic sperm injection. In addition to the clinical problems that accompany the hypogonadism, these men experience increased incidences of autoimmune and endocrine disorders (eg, lupus erythematous, rheumatoid arthritis, and type 2 diabetes mellitus), and they are predisposed to venous diseases, most commonly varicosities.

Although it is rare to identify the etiology for the remainder of men with hypergonadotropic hypogonadism who present with azoospermia, patient 170 represents a recently identified autosomal recessive cause of spermatogenic failure: FSH resistance. This syndrome of gonadotropin resistance was first described in Finnish women who presented with primary amenorrhea, elevated gonadotropin levels, and a seemingly normal number of germ cells within the ovaries, rather than oocyte depletion as was expected. Ultimately, they were identified to be homozygous for mutations within the FSH receptor gene. Their male siblings, who also harbored the same homozygous FSH receptor gene mutations, had normal pubertal development and variable findings at semen analysis. Although most of them had elevated FSH levels, sperm concentrations have varied from near azoospermic to normal.

Oliveira LM, Seminara SB, Beranova M, Hayes FJ, Valkenburgh SB, Schipani E, et al. The importance of autosomal genes in Kallmann syndrome: genotype-phenotype correlations and neuroendocrine characteristics. J Clin Endocrinol Metab 2001;86:1532–8.

Paulsen CA, Gordon DL, Carpenter RW, Gandy HM, Drucker WD. Klinefelter's syndrome and its variants: a hormonal and chromosomal study. Recent Prog Horm Res 1968;24:321–63.

Reutens AT, Achermann JC, Ito M, Ito M, Gu WX, Habiby RL, et al. Clinical and functional effects of mutations in the DAX-1 gene in patients with adrenal hypoplasia congenita. J Clin Endocrinol Metab 1999;84:504–11.

Rucker GB, Mielnik A, King P, Goldstein M, Schlegel PN. Preoperative screening for genetic abnormalities in men with nonobstructive azoospermia before testicular sperm extraction. J Urol 1998;160: 2068–71.

Tapanainen JS, Aittomaki K, Min J, Vaskivuo T, Huhtaniemi IT. Men homozygous for an inactivating mutation of the follicle-stimulating hormone (FSH) receptor gene present variable suppression of spermatogenesis and fertility. Nat Genet 1997;15:205–6.

Appendix A

Table of Normal Values for Laboratory Tests*

Analyte	Conventional Units
Alanine aminotransferase, serum	8–35 U/L
Alkaline phosphatase, serum	15–120 U/L
Menopause	
Amniotic fluid index	3–30 mL
Amylase	20–300 U/L
>60 years old	21–160 U/L
Aspartate aminotransferase, serum	15–30 U/L
Bicarbonate	
Arterial blood	21–27 mEq/L
Venous plasma	23–29 mEq/L
Bilirubin	
Total	0.3–1 mg/dL
Conjugated (direct)	0.1–0.4 mg/dL
Newborn, total	1–10 mg/dL
Blood gases (arterial) and pulmonary function	
Base deficit	<3 mEq/L
Base excess, arterial blood, calculated	−2 to +3 mEq/L
Forced expiratory volume	3.5–5 L
	>80% of predicted value
Forced vital capacity	3.5–5 L
Oxygen saturation (So_2)	95% or higher
Pao_2	≥80 mm Hg
Pco_2	35–45 mm Hg
Po_2	80–95 mm Hg
Peak expiratory flow rate	approximately 450 L/min
pH	7.35–7.45
Pvo_2	30–40 mm Hg
Blood urea nitrogen	
Adult	7–18 mg/dL
>60 years old	8–20 mg/dL
CA 125	<34 U/mL
Calcium	
Ionized	4.6–5.3 mg/dL
Serum	8.6–10 mg/dL
Chloride	98–106 mEq/L
Cholesterol	
Total	
Desirable	140–199 mg/dL
Borderline high	200–239 mg/dL
High	≥240 mg/dL
High-density lipoprotein	40–85 mg/dL
Low-density lipoprotein	
Desirable	<130 mg/dL
Borderline high	140–159 mg/dL
High	>160 mg/dL
Total cholesterol-to-high-density lipoprotein ratio	
Desirable	<3
Borderline high	3–5
High	>5
Triglycerides	<150 mg/dL
<20 years old	35–135 mg/dL

*Values listed are specific for adults or women, if relevant, unless otherwise differentiated.

(continued)

Table of Normal Values for Laboratory Tests* *(continued)*

Analyte	Conventional Units
Cortisol, plasma	
8 AM	5–23 µg/dL
4 PM	3–15 µg/dL
10 PM	<50% of 8 AM value
Creatinine, serum	0.6–1.2 mg/dL
Dehydroepiandrosterone sulfate	60–340 µg/dL
Erythrocyte	
Count	3,800,000–5,100,000/mm^3
Distribution width	10±1.5%
Sedimentation rate	
Wintrobe method	0–15 mm/h
Westergren method	0–20 mm/h
Estradiol-17β	
Follicular phase	30–100 pg/mL
Ovulatory phase	200–400 pg/mL
Luteal phase	50–140 pg/mL
Child	0.8–56 pg/mL
Ferritin, serum	18–160 µg/L
Fibrinogen	150–400 mg/dL
Follicle-stimulating hormone	
Premenopause	2.8–17.2 mIU/mL
Midcycle peak	15–35 mIU/mL
Postmenopause	24–170 mIU/mL
Child	0.1–7 mIU/mL
Glucose	
Fasting	70–105 mg/dL
2-hour postprandial	<120 mg/dL
Random blood	65–110 mg/dL
Hematocrit	36–48%
Hemoglobin	12–16 g/dL
Fetal	<1% of total
Hemoglobin A$_{1c}$ (nondiabetic)	5.5–8.5%
Human chorionic gonadotropin	0–5 mIU/mL
Pregnant	>5 mIU/mL
17α-Hydroxyprogesterone	
Adult	50–300 ng/dL
Child	32–63 ng/dL
25-Hydroxyvitamin D	10–55 ng/mL
Iron, serum	65–165 µg/dL
Binding capacity total	240–450 µg/dL
Lactate dehydrogenase, serum	313–618 U/L
Leukocytes	
Total	5,000–10,000/mm^3
Differential counts	
Basophils	0–1%
Eosinophils	1–3%
Lymphocytes	25–33%
Monocytes	3–7%
Myelocytes	0%
Band neutrophils	3–5%
Segmented neutrophils	54–62%
Lipase	10–140 U/L
>60 years old	18–180 U/L
Luteinizing hormone	
Follicular phase	3.6–29.4 mIU/mL
Midcycle peak	58–204 mIU/mL
Postmenopause	35–129 mIU/mL
Child	0.5–10.3 mIU/mL

*Values listed are specific for adults or women, if relevant, unless otherwise differentiated.

(continued)

Table of Normal Values for Laboratory Tests* (continued)

Analyte	Conventional Units
Magnesium	
Adult	1.6–2.6 mg/dL
Child	1.7–2.1 mg/dL
Newborn	1.5–2.2 mg/dL
Mean corpuscular	
Hemoglobin	27–33 pg
Hemoglobin concentration	33–37 g/dL
Volume	80–100 μm^3
Partial thromboplastin time	30–45 s
Activated	21–35 s
Phosphate, inorganic phosphorus	2.5–4.5 mg/dL
Platelet count	140,000–400,000/mm^3
Potassium	3.5–5.3 mEq/L
Progesterone	
Follicular phase	<3 ng/mL
Luteal phase	2.5–30 ng/mL
On oral contraceptives	0.1–0.3 ng/mL
>60 years old	0–0.2 ng/mL
1st trimester	9–47 ng/mL
2nd trimester	16.8–146 ng/mL
3rd trimester	55–255 ng/mL
Prolactin	0–17 ng/mL
Pregnant	34–386 ng/mL by 3rd trimester
Prothrombin time	10–13 s
Reticulocyte count	Absolute: 25,000–85,000 mm^3
	0.5–2.5% of erythrocytes
Semen analysis, spermatozoa	
Antisperm antibody	% of sperm binding by immunobead technique: >20% = decreased fertility; normal is <20% with adherent particles
Count	≥20 million/mL
Motility	≥60%
Morphology	≥60% normal forms
Sodium	135–145 mEq/L
Testosterone, female	
Total	6–86 ng/dL
Pregnant	3–4 × normal
Postmenopause	1/2 of normal
Free	
20–29 years old	0.9–3.2 pg/mL
30–39 years old	0.8–3 pg/mL
40–49 years old	0.6–2.5 pg/mL
50–59 years old	0.3–2.7 pg/mL
>60 years old	0.2–2.2 pg/mL
Thyroid-stimulating hormone	0.3–3 µU/mL
Thyroxine	
Serum free	0.9–2.3 ng/dL
Total	1.5–4.5 µg/dL
Triiodothyronine uptake	25–35%
Urea nitrogen, blood	
Adult	7–18 mg/dL
>60 years of age	8–20 mg/dL
Uric acid, serum	2.6–6 mg/dL
Urinalysis	
Epithelial cells	0–3/HPF
Erythrocytes	0–3/HPF
Leukocytes	0–4/HPF

*Values listed are specific for adults or women, if relevant, unless otherwise differentiated.

(continued)

Table of Normal Values for Laboratory Tests* *(continued)*

Analyte	Conventional Units
Urinalysis *(continued)*	
Protein (albumin)	
Qualitative	none detected
Quantitative	10–100 mg/24 hours
Specific gravity	
Normal hydration and volume	1.005–1.03
Concentrated	1.025–1.03
Diluted	1.001–1.01

*Values listed are specific for adults or women, if relevant, unless otherwise differentiated.

Appendix B

Markers for Measurement of Biochemical Breakdown Products of Bone Formation or Bone Resorption in Serum and Urine

Bone Formation Serum Markers	Bone Resorption Urine Markers	Bone Resorption Serum Markers
Bone specific alkaline phosphatase*	Hydroxyproline*	Cross-linked C-telopeptide of type 1 collagen
Osteocalcin*	Free and total pyridinolines	
Carboxy-terminal propeptide of type 1 collagen	Free and total deoxypyridinolines	Tartrate-resistant acid phosphatase
	N-telopeptide of collagen cross-links*	
Amino-terminal propeptide of type 1 collagen	C-telopeptide of collagen cross-links*	

*Bone biomarkers that are clinically available for patient management.

Appendix C
Risk Factors for Osteoporosis

Nonmodifiable
- Personal history of fracture as an adult
- History of fracture in first-degree relative
- Advanced age
- Female sex
- Ethnicity (Caucasian or Asian)
- Dementia
- Poor health, frailty
- Impaired eyesight despite adequate correction
- Prolonged immobility

Potentially Modifiable
- Estrogen deficiency
- Low body weight <57.6 kg (<127 lb)
- Current cigarette smoking
- Low calcium intake
- Alcoholism
- Malnutrition
- Inadequate physical activity
- Recurrent falls
- Chronic use of steroids, excessive thyroid hormones, certain anticonvulsants

Data from National Osteoporosis Foundation. Physician's guide to prevention and treatment of osteoporosis. Washington, DC: National Osteoporosis Foundation; 2003.

Appendix D

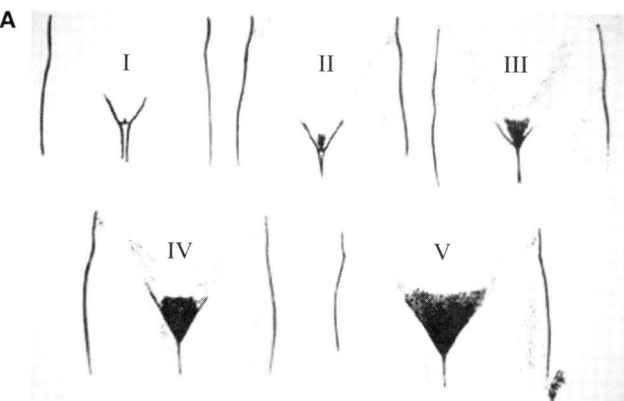

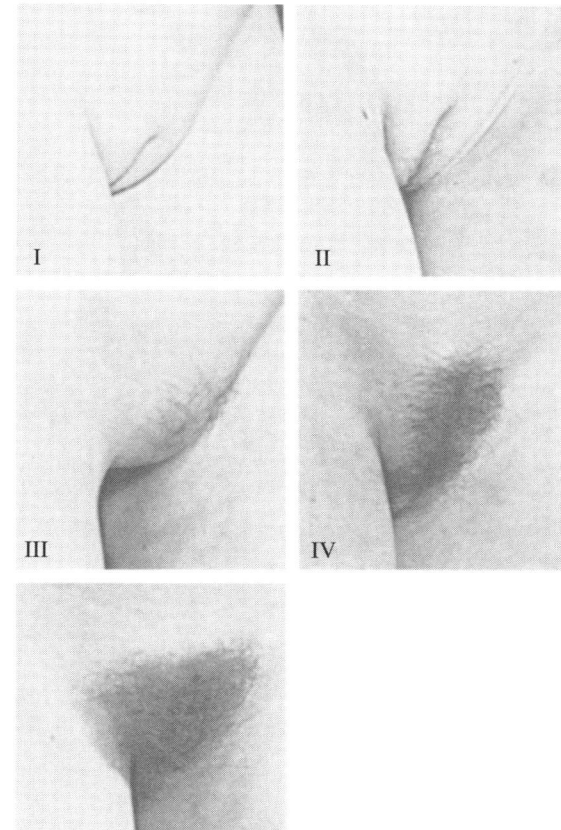

A. Tanner staging of pubic hair development. (Modified from Ross GT, Vandewiele RL, Frantz AG. The ovaries and the breasts. In: Williams RH [ed]. Textbook of endocrinology. 6th ed. Philadelphia [PA]: WB Saunders; 1981, p. 355, as modified from Marshall WA, Tanner JM. Variations in patterns of pubertal changes in girls. Arch Dis Child 1969;44:291–303. Copyright 1981, with permission from Elsevier. Yen SS, Jaffe RB, Barbieri RL, Reproductive endocrinology: physiology, pathophysiology, and clinical management. 4th ed. Baltimore [MD]: Lippincott Williams & Wilkins; p. 393.)

(continued)

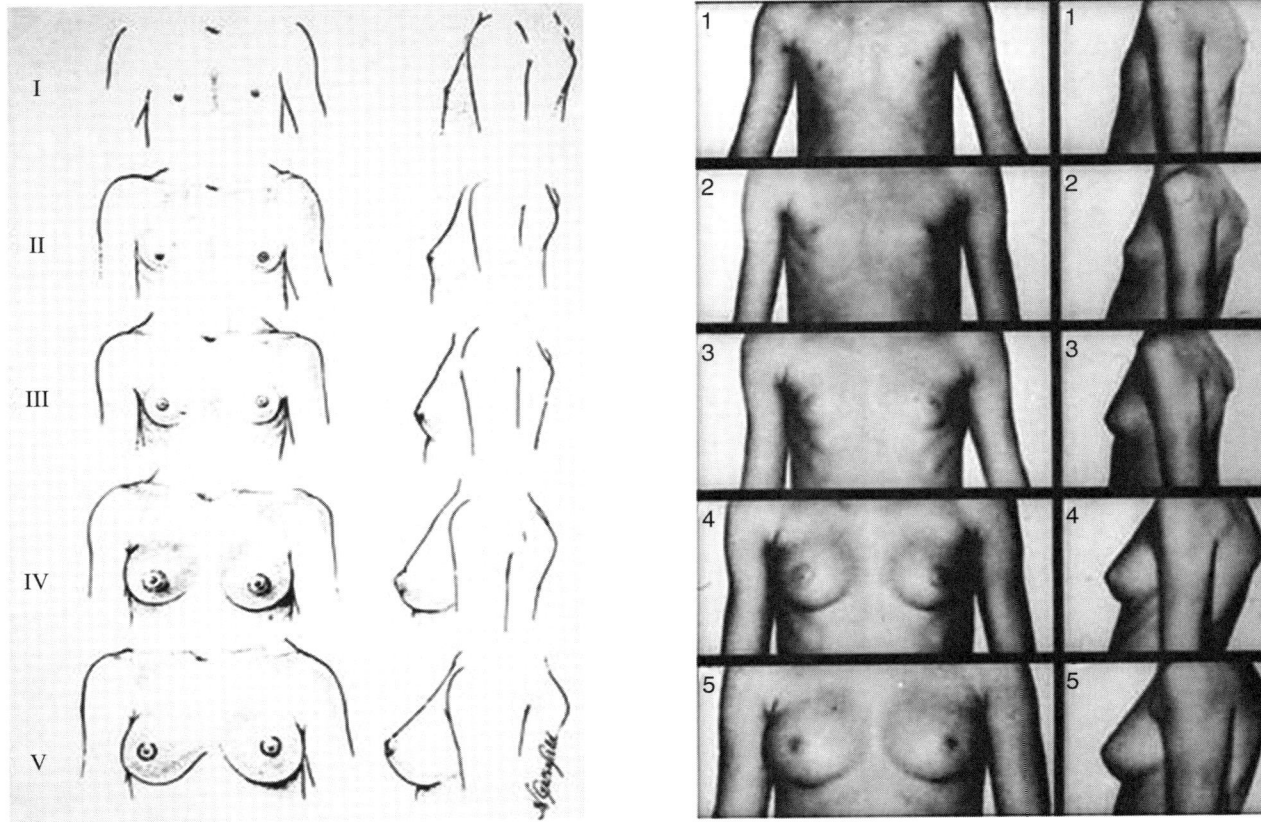

B. Tanner staging of breast development. (Reprinted from Ross GT, Vandewiele RL, Frantz AG. The ovaries and the breasts. In: Williams RH [ed]. Textbook of endocrinology. 6th ed. Philadelphia [PA]: WB Saunders; 1981, p. 355, as modified from Marshall WA, Tanner JM. Variations in patterns of pubertal changes in girls. Arch Dis Child 1969;44:291–303. Copyright 1981, with permission from Elsevier.)

Appendix E

Normal Semen Parameters as Determined by the World Health Organization

Semen Parameters	Normal Values
Volume	≥2 mL
Sperm concentration	≥20 million/mL
Motility	≥50% with forward progression, or ≥25% with rapid progression within 60 minutes of ejaculation
Morphology	≥30% normal forms
	>14% normal forms by strict criteria
White blood cells	<1 million/mL
Immunobead test	<20% spermatozoa with adherent particles
SpermMar test	<10% spermatozoa with adherent particles

Data from World Health Organization. Laboratory manual for the examination of human semen and sperm–cervical mucus interactions. 4th ed. Cambridge (UK): Cambridge University Press; 1999. p. 60–1; and Kruger TF, Menkveld R, Stander FS, Lombard CJ, Van der Merwe JP, van Zyl JA, et al. Sperm morphologic features as a prognostic factor in in vitro fertilization. Fertil Steril 1986;46:1118–23.

Appendix F

The Menopause-Specific Quality of Life (MENQOL) Questionnaire.

INSTRUCTIONS

Each of the items in the questionnaire is in the form of the examples below:

	Not at all bothered	0 1 2 3 4 5 6	Extremely bothered
NIGHT SWEATS	☐ No ☐ Yes →	0 1 2 3 4 5 6	

Indicate whether or not you have experienced this problem in the *last month*.

IF YOU *HAVE NOT* EXPERIENCED THE PROBLEM:

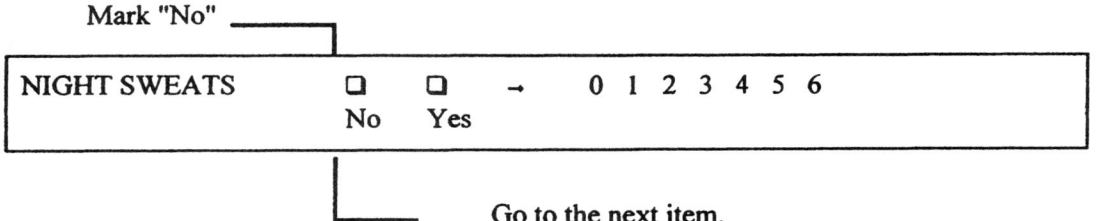

IF YOU *HAVE* EXPERIENCED THE PROBLEM:

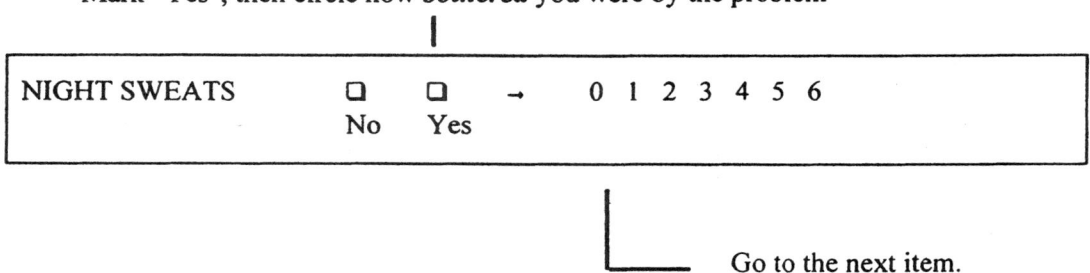

This questionnaire is completely confidential. Your name will not be associated with your responses. However, if for any reason you do not wish to complete an item, please leave it and go on to the next one.

(continued)

The Menopause-Specific Quality of Life (MENQOL) Questionnaire. *(continued)*

For each of the following items, indicate whether you have experienced the problem in the **PAST MONTH**. If you have, rate how much you have been *bothered* by the problem.

		Not at all bothered		0	1	2	3	4	5	6	Extremely bothered
1.	HOT FLUSHES OR FLASHES	☐ No	☐ Yes	→	0	1	2	3	4	5	6
2.	NIGHT SWEATS	☐ No	☐ Yes	→	0	1	2	3	4	5	6
3.	SWEATING	☐ No	☐ Yes	→	0	1	2	3	4	5	6
4.	BEING DISSATISFIED WITH MY PERSONAL LIFE	☐ No	☐ Yes	→	0	1	2	3	4	5	6
5.	FEELING ANXIOUS OR NERVOUS	☐ No	☐ Yes	→	0	1	2	3	4	5	6
6.	EXPERIENCING POOR MEMORY	☐ No	☐ Yes	→	0	1	2	3	4	5	6
7.	ACCOMPLISHING LESS THAN I USED TO	☐ No	☐ Yes	→	0	1	2	3	4	5	6
8.	FEELING DEPRESSED, DOWN OR BLUE	☐ No	☐ Yes	→	0	1	2	3	4	5	6
9.	BEING IMPATIENT WITH OTHER PEOPLE	☐ No	☐ Yes	→	0	1	2	3	4	5	6
10.	FEELINGS OF WANTING TO BE ALONE	☐ No	☐ Yes	→	0	1	2	3	4	5	6
11.	FLATULENCE (WIND) OR GAS PAINS	☐ No	☐ Yes	→	0	1	2	3	4	5	6

(continued)

The Menopause-Specific Quality of Life (MENQOL) Questionnaire. *(continued)*

	Not at all bothered	0	1	2	3	4	5	6	Extremely bothered
12. ACHING IN MUSCLES AND JOINTS	☐ No	☐ Yes	→	0	1	2	3	4	5	6
13. FEELING TIRED OR WORN OUT	☐ No	☐ Yes	→	0	1	2	3	4	5	6
14. DIFFICULTY SLEEPING	☐ No	☐ Yes	→	0	1	2	3	4	5	6
15. ACHES IN BACK OF NECK OR HEAD	☐ No	☐ Yes	→	0	1	2	3	4	5	6
16. DECREASE IN PHYSICAL STRENGTH	☐ No	☐ Yes	→	0	1	2	3	4	5	6
17. DECREASE IN STAMINA	☐ No	☐ Yes	→	0	1	2	3	4	5	6
18. FEELING A LACK OF ENERGY	☐ No	☐ Yes	→	0	1	2	3	4	5	6
19. DRYING SKIN	☐ No	☐ Yes	→	0	1	2	3	4	5	6
20. WEIGHT GAIN	☐ No	☐ Yes	→	0	1	2	3	4	5	6
21. INCREASED FACIAL HAIR	☐ No	☐ Yes	→	0	1	2	3	4	5	6
22. CHANGES IN APPEARANCE, TEXTURE OR TONE OF YOUR SKIN	☐ Yes	☐ No	→	0	1	2	3	4	5	6
23. FEELING BLOATED	☐ No	☐ Yes	→	0	1	2	3	4	5	6

(continued)

The Menopause-Specific Quality of Life (MENQOL) Questionnaire. *(continued)*

		Not at all bothered								Extremely 6 bothered
				0	1	2	3	4	5	6
24.	LOW BACKACHE	☐ No	☐ Yes	→ 0	1	2	3	4	5	6
25.	FREQUENT URINATION	☐ No	☐ Yes	→ 0	1	2	3	4	5	6
26.	INVOLUNTARY URINATION WHEN LAUGHING OR COUGHING	☐ No	☐ Yes	→ 0	1	2	3	4	5	6
27.	CHANGE IN YOUR SEXUAL DESIRE	☐ No	☐ Yes	→ 0	1	2	3	4	5	6
28.	VAGINAL DRYNESS DURING INTERCOURSE	☐ Yes	☐ No	→ 0	1	2	3	4	5	6
29.	AVOIDING INTIMACY	☐ No	☐ Yes	→ 0	1	2	3	4	5	6

(Reprinted from Maturitas, Vol 24, Hilditch JR, Lewis J, Peter A, van Maris B, Ross A, Franssen E, et al. A menopause-specific quality of life questionnaire: development and psychometric properties, Copyright 1996, with permission from Elsevier.)

Index

Abdominal obesity, in metabolic syndrome, 40, 122
Abdominal pain
  bowel injury during endoscopy and, 91
  and granulosa cell tumor, 39
  hematocolpometra and, 62
  and ovarian hyperstimulation syndrome, 60
  and pelvic pain, 44
Abnormal uterine bleeding
  management of, 90
  in menopause transition, 136–138
Abortion
  frequency of, age and, 63
  medical, 95
  spontaneous, after hysterosalpingography, 68
Acanthosis nigricans, 106
Accessory ports, and intraoperative injury, 91
Acne
  antiandrogens for, 123
  oral contraceptives for, 10, 150–151
ACOG. See American College of Obstetricians and Gynecologists
Acquired immunodeficiency syndrome (AIDS), reproduction in individuals with, 12
Acromegaly, with growth hormone secreting tumor, 22
ACTH. See Adrenocorticotropic hormone
Activated protein C (APC) test, 16
Acute adrenal stimulation test, and nonclassic congenital adrenal hyperplasia, 28
Add-back therapy
  with analogs, 120
  to treatment with gonadotropin-releasing hormone agonists, 101, 120
Adenomas
  adrenal, virilizing, 45
  gonadotrope, 84
  gonadotropin-secreting pituitary adenomas, 74
  growth-hormone secreting, 22
  and hyperprolactinemia, 111
  null cell, 84
  prolactin-secreting pituitary microadenoma, 54, 92
Adenomyosis, 2
Adhesions, prevention of, 98
Adiposity, hyperprolactinemia and, 22
Adolescent(s), contraceptive methods for, 108
Adolescent growth spurt, in normal pubertal development, 9
Adolescent pregnancy rate, 126
Adrenal failure/insufficiency
  macroadenomas and, 92
  premature ovarian failure and, 1
  Sheehan's syndrome and, 86
  steroidogenic cell autoimmunity and, 35
Adrenal gland neoplasms, and Cushing's syndrome, 19
Adrenal hyperplasia
  congenital, 59, 96
  and Cushing's syndrome, 19
  late-onset, 28
  nonclassic congenital, 28
Adrenal insufficiency, and hypogonadism, 167–170

Adrenal stimulation test, acute, and nonclassic congenital adrenal hyperplasia, 28
Adrenal tumors
  imaging for, 45
  premature adrenarche and, 59
Adrenarche
  androgen insensitivity syndrome and, 103
  hypogonadotropic hypogonadism and, 109
  in normal pubertal development, 9
  precocious, 59
  premature, 59
  primary amenorrhea and, 3
  Sheehan's syndrome and, 86
Adrenocorticotropic hormone (ACTH), 19, 43, 86
Adrenocorticotropin hormone-(1-24) (Cortrosyn), and acute adrenal stimulation test, 28
African Americans
  incidence of fibroids in, 93
  and inherited thrombophilias, 16
  normal pubertal development, 9
  and premature adrenarche, 59
  and weight gain with depot medroxyprogesterone acetate, 57
African Americans, osteopenia in, 152–154
Age
  advanced maternal, oocyte donor with, 63
  and incidence of trisomy, 63
  median, of menopause, 80
  of oocyte donor, recommendations, 113
  and pregnancy rates with in vitro fertilization, 116
  and risk of in vitro fertilization, 83
AIDS. See Acquired immunodeficiency syndrome
Alcohol consumption
  and fertility, 85
  and metabolic syndrome, 40
Aldosterone antagonist, for hirsutism, 28, 123
Alendronate sodium (Fosamax)
  for glucocorticoid-induced osteoporosis, 41
  markers to monitor therapy with, 115
  for osteoporosis, 65
  for prevention of osteoporosis, 27
Alkaline phosphatase, 15
Alkylating agents
  and male infertility, 129
  and premature ovarian failure, 35, 55
Alloimmunity, and recurrent pregnancy loss, 118
17α-hydroxyprogesterone
  and nonclassic congenital adrenal hyperplasia, 28
  premature ovarian failure and, 35
5α-reductase inhibitor, for hirsutism, 28
Alveolar rupture, in laparoscopy, 163–166
Ambiguous genitalia, 96
Amenorrhea
  after hysteroscopic techniques, 53
  after nonhysteroscopic endometrial ablation, 20
  androgen insensitivity syndrome and, 103
  diagnosis of, 34
  eating disorders and, 4

Amenorrhea (continued)
  evaluation and management of, 84
  hyperprolactinemia and, 22, 32
  hypogonadotropic hypogonadism and, 109
  and osteoporosis, 115
  in perimenopause, 38
  primary, 3, 50, 103, 109, 117
  prolactinomas and, 54
  secondary, 159–162
  Sheehan's syndrome and, 86
American College of Cardiology, on treatment for impotence, 8
American College of Obstetricians and Gynecologists (ACOG)
  mammography guidelines, 152–154
  on oral contraceptives and deep vein thrombosis, 16
  on oral estrogen therapy for osteoporosis, 27
American Diabetes Association, diagnosis of diabetes mellitus, 106
American Gastroenterological Association, on hereditary cancer syndromes, 48
American Heart Association, on treatment for impotence, 8
American Society for Reproductive Medicine (ASRM)
  on assisted reproductive technology and multiple births, 64
  on choice of oocyte donor, 113
  endometriosis classification, 44
  guidelines for oocyte donation, 72, 83
  guidelines for screening sperm donors, 74
  on ovarian hyperstimulation syndrome, 60
Anaphylactoid reactions, to intrauterine insemination, 119
Ancillary surgery, for pelvic pain, 31
Androgen
  absent thelarche and, 3
  and acne, 10
  excess of, 28
  production, suppression of, for hirsutism, 28
Androgen-estrogen, for increasing bone mineral density, 124
Androgen insensitivity syndrome
  management of, 103
  primary amenorrhea and, 117
Androgen-receptor antagonist, for hirsutism, 28, 123
Androgen-secreting tumor, primary amenorrhea and, 117
Androgen therapy, for Klinefelter's syndrome, 69
Aneuploidy, chromosomal abnormalities and, 46
Anorexia nervosa, 4
Anovulation
  chronic, 111
  hypothyroidism and, 78
Anovulatory bleeding, 90
Anterior pituitary, necrosis of, in Sheehan's syndrome, 86
Antiandrogens, cost-effective use of, 123
Antianginal nitrates, and treatment for impotence, 8
Antidepressant drugs, for bulimia, 4
Antiestrogens, use of, 87

NOTE: Numbers refer to questions, not pages.

Antiphospholipid syndrome, 118
Antipsychotic medication
  for bulimia, 4
  hyperprolactinemia and, 32
Antiresorptive therapy for osteoporosis, 65
  evidence of compliance with, 15
  markers to monitor, 115
Antiretroviral agents, for reducing sexual or perinatal transmission of human immunodeficiency virus, 12
Antisperm antibody (ASA), and intrauterine insemination, 119
Antithrombin III deficiency, 16
Antithyroid antibodies, and postpartum thyroiditis, 88, 125
Anus, imperforate, 14
Aortic dilation/dissection/rupture, in Turner's syndrome, 33, 83, 159–162
APC. *See* Activated protein C test
Apoptosis, in müllerian development, 146–149
Appendicitis, ovarian hyperstimulation syndrome versus, 60
Appetite
  depot medroxyprogesterone acetate and, 57
  hormones related to, 57
Arcuate uterus, 139–141
Argon laser, 142–145
Arm span, hypogonadotropic hypogonadism and, 109
ART. *See* Assisted reproductive technology
Arterial embolization, uterine, treatment-related complications of, 25
Artificial donor insemination
  for male infertility, 52
  use of, 74
ASA. *See* Antisperm antibody
Asian Americans, and inherited thrombophilias, 16
ASRM. *See* American Society for Reproductive Medicine
Assisted reproductive technology (ART)
  blastocyst transfer and twinning in, 64
  for Klinefelter's syndrome, 69
  for male infertility, 104
  for males with oligospermia, 52
  and multiple gestations, 112
  and ovarian hyperstimulation syndrome, 60
Autoimmune disorders/diseases
  antiphospholipid syndrome, 118
  and hypothyroidism, 94
  postpartum thyroiditis and, 88, 125
  premature ovarian failure and, 1
  Turner's syndrome and, 33
Autoimmune ovarian failure, 35
Azoospermia, 100
  hypogonadism and, 167–170
  intracycloplasmic sperm injection for, 104
  Klinefelter's syndrome and, 69
AZT. *See* Zidovudine

Balanced reciprocal translocations, 46
Bariatric surgery, 21
Barrier methods, for contraception in menopausal transition, 23
Basal body temperature chart, in menopausal transition, 38
bcl-2 protein, in müllerian development, 146–149
Benign breast disease, oral contraceptives and, 26
Benign ovarian disease, oral contraceptives and, 26

Benztropine mesylate (Cogentin), hyperprolactinemia and, 32
Beta-blockers, for hyperthyroidism, 125
Bicornuate uterus, 14, 24, 139–141
Bicuspid aortic valve, in Turner's syndrome, 33, 83
Bidirectional resorption, in müllerian development, 146–149
Bioabsorbable membrane/antiadhesive (Seprafilm), for prevention of adhesions, 98
Bisphosphonates
  for glucocorticoid-induced osteoporosis, 41
  and osteoporosis, 65
  for prevention of osteoporosis, 27
Black cohosh (Remifemin), for vasomotor symptoms, 17, 124
Bladder, irritative, 44
Blastocyst transfer, and twinning, 64, 112
Bleeding
  abnormal uterine, in menopause transition, 136–138
  continuous vaginal, imaging modality for evaluating, 132–135
  depot medroxyprogesterone acetate and, 105
  with medical abortion, 95
Blepharophimosis-ptosis-epicanthus inversus syndrome, 35
Blood pressure
  classification of, 18
  insulin resistance and, 122
  and metabolic syndrome, 122
  serum lipids and, 122
Blood urea nitrogen (BUN) levels, for identification of injury from pelvic surgery, 37
BMD. *See* Bone mineral density
BMI. *See* Body mass index
Body mass index (BMI)
  and obesity definitions, 21
  and ovulation induction, 111
Body weight, and bulimia versus anorexia, 4
Bone, normal physiology of, 109
Bone age imaging
  in hypogonadotropic hypogonadism, 109
  for precocious thelarche, 39
  in precocious thelarche, 75
Bone growth
  hypogonadotropic hypogonadism and, 109
  and precocious thelarche, 39
Bone loss
  gonadotropin-releasing hormone agonists and, 45
  with or following hormone therapy, 66
Bone markers, for osteoporosis, 15, 115
Bone mineral density (BMD)
  androgen-estrogen for increasing, 124
  biochemical hyperthyroidism and, 79
  diagnostic tests for determining, 130
  dual-energy X-ray absorptiometry to determine, 66
  and fracture risk, 102
  glucocorticoids and, 41
  guidelines for testing, 102
  hormone therapy and, 66
  hyperprolactinemia and, 32
  and selective estrogen receptor modulators, 6
Bowel injury
  during endoscopy, 91
  during pelvic surgery, 37
Bowel obstruction, after endoscopy, 91
Bradyarrhythmias, in laparoscopy, 163–166
Brain development, hypothyroidism and, 94

BRCA-positive patients
  breast cancer in, 13
  cancer risk in, 48
  hormone therapy for, 152–154
Breast cancer
  alternative therapies for menopausal symptoms after, 17
  in *BRCA*-positive patients, 13
  diethylstilbestrol exposure and, 128
  hormone therapy and, 56, 152–154
  oral contraceptive therapy and, 26
  raloxifene and, 27
  selective estrogen receptor modulators and, 6
  tamoxifen and, 27
Breast development
  absent, primary amenorrhea and, 3
  androgen insensitivity syndrome and, 103
  in normal pubertal development, 9
  premature, 39, 75
  Turner's syndrome and, 33
Breast engorgement, failure, Sheehan's syndrome and, 43
Bromocriptine mesylate (Parlodel)
  for hyperprolactinemia, 32, 54
  for ovulation induction, 111
  for treatment of macroadenomas, 92
Bulimia, 4
BUN. *See* Blood urea nitrogen levels
Buserelin acetate (Suprefact), 67

Cabergoline (Dostinex)
  for hyperprolactinemia, 54
  for ovulation induction, 111
  for treatment of macroadenomas, 92
Caffeine intake, and fertility, 85
CAH. *See* Congenital adrenal hyperplasia
Calcaneus, ultrasonographic measurement of, 115, 130
Calcitonin, for osteoporosis, 41
Calcium
  supplementation, for osteoporosis, 27
  urinary, and antiresorptive therapy, 115
Cancer, treatment for, and premature ovarian failure, 35
Carbon-dioxide laser, 142–145
Cardiopulmonary disease, and risks of laparoscopy, 163–166
Cardiovascular abnormalities
  in Marfan syndrome, 83
  in Turner's syndrome, 33, 83
Cardiovascular disease (CVD)
  and hormone therapy, 18, 152–154
  metabolic syndrome and, 40
  Turner's syndrome and, 33, 83
Cardiovascular events, oral contraceptives and, 89
Caseating cervicitis, and genital tuberculosis, 34
CAT. *See* Computerized axial tomography scan
Caucasians
  incidence of fibroids in, 93
  and inherited thrombophilias, 16
  normal pubertal development in, 9
Centers for Disease Control and Prevention
  on assisted reproductive technology and multiple births, 64
  on osteoporosis, 66
  and pregnancies of older women, 83
Central nervous system lesions
  hyperprolactinemia and, 22
  and secondary amenorrhea, 159–162
Central nervous system tumors, and precocious thelarche, 75

NOTE: Numbers refer to questions, not pages.

Cervical atresia, 62
Cervicitis, caseating, 34
Cervix
    absent, 14
    and genital tuberculosis, 34
Cetrorelix (Cetrotide), 67
Chemotherapy
    alternative therapies for menopausal symptoms after, 17
    conservation of ovarian function before, 67
    and male infertility, 129
    and premature ovarian failure, 35, 55, 67, 113
Chest pains, and treatment for impotence, 8
Cholesterol
    and hormone therapy, 5
    raloxifene hydrochloride (Evista) and, 6
Choriocarcinoma, and serum human chorionic gonadotropin levels, 82
Chromosomal abnormalities
    and oligospermia, 100
    recurrent abortion and, 46
    secondary amenorrhea and, 159–162
Chromosome 8, defects in, 146–149
Chromosome translocation, 46
Chromotubation, for patients with infertility, 93
Chronic anovulation, 111
Chronic autoimmune thyroiditis, postpartum thyroiditis and, 125
Chronic labial agglutination, 58
Chronic pelvic pain
    evaluation of, 44, 101
    surgery for, 2
Cigarette smoking
    and cardiovascular disease, 18
    cessation, for metabolic syndrome, 40
    and contraception in menopausal transition, 23
    and fertility, 85
    and risk of stroke, 121
    and sperm count, 51
    and sperm donation, 74
Cimetidine (Tagamet), and treatment for impotence, 8
Classical premature thelarche, 75
Clear cell adenocarcinoma, diethylstilbestrol exposure and, 128
Clomiphene citrate (Clomid, Serophene)
    challenge test, to evaluate ovarian reserve, 97
    and ectopic pregnancy, 30
    for idiopathic infertility, 7
    for male infertility, 52
    for osteoporosis, 27
    and ovarian cancer, 73
    ovarian cyst management during use of, 36
    use of, 87
Clonidine (Catapres-TTS)
    for menopausal symptoms, 17
    for vasomotor symptoms, 124
Clozapine (Clozaril), 32
Coagulopathy, inherited, and deep vein thrombosis with oral contraceptives, 16
Coarctation of aorta, Turner's syndrome and, 33
Cognitive–behavioral therapy, for bulimia, 4
College of American Pathologists, on oral contraceptives and deep vein thrombosis, 16
Colonoscopy, for bowel injury during endoscopy, 91
Colorectal cancer, hereditary nonpolyposis, 48

Combination oral contraceptives
    for emergency contraception, 11
    for fertility preservation before chemotherapy, 67
    in menopausal transition, 80
Computerized axial tomography (CAT) scan
    for bowel injury during endoscopy, 91
    for identification of injury from pelvic surgery, 37
    to screen for adrenal tumor, 45
Condoms, 108
Congenital adrenal hyperplasia (CAH), 96
    late-onset, 45
    nonclassic, 28
    premature adrenarche and, 59
Congenital adrenal insufficiency, and hypogonadism, 167–170
Congenital anomalies
    of female reproductive tract, and primary amenorrhea, 117
    of müllerian system, 14, 114, 139–141
Congenital bilateral absence of vas deferens, 100, 104, 127
Congenital hypothyroidism, 94
Congenital uterine anomalies, 14, 24, 114, 139–141
Consent
    for gonadectomy, in androgen insensitivity syndrome, 72
    for oocyte donation, 72
Continuous oral contraceptives
    for dysmenorrhea, 81
    for menorrhagia, 90
    for menstrual migraine, 121
Contraception
    for adolescents, 108
    in menopausal transition, 23
    method comparison, 49, 110
Controlled ovarian stimulation cycle, and ovarian hyperstimulation syndrome, 60
Corneal injury, lasers and, 142–145
Coronary disease events, raloxifene and, 27
Corpus luteum, and maintenance of pregnancy, 76
Corticosteroids, for Sheehan's syndrome, 43
Corticotropin, and Cushing's syndrome, 19
Corticotropin-releasing hormone (CRH), 19
Cortisol
    and Cushing's syndrome, 19
    premature ovarian failure and, 1
    and Sheehan's syndrome, 43, 86
Cortisone acetate, for Sheehan's syndrome, 43
Craniopharyngioma, 22, 50
CRH. See Corticotropin-releasing hormone
Cryopreservation
    oocyte, for preservation of fertility, 55
    of ovarian cortical strips, 55
    sperm, 129
Cryptorchidism, ambiguous genitalia with, 96
Crystalloid solution, intraperitoneal, for prevention of adhesions, 98
Cushing's disease, 19
Cushing's syndrome, 19
    adrenal tumors and, 45
    hyperprolactinemia and, 22
    weight gain and, 57
CVD. See Cardiovascular disease
Cystectomy, ovarian, for endometrioma, 29
Cystic fibrosis, and obstruction of vas deferens, 100, 104
Cystic thyroid, 78
Cystitis, interstitial, chronic pelvic pain and, 44

Danazol (Danocrine)
    for chronic pelvic pain, 101
    for fertility preservation before chemotherapy, 67
    and idiopathic infertility, 7
DAX-1 gene mutation, 167–170
Death, leading causes of, 18, 21
Deep inferior epigastric vessels, injury with laparoscopy, 47
Deep vein thrombosis (DVT), oral contraceptives and, 16
Delayed puberty
    definition of, 9
    diagnosis and management of, 33
Deoxypyridinoline, 15
Depot medroxyprogesterone acetate
    and abnormal bleeding, 105
    and appetite, 57
    for chronic pelvic pain, 101
    for contraception in menopausal transition, 23
    for dysmenorrhea secondary to endometriosis, 81
    for fertility preservation before chemotherapy, 67
    for menorrhagia, 90
    for menstrual migraine, 121
    and weight gain, 108
DES. See Diethylstilbestrol exposure
Dexamethasone (Decadron)
    intraperitoneal, for prevention of adhesions, 98
    for ovulation induction, 111
Dexamethasone suppression tests, 19
Dextran 70 (Hyskon), for prevention of adhesions, 98
Diabetes mellitus
    diagnosis of, 106
    hormone therapy and, 152–154
    metabolic syndrome and, 122
    oral contraceptive therapy and, 26
    polycystic ovary syndrome and, 106
    premature adrenarche and, 59
    premature ovarian failure and, 1
    and retrograde ejaculation, 127
    Turner's syndrome and, 33
Diagnostic studies
    for identification of injury from pelvic surgery, 37
    of pelvic anatomy, 132–135
Diaphragm and spermicide, for contraception in menopausal transition, 23
Didelphys uterus, 139–141
Diethylstilbestrol (DES) exposure, 61, 128
Dihydrotestosterone, 123
Dilation and curettage, with medical abortion, 95
Distention media, in hysteroscopic procedures, 20, 99
Dizygotic twins, monozygotic twinning versus, 112
DNA repair enzymes, and hereditary cancer syndromes, 48
Donor oocyte
    choice of donor for, 113
    in older patient, 63
    pregnancy and Turner's syndrome, 83
Donor sperm insemination, for male infertility, 52, 74
Dopamine, and prolactin secretion, 54
Dopamine agonists
    for nonprolactin secreting adenoma, 84
    for ovulation induction, 111
    for treatment of macroadenomas, 92

NOTE: Numbers refer to questions, not pages.

Dopamine receptor agonists, for prolactinomas, 54
Dopamine receptor antagonists, hyperprolactinemia and, 32
Down syndrome, 46
Dual-energy X-ray absorptiometry (DXA) scan, 15, 130
  for assessment of fracture risk, 115
  biochemical hyperthyroidism and, 79
  for diagnosis of osteoporosis, 66
  for hyperprolactinemia, 32
DVT. *See* Deep vein thrombosis
DXA. *See* Dual-energy X-ray absorptiometry scan
Dyslipidemia, insulin resistance and, 122
Dysmenorrhea, 81
  ancillary surgery for pain relief in, 31
  evaluation of, 44
  oral contraceptive therapy for, 26
Dyspareunia, evaluation of, 44
Dysrhythmias, in laparoscopy, 163–166
Dysuria, labial adhesions and, 58

Eating disorders, 4
Echocardiography, in secondary amenorrhea, 159–162
Ectopic adrenocorticotropic hormone syndrome, 22
Ectopic kidney, 14
Ectopic pregnancy
  diagnosis of, 30
  ovarian hyperstimulation syndrome versus, 60
  and serum human chorionic gonadotropin levels, 82
  tubal ligation reversal and, 42
Ejaculation, retrograde, 127
Ejaculatory dysfunction, 127
Electrosurgical approach, to hysteroscopy, 99
Emergency contraception therapy, 11
Endometrial ablation, 2
  complications of, 99
  hysteroscopic, 53
  for menorrhagia, 90
  nonhysteroscopic, 20
Endometrial biopsy, in postmenopausal women, 136–138
Endometrial cancer
  hereditary nonpolyposis colorectal cancer and, 48
  oral contraceptives and, 26
  in postmenopausal women, 136–138
Endometrial hyperplasia, evaluation of, 136–138
Endometrial receptivity, hydrosalpinges and, 107
Endometrial thickness, evaluation of, in postmenopausal women, 136–138
Endometrioma, ruptured, management of, 29
Endometriosis
  ancillary surgery for pelvic pain of, 31
  and chronic pelvic pain, 44, 101
  dysmenorrhea secondary to, 81
  fertility and, 155–158
  long-term pain relief for, 2
  minimal, and infertility, 7
Endometritis, tuberculosis, 34
Endometrium, 90
Endoscopic surgery
  bowel injury during, 91
  risks of, 163–166
Epigastric vessels, injury with laparoscopy, 47

Erectile dysfunction, treatment for, 8
Erection-enhancing drugs, chest pains and, 8
Erythromycin, and treatment for impotence, 8
Estradiol levels, and precocious thelarche, 39
Estradiol ring (Estring), 27
Estrogen cream, for labial adhesions, 58
Estrogen deficiency. *See* Hypoestrogenism
Estrogen therapy
  for androgen insensitivity syndrome, 103
  for bone growth, 109
  and breast cancer, 6, 56
  for hyperprolactinemia, 32
  and lipid profile, 5
  for menopausal symptoms, 17
  for menstrual migraine, 121
  oral, for osteoporosis, 27
  and reduction in ovarian reserve, 97
  and thyroid hormone therapy, 79
  for Turner's syndrome, 33
  vaginal, 27
Estrone sulfate, for bleeding with depot medroxyprogesterone acetate, 105
Ethinyl estradiol
  for bleeding with depot medroxyprogesterone acetate, 105
  for contraception in menopausal transition, 23
  for emergency contraception, 11
  mechanism of action of, 150–151
Exercise
  and cardiovascular disease, 18
  for metabolic syndrome, 40
Exudative salpingitis, 34
Eye injuries, lasers and, 142–145

Facial hair growth. *See* Hirsutism
Factor V Leiden mutation, 16
Fallopian tubes
  distal obstruction in, 107, 155–158
  evaluation of patency, 131, 132–135
  occlusion of, 131
Familial adenomatous polyposis syndrome, 48
Fasting plasma glucose, 40
Female pseudohermaphroditism, 96
Feminizing childhood ovarian tumors, 39
Fertility
  bilateral tubal ligation and, 116
  lifestyle factors and, 85
  with premature ovarian failure, 113
  preservation of, before chemotherapy or irradiation, 55
Fertility drugs/treatments
  and heterotopic pregnancy, 30
  and ovarian cancer, 73
  ovarian cyst management during use of, 36
Fetal death, hypothyroidism and, 94
Fibroids
  management of, in infertile women, 93
  necrotic, after uterine arterial embolization, 25
Finasteride, for hirsutism, 28
Fluoxetine, for menopausal symptoms, 17
Flutamide (Eulexin), for hirsutism, 28, 123
Follicle-stimulating hormone (FSH)
  day 3 test, 79
  deficiency, in Sheehan's syndrome, 43
  and evaluation of amenorrhea, 84
  gene mutation, 167–170
  and gonadotrope adenomas, 84
  gonadotropin-releasing hormone and, 67
  hypogonadotropic hypogonadism and, 109
  in infants, and premature thelarche, 75

Follicle-stimulating hormone (FSH) *(continued)*
  in menopausal transition, 38, 80
  primary amenorrhea and, 117
  secreting tumors, 70
  Sheehan's syndrome and, 86
  in stages of reproductive aging, 38
Fracture risk
  assessment of, 115
  gonadotropin-releasing hormone agonists and, 65
  indicators of, 102
  osteoporosis and, 66
  peripheral bone mineral density and, 130
Fragile X premutation, 35, 83
Fragile X syndrome, 14, 35
Frank method, versus vaginoplasty, for müllerian aplasia, 77
FSH. *See* Follicle-stimulating hormone

Galactorrhea
  evaluation and management of, 84
  hyperprolactinemia and, 32
  hypothyroidism and, 71
  prolactinomas and, 54
Ganirelix acetate (Antagon), 67
G20210A prothrombin mutation, 16
Gastric bypass, 21
Gastrointestinal system, symptoms after pelvic surgery, 37
Genes, and hereditary cancer syndromes, 48
Genetic diagnosis, preimplantation, 63
Genetic mutations
  BRCA, 13, 48
  and familial adenomatous polyposis syndrome, 48
  of fragile X gene, 35
  G20210A prothrombin mutation, 16
  and hereditary cancer syndromes, 48
  and hypogonadism in males, 167–170
  of leptin gene, 40, 57
  MSH2, 48
  pituitary insufficiency and, 3
  and premature ovarian failure, 35
Genital, renal, ear, skeletal syndrome, 146–149
Genital atrophy, 27
Genitalia
  ambiguous, 96
  in androgen insensitivity syndrome, 103
Genital tuberculosis, 34
Gestational trophoblastic neoplasia (GTN), and serum human chorionic gonadotropin levels, 82
GH. *See* Growth hormone secreting tumor
Ghrelin, 57
Glucocorticoid-induced osteoporosis, 41, 152–154
Glycine, as distention medium in hysteroscopy, 99
GnRH. *See* Gonadotropin-releasing hormone
Goldman perimetry visual fields testing, for macroadenomas, 92
Gonadal dysgenesis
  diagnosis and management of, 33
  and premature ovarian failure, 35
  and secondary amenorrhea, 159–162
Gonadectomy, for androgen insensitivity syndrome, 103
Gonadotoxins, 129
Gonadotrope adenomas, 84

NOTE: Numbers refer to questions, not pages.

Gonadotropin
- for idiopathic infertility, 7
- in infants, and premature thelarche, 75
- and precocious thelarche, 39
- Sheehan's syndrome and, 86

Gonadotropin-releasing hormone (GnRH), 67
- analogs, and idiopathic infertility, 7
- antiestrogens and, 87
- challenge test, for precocious thelarche, 39, 75
- in hypogonadotropic hypogonadism, 109
- in infants, and premature thelarche, 75
- receptor gene mutation, 167–170

Gonadotropin-releasing hormone agonists, 67
- add-back therapy with, 120
- for chronic pelvic pain, 101
- for dysmenorrhea secondary to endometriosis, 81
- for hirsutism, 28, 123
- for menorrhagia, 90
- and osteoporosis, 65
- for prevention of chemotherapy-induced ovarian failure, 55

Gonadotropin-releasing hormone antagonists, 67
- for conservation of ovarian function, 67
- for endometriosis with pelvic pain, 120

Gonadotropin-secreting tumors, diagnosis of, 70

Goserelin (Zoladex), 67

Granulosa cell tumor
- and precocious thelarche, 75
- precocious thelarche and, 39

Graves' disease, Turner's syndrome and, 33

Greene Climacteric Scale questionnaire, 152–154

Growth
- in normal pubertal development, 9
- precocious adrenarche and, 59

Growth hormone (GH) secreting tumor, 22

Growth hormone therapy, for Turner's syndrome, 33

GTN. See Gestational trophoblastic neoplasia

Haloperidol decanoate (Haldol), hyperprolactinemia and, 32

Hashimoto's thyroiditis, postpartum thyroiditis and, 125

hCG. See Human chorionic gonadotropin

HDL. See High-density lipoprotein cholesterol

Headaches
- and hormonal contraception, 26, 121
- macroadenomas and, 92

Heartburn symptoms, 5

Heavy metals, and sperm count, 51

Height
- precocious adrenarche and, 59
- reduction in, biochemical hyperthyroidism and, 79
- Turner's syndrome and, 33

Hematocolpometra, 62, 139–141

Hematosalpinges, 139–141

Hemivagina, obstructed, 139–141

Hemorrhagic stroke, oral contraceptives and, 89

Heparin, for antiphospholipid syndrome, 118

Heparin-induced osteoporosis, 41

Hereditary cancer syndromes, 48

Hereditary nonpolyposis colorectal cancer, 48

Hernias, incisional, laparoscopic-related, 91

Heterotopic pregnancy, 30

High-density lipoprotein (HDL) cholesterol
- and hormone therapy, 5
- and metabolic syndrome, 40
- metabolic syndrome and, 122
- raloxifene hydrochloride (Evista) and, 6

Hilus cell tumors, 45

Hip fractures
- bisphosphonates and, 41
- hip bone mass and risk of, 66
- raloxifene and, 27

Hirsutism
- antiandrogens for, 123
- evaluation and management of, 28
- hyperprolactinemia and, 22
- oral contraceptives for, 150–151
- ovarian androgen-secreting tumors and, 45

Hispanic Americans, and inherited thrombophilias, 16

HIV. See Human immunodeficiency virus

Hormonal contraceptive methods
- choices of, 126
- migraines and, 121
- and weight gain, 108

Hormone therapy (HT)
- bone loss with or following, 66
- and breast cancer, 6, 56
- cardiovascular disease and, 18
- evaluation of bleeding with, 136–138
- lipids and, 5
- in menopausal transition, 80
- screening before, 152–154
- tapering off, 56

Horseshoe kidney, Turner's syndrome and, 33

Hot flushes, alternative therapies for, 17

HSG. See Hysterosalpingography

HT. See Hormone therapy

Human chorionic gonadotropin (hCG)
- ectopic pregnancy after tubal reversal and, 42
- false positive (phantom) titers, 82
- serum levels of, 82

Human Gene Mutation Database, 48

Human immunodeficiency virus (HIV)
- condoms and, 108
- reproduction in individuals with, 12, 119
- screening for, in sperm donors, 74

Human parathyroid hormone 1-34 (Forteo), for osteoporosis, 65

Hydatidiform mole, and serum human chorionic gonadotropin levels, 82

Hydrosalpinges, 107, 155–158

17-Hydroxylase deficiency, primary amenorrhea and, 3

21-Hydroxylase deficiency, 59, 96

17-Hydroxyprogesterone, and congenital adrenal hyperplasia, 96

Hydroxyproline, 15

Hymen
- imperforate, versus transverse vaginal septum, 62
- microperforate, 62

Hyperandrogenic anovulation. See Polycystic ovary syndrome

Hyperandrogenism, primary amenorrhea and, 117

Hypercapnia, in laparoscopy, 163–166

Hypercoagulable state, 16

Hypercorticolism, 19

Hypergonadotropic gonadal failure, 100

Hypergonadotropic hypogonadism, 35
- diagnosis and management of, 33
- and male infertility, 69, 167–170
- primary amenorrhea and, 117

Hyperinsulinemia, 122
- in metabolic syndrome, 40
- in polycystic ovary syndrome, 106

Hyperlipidemia, metabolic syndrome and, 40

Hyperpigmentation, hyperprolactinemia and, 22

Hyperprolactinemia
- and chronic anovulation, 111
- with craniopharyngiomas, 50
- evaluation of, 22
- hypothyroidism and, 71, 78
- with nonprolactin-secreting pituitary tumor, 84
- and ovulation induction, 111
- prolactin-secreting pituitary microadenoma and, 54
- therapy for, 32, 54

Hypertension
- and cardiovascular disease, 18
- insulin resistance and, 122
- oral contraceptive therapy and, 26, 89

Hyperthecosis of ovaries, postmenopausal, 45

Hyperthyroidism, 125
- biochemical, and osteoporosis, 79
- postpartum thyroiditis and, 88
- Turner's syndrome and, 33

Hypertriglyceridemia, 122

Hypocorticolism, in Sheehan's syndrome, 43

Hypoestrogenism
- and bone growth, 109
- gonadotropin-releasing hormone agonists and, 65
- hyperprolactinemia and, 32
- in hypogonadotropic hypogonadism, 109
- induced, for treatment of chronic pelvic pain, 101
- and osteoporosis, 65, 66, 115
- and secondary amenorrhea, 159–162

Hypogonadotropic hypogonadism, 109
- macroadenomas and, 92
- and male infertility, 167–170
- primary amenorrhea and, 117

Hyponatremia, in Sheehan's syndrome, 86

Hypopituitarism
- causes of, 3
- primary amenorrhea and, 3
- with prolactinoma, 50
- in Sheehan's syndrome, 43

Hypothalamic tumor, and Cushing's syndrome, 19

Hypothalamus, antiestrogens and, 87

Hypothyroidism
- after postpartum thyroiditis, 125
- congenital, 94
- diagnosis of, 94
- hyperprolactinemia and, 22, 71
- and ovulation induction, 111
- postpartum thyroiditis and, 88
- and pregnancy, 94
- premature ovarian failure and, 1
- subclinical, 78, 94
- testing for, 78
- Turner's syndrome and, 33
- weight gain and, 57

Hypoxemia, in laparoscopy, 163–166

Hysterectomy, 53
- for menorrhagia, 20
- for uterine anomalies, 24

Hysterosalpingography (HSG)
- after ectopic pregnancy, 42
- complications of, 68
- and occlusion of fallopian tubes, 131
- for patients with infertility, 93
- of salpingitis isthmica nodosa, 61

NOTE: Numbers refer to questions, not pages.

Hysterosalpingography (HSG) (continued)
   for septate uterus, 114
   of tubal tuberculosis, 34
   of uterine cavity with congenital anomaly, 24
   versus sonohysterography, 132–135
Hysteroscopy, 132–135
   distention medium with, 20, 99
   electrosurgical approach to, 99
   endometrial ablation, 53, 99
   to evaluate endometrium, 136–138
   to evaluate tubal patency, 131
   for patients with infertility, 93
   for septate uterus, 114

Ibuprofen, for menstrual disturbances, 105
ICSI. See Intracytoplasmic sperm injection
Idiopathic infertility, 7
Idiopathic premature ovarian failure, 1
Imaging modalities, for pelvic anatomy, 132–135
Immune function, and postpartum thyroiditis, 88
Immunoglobulin, intravenous, for recurrent pregnancy loss, 118
Imperforate anus, 14
Imperforate hymen, versus transverse vaginal septum, 62
Implantation
   hydrosalpinges and, 107
   rates, with in vitro fertilization, 64
Impotence, treatment for, 8
Incisional hernias, laparoscopic-related, 91
Indomethacin (Indocin), for prevention of adhesions, 98
Infants, gonadotropin levels in, and premature thelarche, 75
Infertility
   genital tuberculosis and, 34
   imaging modality for evaluating, 132–135
   male, 8, 52
   management of fibroids in patients with, 93
   minimal endometriosis and, 7
   ovulation induction for, 36
   ovulation induction selection for, 97
   refractory, nulligravid women with, and ovarian cancer, 73
   tubal factor, 155–158
Informed consent
   for gonadectomy, in androgen insensitivity syndrome, 72
   for oocyte donation, 72
Ingram method, for müllerian aplasia, 77
Inhibin, and feminizing childhood ovarian tumors, 39
Insulin resistance
   in polycystic ovary syndrome, 106
   premature adrenarche and, 59
   Turner's syndrome and, 33
Insulin resistance syndrome. See Metabolic syndrome
Insulin-sensitizing agent, for insulin-resistant polycystic ovary syndrome, 106
Insulin tolerance test, for macroadenomas, 92
International Headache Society, menstrual migraine, 121
Interstitial cystitis, chronic pelvic pain and, 44
Interstitial Cystitis Symptoms Index and Problem Index, 44
Intracytoplasmic sperm injection (ICSI)
   for Klinefelter's syndrome, 69
   for male infertility, 52, 104
   risks of, 100

Intraoperative injury, 91
Intrauterine device (IUD)
   and adolescents, 108
   for contraception in menopausal transition, 23
   hypertension and, 89
   levonorgestrel-releasing, 49, 110, 126
   progestin-releasing, for contraception in menopausal transition, 23
   versus depot medroxyprogesterone acetate, 57
Intrauterine insemination (IUI)
   complications of, 119
   decreasing risk of human immunodeficiency virus transmission in, 12
   and ectopic pregnancy, 30
   for idiopathic infertility, 7
   for male infertility, 52
Intravenous immunoglobulin, for recurrent pregnancy loss, 118
In vitro fertilization (IVF)
   after pelvic irradiation, 55
   blastocyst transfer and twinning in, 64
   hydrosalpinges and success of, 107
   for idiopathic infertility, 7
   for Klinefelter's syndrome, 69
   lifestyle factors and success of, 85
   for male infertility, 52, 104
   and ovarian cancer, 73
   salpingectomy with, 42
   for salpingitis isthmica nodosa, 61
   versus surgery, 155–158
In vitro fertilization with embryo transfer (IVF-ET), for tubal factor infertility, 116
Iodine deficiency, and hypothyroidism, 94
Irradiation
   conservation of ovarian function before, 67
   and premature ovarian failure, 55
Irritable bowel syndrome, chronic pelvic pain and, 44
Ischemic stroke, oral contraceptives and, 89
Isolated precocious thelarche, 39
IUD. See Intrauterine device
IUI. See Intrauterine insemination
IVF. See In vitro fertilization
IVF-ET. See In vitro fertilization with embryo transfer

Joint National Committee on Prevention, Detection, Evaluation, and Treatment of High Blood Pressure, 18

Kallmann syndrome, and hypogonadism, 167–170
Karyotype
   congenital adrenal hyperplasia and, 96
   and premature ovarian failure, 1
   primary amenorrhea and, 117
   in secondary amenorrhea, 159–162
   45,X, 35
   47,XXY, 69, 100, 104, 167–170
   46,XY, 35, 103
   46,XY/47,XXY, 69, 167–170
Ketoconazole (Nizoral), for hirsutism, 123
Kidney(s)
   ectopic, 14
   malformation of, Turner's syndrome and, 33
Klinefelter's syndrome, 69
   and hypogonadism, 167–170
   intracycloplasmic sperm injection and, 100, 104
KTP laser, 142–145

Labial agglutination, chronic, 58
Laboratory studies
   premature ovarian failure and, 1
   of primary hypercoagulable states, 16
Lactation, failure, Sheehan's syndrome and, 43, 86
Lactotrope cells, 54, 111
Langerhans giant cells, 34
Laparoscopic gastric banding (Lap-Band), 21
Laparoscopic transposition of ovaries, 55
Laparoscopic uterine nerve ablation, for pelvic pain, 31
Laparoscopy
   for ablation or excision of endometriotic lesions, 2
   bowel injury during, 91
   for diagnosis and management of endometriosis, 44
   for patients with infertility, 93
   risks of, 163–166
   vascular injury with, 47
   with versus without treatment of endometriotic lesions, in idiopathic infertility, 7
Lasers, characteristics and safety of, 142–145
Late-onset congenital adrenal hyperplasia, 28, 45
Lateral spine radiography, 115, 130
Laurence-Moon syndrome, and hypogonadism, 167–170
L-carnitine (Proxeed), for impotence, 8
LDL. See Low-density lipoprotein cholesterol
Lead, and sperm count, 51
Lee-Frankenhaeuser plexus, and pelvic pain, 31
Leptin, 40, 57
Leuprolide acetate (Lupron), 67, 90
Leuprolide acetate, for chronic pelvic pain, 101
Levonorgestrel, for emergency contraception, 11
Levonorgestrel implants (Norplant), and menstrual disturbances, 105
Levonorgestrel-releasing intrauterine device (Mirena), 49, 110, 126
   and acne, 10
   for contraception in menopausal transition, 23
   for menorrhagia, 20, 90
Levothyroxine sodium (Synthroid)
   for hypothyroidism, 78
   for postpartum thyroiditis, 125
LH. See Luteinizing hormone
Libido, androgen-estrogen and, 124
Lifestyle factors/modifications
   and cardiovascular disease, 18
   and fertility, 85
   for metabolic syndrome, 40
Li-Fraumeni syndrome, 48
Lipids
   and hormone therapy, 5
   metabolic syndrome and, 122
   raloxifene hydrochloride (Evista) and, 6
Live birth rate, donor oocyte and, 63
Liveborn children, of parents with chromosome translocations, 46
Loop diuretics, thiazide diuretics versus, 41
Lorazepam (Ativan), hyperprolactinemia and, 32
Low-density lipoprotein (LDL) cholesterol
   and hormone therapy, 5
   raloxifene hydrochloride (Evista) and, 6
L-thyroxine, in pregnancy, 94
Lumbar spinal disease, chronic pelvic pain and, 44
Lupus erythematosus, premature ovarian failure and, 35

NOTE: Numbers refer to questions, not pages.

Luteal phase deficiency, and recurrent pregnancy loss, 118
Luteal phase support, 76
Luteal-placental shift, 76
Luteectomy, luteal phase support for pregnancy after, 76
Luteinizing hormone (LH)
　deficiency, in Sheehan's syndrome, 43
　gonadotrope adenomas and, 84
　gonadotropin-releasing hormone and, 67
　hypogonadotropic hypogonadism and, 109
　in infants, and premature thelarche, 75
　in menopausal transition, 38, 80
　oral contraceptives and, 10
　secreting tumors, 70
　Sheehan's syndrome and, 86
Lynch II syndrome, 48

Macroadenoma, pituitary
　nonprolactin-secreting, 84
　prolactin-secreting, 54
　treatment of, 92
Macroprolactinomas, 92
Magnetic resonance imaging (MRI)
　for macroadenomas, 92
　of sella turcica, 84
Male infertility, 8, 52
　chemotherapy and, 129
　environmental toxicity and, 51
　and hypergonadotropic hypogonadism, 69
　hypogonadism and, 167–170
　intracytoplasmic sperm injection for, 52, 104, 155–158
　retrograde ejaculation, 127
Male pseudohermaphroditism, 96
Male reproductive function, environmental toxicity and, 51
Marfan syndrome, risk of pregnancy in, 83
Marijuana, and sperm count, 51
Mastectomy, prophylactic, for *BRCA*-positive patients, 13
Maternal mortality, ectopic pregnancy and, 30
Maternal mortality rate, Turner's syndrome and, 83
Mayer-Rokitansky-Küster-Hauser syndrome, 146–149
McCune-Albright's syndrome, 39
McIndoe technique, for müllerian aplasia, 77
Medroxyprogesterone acetate
　and abnormal bleeding, 105
　and appetite, 57
　for chronic pelvic pain, 101
　for contraception in menopausal transition, 23
　for dysmenorrhea secondary to endometriosis, 81
　for fertility preservation before chemotherapy, 67
　in menopausal transition, 80
　for menorrhagia, 90
Megestrol acetate, for menopausal symptoms, 17
Meiosis, of oocytes, 63
Menarche, 9, 117
Menopausal symptoms, 17, 80
Menopausal transition
　changes in, 80
　contraception in, 23
　diagnosis of, 38
　normal versus abnormal uterine bleeding in, 136–138
Menopause, definition of, 38

Menopause-Specific Quality of Life (MENQOL) questionnaire, 152–154
Menorrhagia, 20
　management of, 90
　oral contraceptive therapy for, 26
Menstrual disturbances, depot medroxyprogesterone acetate and, 105
Menstrual migraine, 121
Menstruation, obstructed, 62
Mestranol, 11
Metabolic syndrome, 40
　medical management of, 122
　premature adrenarche and, 59
Metalloproteinases, 90
Metastatic gestational trophoblastic neoplasia, and serum human chorionic gonadotropin levels, 82
Metformin (Glucophage)
　for insulin-resistant polycystic ovary syndrome, 106
　for ovulation induction, 111
Methotrexate, for ectopic pregnancy after tubal reversal, 42
Methyltestosterone (Estratest), for increasing bone mineral density, 124
Metroplasty, hysteroscopic, for septate uterus, 114
Microadenoma
　management of, 84
　pituitary, prolactin-secreting, 54
Microdeletions of Y chromosome, 100
Micromanipulation, monozygotic twinning and, 112
Micronized estradiol (Vagifem), 27
Microperforate hymen, 62
Mifepristone (Mifeprex), 11, 95
Migraines, and hormonal contraception, 26, 121
Million Women Study
　on breast cancer, 13
　on hormone therapy and breast cancer, 56
Miscarriage
　after hysterosalpingography, 68
　frequency of, age and, 63
Misoprostol, and pregnancy termination, 95
Mittelschmerz, 14
Monetary compensation, for oocyte donation, 72
Monozygotic twinning, blastocyst transfer and, 112
Mood changes, in menopausal transition, 38
Morbid obesity, bariatric surgery for, 21
Mosaicism, 46
Mosaic Klinefelter's syndrome, 69, 167–170
MSH2 gene mutation, 48
Müllerian, renal, cervical spine association, 14
Müllerian agenesis/aplasia
　definition of, 146–149
　primary amenorrhea and, 117
　vaginoplasty versus Frank method for, 77
Müllerian anomalies, 14, 114, 139–141
Müllerian system, development of, 14, 114, 146–149
Multicystic ovaries, 70
Multiple endocrine neoplasia, 48
Multiple gestations
　blastocyst transfer and, 64, 112
　and pregnancies of older women, 83
Multiple Outcomes of Raloxifene Evaluation Trial (MORE), 27
Mutations. See Genetic mutations
Myocardial infarction
　hormone therapy and, 5, 152–154
　oral contraceptives and, 89

Myomas, uterine arterial embolization for, 25
Myomectomy
　for patients with infertility, 93
　prevention of adhesions following, 98

Nafarelin (Synarel), 67
National Cholesterol Education Program Adult Treatment Panel III (NCEP ATP III), 5, 122
National Institute of Diabetes and Digestive and Kidney Diseases, diagnostic criteria for interstitial cystitis, 44
National Institute of Health
　diagnostic criteria for interstitial cystitis, 44
　on obesity, 21
National Osteoporosis Foundation
　guidelines for bone mineral density testing, 102
　on hormone therapy for osteoporosis, 66
　medical therapy for prevention and treatment of osteoporosis, 27
National Osteoporosis Risk Assessment study, 152–154
2001 National Summary of Fertility Clinic Reports, on assisted reproductive technology and multiple births, 64
Native Americans, and inherited thrombophilias, 16
Nausea, bowel injury during endoscopy and, 91
nd:YAG. See Neodymium:yttrium-aluminum-garnet laser
Necrotic fibroid, after uterine arterial embolization, 25
Neodymium:yttrium-aluminum-garnet (nd:YAG) laser, 142–145
Neovagina, creation of, 77
Nicotine, and cardiovascular disease, 18
Nitroglycerin, and treatment for impotence, 8
Nodular thyroid, 78
Nonclassic congenital adrenal hyperplasia, 28
Nonfunctioning pituitary adenoma, 92
Nonprolactin secreting pituitary tumor, diagnosis of, 84
Norethindrone, mechanism of action of, 150–151
NovaSure, 20
N-telopeptides, 15, 115
Null cell adenomas, 84

Obesity
　bariatric surgery for, 21
　and cardiovascular disease, 18
　depot medroxyprogesterone acetate and, 57
　hormones related to, 57
　hyperprolactinemia and, 22
　and insulin-resistant polycystic ovary syndrome, 106
　and metabolic syndrome, 40
Obstetric hemorrhage, Sheehan's syndrome and, 43
Obstructed reproductive tract, 62, 117
Octreotide acetate (Sandostatin), for nonprolactin-secreting tumors, 84
Olanzapine (Zyprexa), 32
Oligoasthenospermia, environmental toxicity and, 51
Oligospermia
　hypogonadism and, 167–170
　intracycloplasmic sperm injection for, 100, 104
　treatment for, 8

NOTE: Numbers refer to questions, not pages.

Oocyte cryopreservation, for preservation of fertility, 55
Oocyte donation
　choice of donor for, 113
　fragile X premutation and, 35
　guidelines for, 72
　for older patient, 63
　risk of pregnancy by, in patients with Turner's syndrome, 83
　to women with premature ovarian failure, 113
Oocytes
　age-related changes in, 63
　and reduction in ovarian reserve, 97
Oophorectomy
　androgen-estrogen therapy after, 124
　for endometrioma, 29
　for hilus cell tumors, 45
　prophylactic, for *BRCA*-positive patients, 13
Optic chiasm
　macroadenomas and, 92
　pituitary tumors and, 84
Oral contraceptives
　for acne, 10
　antiandrogenic effects of, 10
　and cardiovascular events, 89
　for chronic pelvic pain, 101
　for contraception in menopausal transition, 23
　contraindications to, 26
　and deep vein thrombosis, 16
　for dysmenorrhea, 81
　for fertility preservation before chemotherapy, 67
　for hirsutism, 28
　hypertension and, 89
　macroadenomas and, 92
　mechanism of action of, 150–151
　in menopausal transition, 80
　for menorrhagia, 90
　migraines and, 26, 121
　for osteopenia, 32
　for osteoporosis, 32, 65
　and preexisting conditions, 89
　and risk of stroke, 121
　and weight gain, 108
Oral estrogen therapy, for osteoporosis, 27
Osteocalcin, 15
Osteopenia, 66, 102, 152–154
Osteoporosis
　biochemical hyperthyroidism and, 79
　bisphosphonates and, 65
　bone markers for, 15
　glucocorticoid-induced, 41
　heparin-induced, 41
　hormone therapy and, 66, 152–154
　hyperprolactinemia and, 32
　markers for, 115
　with or following hormone therapy, 66
　premenopausal, 65
　in reproductive-aged women, 115
　risk factors for, 102
　and selective estrogen receptor modulators, 6, 27, 65
Outflow tract disorders, and primary amenorrhea, 117
Ovarian androgen-secreting tumors, 45
Ovarian autoimmune disease, 35
Ovarian cancer
　and *BRCA*-positive patients, 13
　fertility drugs and, 73
　hereditary nonpolyposis colorectal cancer and, 48
　oral contraceptives and, 26

Ovarian cortical strips, cryopreservation of, 55
Ovarian cyst(s)
　and controlled ovarian stimulation, 60
　and gonadotropin-secreting tumors, 70
　management during ovulation induction, 36
　transvaginal aspiration of, 36
Ovarian cystectomy
　for endometrioma, 29
　luteal phase support of pregnancy after, 76
Ovarian failure
　autoimmune, 35
　chemotherapy-induced, 55
　premature. See Premature ovarian failure
　primary amenorrhea and, 117
　secondary amenorrhea and, 159–162
　in Turner's syndrome, and risk of in vitro fertilization, 83
Ovarian hyperstimulation, gonadotropin-secreting tumor and, 70
Ovarian hyperstimulation syndrome, 60
Ovarian reserve, evaluation of, 97
Ovarian stimulation
　and ovarian cancer, 73
　and ovarian hyperstimulation syndrome, 60
Ovarian torsion, and controlled ovarian stimulation, 60
Ovarian tumors
　feminizing childhood, 39
　and precocious thelarche, 39, 75
　premature adrenarche and, 59
Ovaries
　laparoscopic transposition of, 55
　multicystic, 70
　postmenopausal hyperthecosis of, 45
　streak, 35
Ovulation induction
　choice of agent in, 111
　ovarian cyst management during, 36
　ovarian reserve and, 97
Oxandrolone, for Turner's syndrome, 33
Oxidized regenerated cellulose (Interceed), for prevention of adhesions, 98

Pain, of dysmenorrhea, 81. See also Abdominal pain; Pelvic pain
Pancreatic β-cell dysfunction, in polycystic ovary syndrome, 106
Pancreatitis, hormone therapy and, 5
Paranoid schizophrenia, hyperprolactinemia and, 32
Paroxetine (Paxil), for menopausal symptoms, 17
Partial trisomy 8 mosaicism, 146–149
PCBs. See Polychlorinated biphenyl hydrocarbons
PCOS. See Polycystic ovary syndrome
Pediatric Research in Office Settings Network Study, of normal pubertal development, 9
Pelvic adhesions, prevention of, 98
Pelvic inflammatory disease, imaging modality for evaluating, 132–135
Pelvic pain
　ancillary surgery for, 31
　endometrioma and, 29
　genital tuberculosis and, 34
　hematocolpometra and, 62
　imaging modality for evaluating, 132–135
Pelvic surgery, injury during, 37
Perimenopause. See Menopausal transition
Perioophoritis, in genital tuberculosis, 34
Peripheral bone mineral density, and fracture risk, 130

Phallic structure, in congenital adrenal hyperplasia, 96
Phantom human chorionic gonadotropin titers, 82
Phenothiazine, for bulimia, 4
Phosphodiesterase inhibitors, for impotence, 8
Physical abuse, and pelvic pain, 2
Phytoestrogens, for menopausal symptoms, 17
Pituitary adenoma
　and hyperprolactinemia, 111
　nonfunctioning, 92
　nonprolactin-secreting macroadenoma, 54
　prolactin-secreting microadenoma, 54
　treatment of, 92
Pituitary apoplexy, 92
Pituitary insufficiency. See Hypopituitarism
Pituitary necrosis
　postpartum, 43
　in Sheehan's syndrome, 86
Pituitary stalk compression
　with craniopharyngiomas, 50
　with macroadenomas, 92
Pituitary stimulation testing, in hypogonadotropic hypogonadism, 109
Pituitary tumors
　follicle-stimulating hormone-secreting, 70
　and hyperprolactinemia, 111
　hypothyroidism and, 78
　and optic chiasm, 84
　prolactin-secreting microadenoma, 54
　secondary amenorrhea and, 159–162
Placenta, progesterone production in, luteal phase support and, 76
Plan B, 11
Polychlorinated biphenyl hydrocarbons (PCBs), and semen quality, 51
Polycystic ovary syndrome (PCOS), 90
　hirsutism and, 28
　hyperprolactinemia and, 22
　insulin resistance in, 106
　metabolic syndrome and, 40
　premature adrenarche and, 59
Polytetrafluoroethylene (Gore-Tex), for prevention of adhesions, 98
Postembolization syndrome, 25
Postmenopausal Estrogen/Progestin Interventions (PEPI) trial, 6, 66, 136–138
Postmenopausal hyperthecosis of ovaries, 45
Postpartum depression, and thyroid autoantibodies, 88
Postpartum hemorrhage, and Sheehan's syndrome, 86
Postpartum pituitary necrosis, 43
Postpartum thyroiditis, 88, 125
Potassium sensitivity test, for interstitial cystitis, 44
Prader-Willi, and hypogonadism, 167–170
Precocious adrenarche, 59
Precocious puberty, 9
　precocious thelarche and, 39, 75
　premature adrenarche and, 59
Precocious thelarche, 39
Prednisone
　and osteoporosis, 41
　for Sheehan's syndrome, 43
Pregnancy
　discovered by hysterosalpingography, 68
　and hypothyroidism, 94
　imaging modality for evaluating, 132–135
　luteal phase support in, 76
　prevention with emergency contraception, 11
　success rates, after tubal ligation reversal, 42
　treatment of hyperthyroidism in, 125

NOTE: Numbers refer to questions, not pages.

Pregnancy loss
  frequency of, age and, 63
  recurrent, 118
  and uterine anomalies, 24
Pregnancy rates
  adolescent, 126
  and clomiphene challenge test, 97
  for different contraceptive methods, 126
Pregnancy termination, mifepristone (Mifeprex) and, 95
Pregnancy test, before hysterosalpingography, 68
Prehypertensive, 18
Premature breast development, evaluation of, 75
Premature ovarian failure, 1, 35
  achieving fertility with, 113
  after uterine arterial embolization, 25
  chemotherapy and, 55, 67, 113
  fragile X premutation and, 35, 83
  irradiation and, 55
Premature testicular failure, 67, 100
Premature thelarche, evaluation of, 75
Premenopausal osteoporosis, 65
Presacral neurectomy
  for chronic pelvic pain, 2
  for pelvic pain, 31
Preterm birth rate, multiple gestation and, 112
Preven emergency contraceptive kit, 11
Primary amenorrhea, 3, 117
  androgen insensitivity syndrome and, 103
  congenital anomalies and, 14
Primary dysmenorrhea, 81
Progesterone, for luteal phase deficiency, 118
Progesterone therapy, for luteal phase support in pregnancy, 76
Progestin(s)
  for acne, 150–151
  add-back therapy, with, gonadotropin-releasing hormone agonists, 120
  and breast cancer, 56
  for menopausal symptoms, 17
Progestin challenge test, for secondary amenorrhea, 159–162
Progestin-only contraceptives, 49
  and acne, 10
  for adolescents, 108
  and breast cancer in *BRCA*-positive patients, 13
  for contraception in menopausal transition, 23
  for emergency contraception, 11
  hypertension and, 89
  menstrual disturbances with, 105
Progestin-releasing intrauterine device, for contraception in menopausal transition, 23
Prolactin
  deficiency, in Sheehan's syndrome, 43
  and evaluation of amenorrhea, 84
  excess levels of. *See* Hyperprolactinemia
Prolactin-secreting adenoma, treatment of, 92
Prolactin-secreting pituitary microadenoma, 54, 92
Prolactinomas, 22, 50, 54
  secondary amenorrhea and, 159–162
  versus nonprolactin-secreting pituitary tumor, 84
Prophylactic mastectomy, for *BRCA*-positive patients, 13
Prostaglandins, and dysmenorrhea, 81
Protein C deficiency, 16
Protein S deficiency, 16
Proto-oncogenes, and hereditary cancer syndromes, 48

Proximal tube occlusion, 131
Pseudogestational sac, 30
Pseudohermaphroditism, 96
Psychiatric illnesses, hyperprolactinemia and, 32
Psychologic evaluation, for donor insemination, 74
Psychologic counseling, for androgen insensitivity syndrome, 103
Pubarche, hypogonadotropic hypogonadism and, 109
Puberty
  development, evaluation of, in primary amenorrhea, 117
  normal development, 9
  precocious, 9, 59
Pubic hair growth
  androgen insensitivity syndrome and, 103
  hypogonadotropic hypogonadism and, 109
  in normal pubertal development, 9
  precocious, 59
  premature, 59
  primary amenorrhea and, 3
  Sheehan's syndrome and, 86
Pulmonary embolus, oral contraceptives and, 16
Pulmonary function testing, in laparoscopy, 163–166
Pyocolpos, 62
Pyridinoline, 15

Quarantine, of frozen sperm donation, 74
Quetiapine (Seroquel), 32

Race
  and incidence of fibroids, 93
  and inherited thrombophilias, 16
  and normal pubertal development, 9
  and premature adrenarche, 59
  and weight gain with depot medroxyprogesterone acetate, 57
Radiation
  in hysterosalpingography, 68
  and premature ovarian failure, 35
  sperm count and, 51
Radioactive iodine therapy, for hyperthyroidism, 125
Radioactive iodine uptake, and postpartum thyroiditis, 88
Radiography
  for identification of injury from pelvic surgery, 37
  lateral spine, 115, 130
Raloxifene hydrochloride (Evista)
  and breast cancer, 6
  for menstrual disturbances, 105
  for osteoporosis, 27, 41, 65
Raloxifene Use for the Heart study, 27
Recurrent pregnancy loss, 118
  septate uterus and, 114
  and uterine anomalies, 24
Renal agenesis/anomalies, 14, 139–141
Reproductive aging, staging system for, 38
Reproductive history, chromosomal abnormalities and, 46
Resistant ovary syndrome, 35
Retinal damage, lasers and, 142–145
Retrograde ejaculation, 127
Risedronate sodium (Actonel)
  for glucocorticoid-induced osteoporosis, 41
  for osteoporosis, 65
Robertsonian translocation, 46
Rudimentary horn, of uterus, 24

Saline, as distention medium in hysteroscopy, 99
Salmon calcitonin (Miacalcin), for osteoporosis, 65
Salpingectomy
  for ectopic pregnancy after tubal reversal, 42
  for hydrosalpinges before in vitro fertilization, 107, 155–158
  with in vitro fertilization, 42
Salpingitis
  exudative, 34
  tuberculous, 34, 61
Salpingitis isthmica nodosa, 61
Salpingostomy, for ectopic pregnancy after tubal reversal, 42
Salt wasting, congenital adrenal hyperplasia and, 96
Savage syndrome, 35
Scoliosis, congenital anomalies and, 14
Seasonale
  for dysmenorrhea, 81
  for menstrual migraine, 121
Secondary amenorrhea, 159–162
Secondary dysmenorrhea, 81
Secondary sex characteristics
  in normal pubertal development, 9
  Turner's syndrome and, 33
Selective estrogen receptor modulators (SERMs)
  and breast cancer, 6, 13
  for osteoporosis, 27, 41, 65
Selective progesterone receptor modulators, and breast cancer in *BRCA*-positive patients, 13
Selective serotonin reuptake inhibitors (SSRIs)
  for bulimia, 4
  for increasing bone mineral density, 124
  for menopausal symptoms, 17
Sella turcica, magnetic resonance imaging of, 84
Semen analysis, 127
Semen parameters, 52
Septate uterus
  surgical repair of, 24
  surgical therapy for, 114
Septic uterine necrosis, versus severe ischemic injury, after uterine arterial embolization, 25
SERMs. *See* Selective estrogen receptor modulators
Sertoli-Leydig cell tumor, precocious thelarche and, 39
Serum creatinine, for identification of injury from pelvic surgery, 37
Sex assignment, in congenital adrenal hyperplasia, 96
Sex hormone-binding globulin, oral contraceptives and, 150–151
Sexual abuse, and pelvic pain, 2
Sexual intercourse, and neovagina, 77
Sexually transmitted diseases (STDs)
  condoms and, 108
  screening for, in sperm donors, 74
Sheehan's syndrome, 43, 86
Short stature, in Turner's syndrome, 33
Sildenafil citrate (Viagra), for impotence, 8
Skeletal growth, hypogonadotropic hypogonadism and, 109
Smell, sense of, hypogonadotropic hypogonadism and, 109
Smoking. *See* Cigarette smoking
Society for Assisted Reproductive Technology
  guidelines for embryo transfer, 64
  on male infertility, 104

NOTE: Numbers refer to questions, not pages.

Sonocolpography, 62
Sonohysterography
　for evaluation of tubal patency, 131
　hysterosalpingography versus, 132–135
　for patients with infertility, 93
Sorbitol, as distention medium in hysteroscopy, 99
Soy, for menopausal symptoms, 17
Spermatogenesis, 129
Spermatogonium, 129
Sperm count
　environmental toxicity and, 51
　hypogonadism and, 167–170
　Klinefelter's syndrome and, 69
Sperm cryopreservation, 129
Sperm donation, 52, 74
Sperm harvest procedures, 127
Sperm morphology, intracytoplasmic sperm injection and, 104
Sperm physiology, 129
Sperm washing
　for intrauterine insemination, 119
　for reducing sexual transmission of human immunodeficiency virus, 12, 119
Spindle fiber damage, 63
Spine fractures. See Vertebral fractures
Spironolactone, for hirsutism, 28, 123
Spotting, in menopause transition, 136–138
SSRIs. See Selective serotonin reuptake inhibitors
Stages of Reproductive Aging Workshop (STRAW), staging system for reproductive aging, 38
STDs. See Sexually transmitted diseases
Sterilization, tubal, and future fertility, 116, 155–158
Sterilization reversal, 42, 116, 132–135, 155–158
Steroidogenic cell autoimmunity, 35
Stomach stapling, 21
Strassman metroplasty, 24
Streak ovaries, 35
Stress reduction, for idiopathic infertility, 7
Stroke risk
　and migraine headaches, 121
　oral contraceptives and, 26, 89, 121
Study of Tamoxifen and Raloxifene trial, 6, 27
Subclinical hypothyroidism, 78, 94
Subtotal thyroidectomy, for hyperthyroidism, 125
Superficial epigastric vessels, injury with laparoscopy, 47
Superovulation
　for idiopathic infertility, 7
　ovarian cyst management during, 36
Surgery, for chronic pelvic pain, 2
Swyer syndrome, and premature ovarian failure, 35

T_4. See Thyroxine
Tachyarrhythmias, in laparoscopy, 163–166
Tadalafil (Cialis), for impotence, 8
Tamoxifen citrate (Nolvadex)
　and breast cancer, 6, 13
　for osteoporosis, 27
Tanner stages
　of breast development, 9
　of pubic hair development, 9
Technetium uptake, and postpartum thyroiditis, 88
Testes, in androgen insensitivity syndrome, 103
Testicular cancer, gonadotoxicity of treatment for, 129
Testicular failure, premature, 100
Testosterone
　androgen insensitivity syndrome and, 103
　oral contraceptives and, 10, 150–151
　postmenopausal production of, 124
　primary amenorrhea and, 117
　production in women, 123
Tetrahydrocannabinol, and sperm count, 51
Thelarche
　absent, primary amenorrhea and, 3
　androgen insensitivity syndrome and, 103
　in normal pubertal development, 9
　premature, 39, 75
　Turner's syndrome and, 33
Thermal balloons, for endometrial ablation, 20
Thiazide diuretic
　for glucocorticoid-induced osteoporosis, 41
　for hypertension, 18
　versus loop diuretics, 41
Thrombophilia, inherited, and deep vein thrombosis with oral contraceptives, 16
Thyroid autoantibodies, and postpartum thyroiditis, 88
Thyroid dysfunction, testing for, 78
Thyroidectomy, subtotal, for hyperthyroidism, 125
Thyroid hormone therapy
　for hypothyroidism, 78
　and osteoporosis, 79
　in Sheehan's syndrome, 43
Thyroiditis
　autoimmune, Turner's syndrome and, 33
　postpartum, 88, 125
Thyroid-stimulating hormone (TSH)
　deficiency, in Sheehan's syndrome, 43
　and evaluation of amenorrhea, 84
　guidelines for screening of, 94
　and hyperprolactinemia, 54, 71
　and pregnancy, 94
　and prolactin secretion, 54
　and testing for thyroid dysfunction, 78
Thyrotoxicosis, in postpartum thyroiditis, 125
Thyrotropin-releasing hormone (TRH), and hyperprolactinemia, 71
Thyroxine (T_4), in Sheehan's syndrome, 43
Tompkins metroplasty, 24
Total abdominal hysterectomy, and bilateral salpingo-oophorectomy, 2
Transdermal contraceptive patch (Ortho Evra), 49
　for acne, 10
　for Turner's syndrome, 33
　versus vaginal ring, 110
Transdermal estradiol patch, in menopausal transition, 80
Transposition of ovaries, laparoscopic, 55
Transvaginal ovarian cyst aspiration, 36
Transvaginal ultrasonography, 132–135
　to evaluate endometrial thickness, 136–138
　of normal gestational sac versus pseudogestational sac, 30
　for persistently infertile women, 73
Transverse vaginal septum, imperforate hymen versus, 62
TRH. See Thyrotropin-releasing hormone
Triglycerides
　and hormone therapy, 5
　metabolic syndrome and, 122
　raloxifene hydrochloride (Evista) and, 6
Triiodothyronine, and diagnosis of thyroid dysfunction, 78
Triptorelin pamoate (Trelstar), 67
Trisomy 14, 46
Trisomy 21, 46, 69
Trisomy, incidence of, and maternal age, 63
Trocars
　and intraoperative injury, 91
　vascular injury and, 47
TSH. See Thyroid-stimulating hormone
Tubal anastomosis, 42, 116
Tubal ligation
　laparoscopic bilateral, for contraception, 49
　risks of, 163–166
Tubal ligation reversal, 42, 116, 132–135, 155–158
Tubal tuberculosis, 34, 61
Tuberculosis, genital, 34
Tuberculosis endometritis, 34
Tuberculous salpingitis, 61
Tumor markers, for feminizing childhood ovarian tumors, 39
Tumors
　and Cushing's syndrome, 19
　and primary amenorrhea, 50
Tumor suppressors, and hereditary cancer syndromes, 48
Turner's syndrome
　diagnosis and management of, 33
　and offspring with trisomy 21, 69
　and premature ovarian failure, 35
　primary amenorrhea and, 117
　risk of in vitro fertilization in, 83
　secondary amenorrhea and, 159–162
Twinning, blastocyst transfer and, 64, 112

Ultrasonography
　for bowel injury during endoscopy, 91
　of calcaneus, for assessing bone mineral density, 115, 130
　to evaluate endometrium of postmenopausal women, 136–138
　gynecologic uses of, 132–135
　for identification of injury from pelvic surgery, 37
　with medical abortion, 95
　of nodular or cystic thyroid, 78
　of normal gestational sac versus pseudogestational sac, 30
　for persistently infertile women, 73
Umbilical ligaments, and avoidance of vascular injury with laparoscopy, 47
Umbilical port, and incisional hernias, 91
Unicornuate uterus, 139–141
Upper gastrointestinal series, with small bowel follow-through, for identification of injury from pelvic surgery, 37
Ureters
　anomalies of, 14
　injury during pelvic surgery, 37
Urinary frequency, in interstitial cystitis, 44
Urinary tract
　abnormalities, 14
　infections, labial adhesions and, 58
　injury during pelvic surgery, 37
　symptoms, of interstitial cystitis, 44
Urine analysis, for retrograde ejaculation, 127
U.S. Food and Drug Administration
　on emergency contraception, 11
　on oral estrogen therapy for osteoporosis, 27
U.S. Preventive Services Task Force, on selective estrogen receptor modulators and breast cancer, 6

NOTE: Numbers refer to questions, not pages.

Uterine adenomyosis, salpingitis isthmica nodosa and, 61
Uterine arterial embolization, treatment-related complications of, 25
Uterine bleeding, abnormal, management of, 90
Uterine contraction, intrauterine insemination and, 119
Uterine didelphys, 139–141
Uterine leiomyomata
  management of, in infertile women, 93
  oral contraceptive therapy and, 26
Uterine polyps, 136–138
Uterine unification procedures, 24
Uterosacral ligament transection, 37
Uterosacral nerve ablation
  for chronic pelvic pain, 2
  for pelvic pain, 31
Uterotubal junction occlusion, 131
Uterus
  arcuate, 139–141
  bicornuate, 14, 24, 139–141
  congenital anomalies of, 14, 114, 139–141
  didelphys, 139–141
  septate, 24, 114, 139–141
  severe ischemic injury to, after uterine arterial embolization, 25
  unicornuate, 139–141

Vagina
  absence of, 77
  blind ending, 14, 62
  congenital adrenal hyperplasia and, 96
  hypoestrogenic changes in, 27
  nonsurgical creation of, 103
  transverse septum, versus imperforate hymen, 62
Vaginal contraceptive ring (NuvaRing), transdermal contraceptive patch versus, 110
Vaginal cytology, for secondary amenorrhea, 159–162
Vaginal dilators
  for androgen insensitivity syndrome, 103
  for müllerian aplasia, 77
Vaginal dryness, 27
Vaginal estrogen, 27
Vaginal smear, in secondary amenorrhea, 159–162
Vaginoplasty
  for androgen insensitivity syndrome, 103
  versus Frank method, for müllerian aplasia, 77
Vardenafil (Levitra), for impotence, 8
Varicocele, 52
Vascular embolization, uterine artery, treatment related complications of, 25
Vas deferens
  absence of, 100, 127
  obstruction of, 100
Vasomotor symptoms, 80
  add-back therapy for, 120
  alternative therapies for, 17
  hormone therapy for, 152–154
  in menopausal transition, 38
  Sheehan's syndrome and, 86
  treatment for, 124
Vasopressin, Sheehan's syndrome and, 86
Vechietti procedure, 77
Venlafaxine hydrochloride (Effexor), for menopausal symptoms, 17, 124
Venous thromboembolism, oral contraceptives and, 89
Vertebrae, bone mass and fracture risk, 66
Vertebral anomalies, 14
Vertebral fractures
  biochemical hyperthyroidism and, 79
  bisphosphonates and, 41
  bone mass and, 66
  indicators of risk for, 102
  raloxifene and, 27
Virilization
  in congenital adrenal hyperplasia, 96
  ovarian androgen-secreting tumors and, 45
  premature adrenarche and, 59
  primary amenorrhea and, 117
Visual field
  defects, macroadenomas and, 92
  testing, for nonprolactin-secreting tumors, 84
Vitamin D supplementation, for osteoporosis, 27
Vitamin E, for menopausal symptoms, 17
Vulvar pain, labial adhesions and, 58

Waist circumference, and metabolic syndrome, 40, 122
Wedge resection method of repair, of septate uterus, 24
Weight, precocious adrenarche and, 59
Weight-control behavior, eating disorders and, 4
Weight gain
  depot medroxyprogesterone acetate and, 57
  hormonal contraception and, 108
  and metabolic syndrome, 40
Weight reduction
  by bariatric surgery, 21
  for metabolic syndrome, 40
Women's Health Initiative (WHI) trial
  on breast cancer and hormone therapy, 13, 56
  on cardiovascular disease and hormone therapy, 18
  on lipids and hormone therapy, 5
  on oral estrogen therapy for osteoporosis, 27
World Health Organization
  Collaborative Study of Cardiovascular and Steroid Hormone Contraception, 89
  criteria for defining osteoporosis, 152–154
  definition of perimenopause, 38
  on depot medroxyprogesterone acetate and bleeding, 105
  male infertility, 52
  perimenopause definition, 80

X chromosome mosaicism, 46
X-linked laterality sequence, 146–149

Y chromosome, microdeletions of, 100, 104
Yohimbine, for vasomotor symptoms, 124

Zidovudine (AZT), for reducing perinatal transmission of human immunodeficiency virus, 12
Zuclomiphene, 87

NOTE: Numbers refer to questions, not pages.

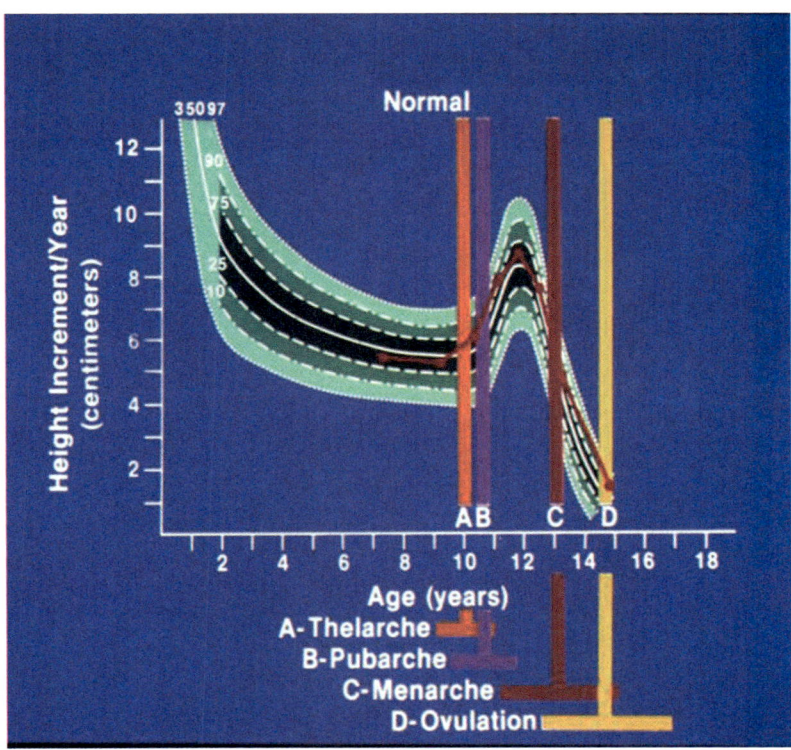

FIG. 9-1. Pubertal development chart. (Data from Reindollar RH, Tho SP, McDonough PG. When sexual development is delayed. Contemp Obstet Gynecol 1981;17:95–115.)

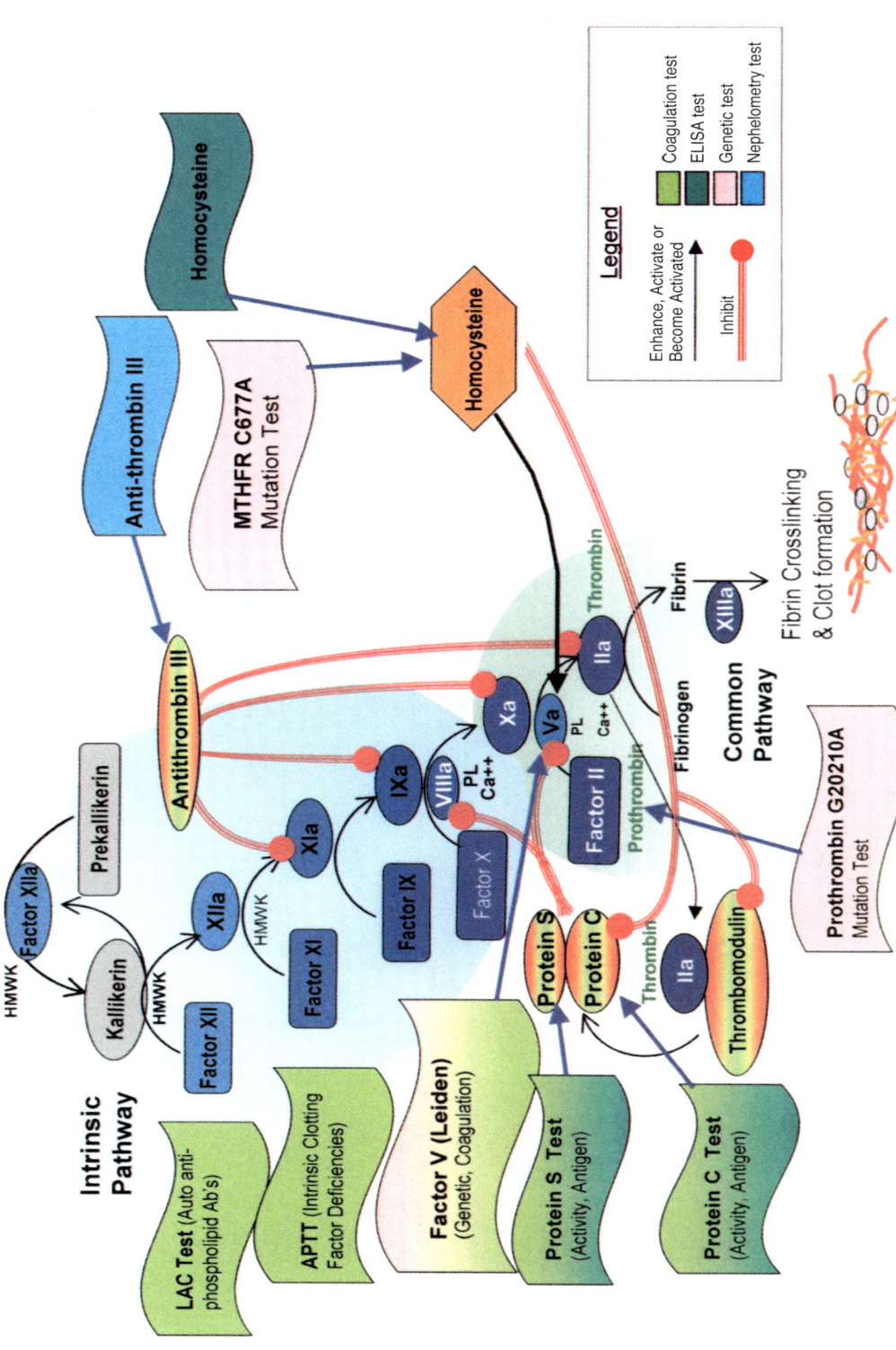

FIG. 16-1. Thrombophilia test graph. Coagulation cascade necessary to form a clot and location of genetic tests for inherited thrombophilias. The goal of the cascade is to form fibrin, which forms a mesh within the platelet aggregate to stabilize the clot. All of the factors have an inactive and an active form (active form is here designated by "a"). Once activated, the factor will serve to activate the next factor in the sequence until fibrin is formed. The coagulation cascade takes place at the site of a break in a blood vessel where platelets aggregate. Tissue factor and factor VIIa activate factor X to form factor Xa. Factor Xa is then able to activate prothrombin (also known as factor II) to form thrombin (factor IIa). Thrombin converts fibrinogen (factor I) to fibrin (factor Ia). The fibrin mesh is further stabilized by factor XIII, which "cross-stitches" the strands of fibrin together. Several factors accelerate clot formation (denoted by arrows). Factor VIII accelerates the conversion of factor X to factor Xa by factor IXa, and Factor V accelerates the conversion of prothrombin to thrombin as done by factor Xa. Other factors slow down clot formation (denoted by filled circles). Protein C, protein S, and thrombomodulin form a complex of proteins that can inactivate factor VIII and factor V. This complex is activated by thrombin. Antithrombin III serves to block the actions of multiple clotting factors. Tissue factor pathway inhibitor works to inhibit the formation of factor Xa. All of the above interactions are required to maintain hemostatic balance and to prevent excessive bleeding or clotting (HMWK = high molecular weight kininogen). (Reprinted with permission from Repromedix Inc. Copyright © 2004.)

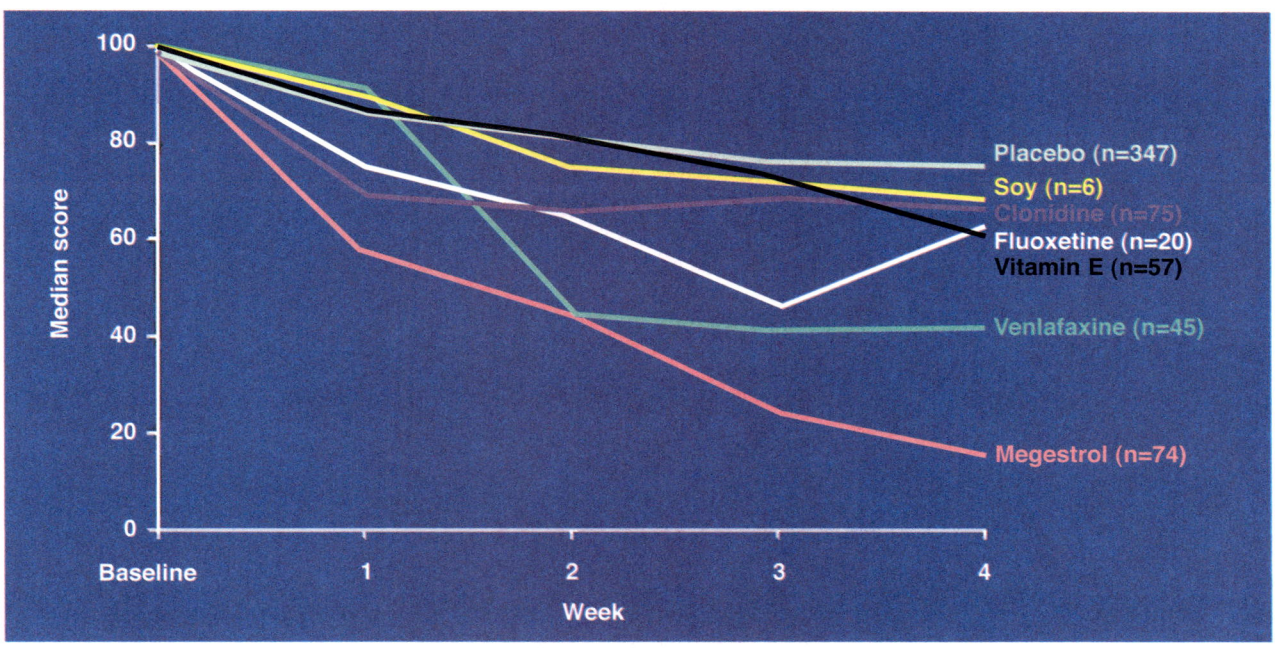

FIG. 17-1. Relative effectiveness of different compounds for the treatment of vasomotor symptoms. (Data from Loprinzi CL, Michalak JC, Quella SK, O'Fallon JR, Hatfield AK, Nelimark RA, et al. Megestrol acetate for the prevention of hot flashes. N Engl J Med 1994;331:347–52.)

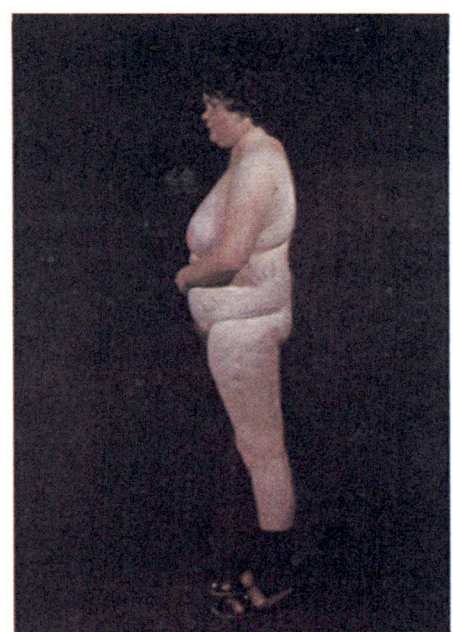

FIG. 19-1. Patient with Cushing's syndrome showing obesity with distribution of fat, particularly of the trunk with characteristic "buffalo hump." (Yen SS, Jaffe RB, Barbieri RL, Reproductive endocrinology: physiology, pathophysiology, and clinical management. 4th ed. Baltimore [MD]: Williams & Wilkins. p. 529.)

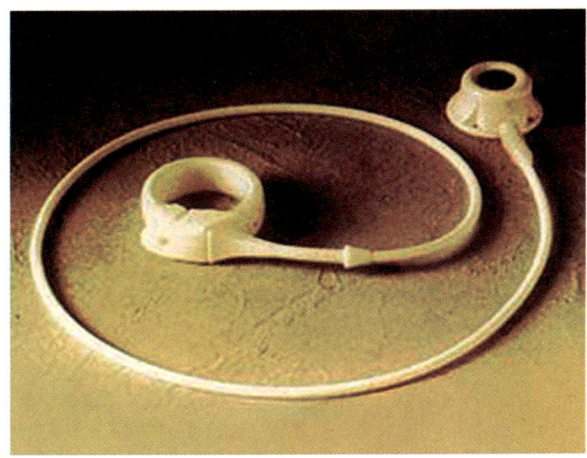

FIG. 21-1. Lap-Band Prosthesis. (Courtesy of INAMED Health Corporation.)

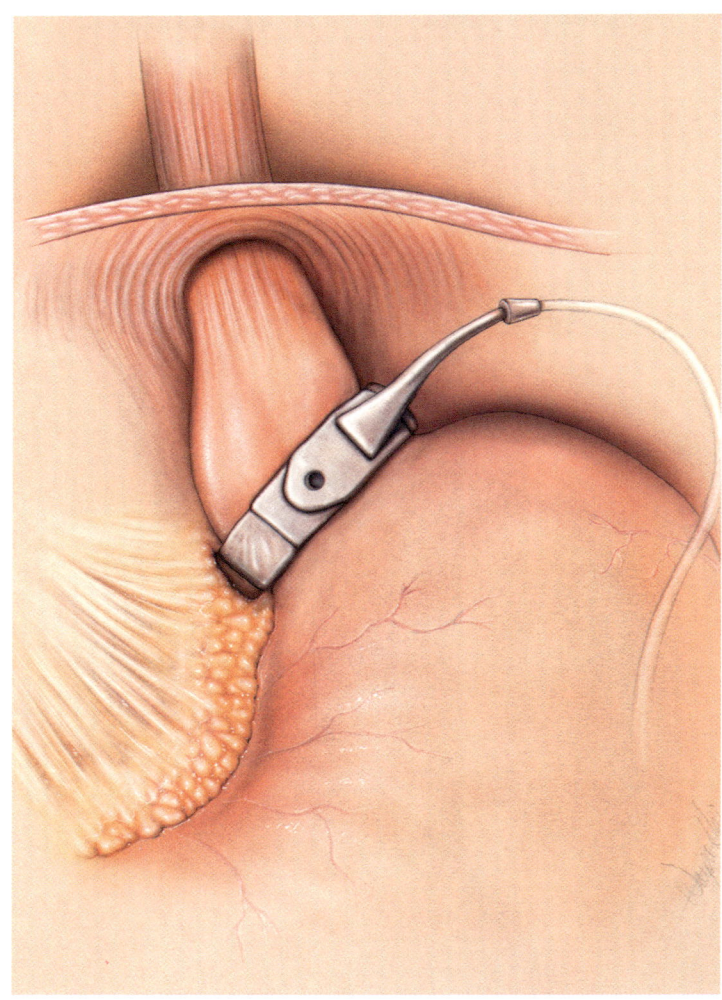

FIG. 21-2. The silicone-adjustable band component of the Lap-Band Prosthesis is placed around the upper part of the stomach. This forms a small gastric pouch to control the amount of food eaten by the patient and slow the emptying of the stomach into the intestines. (Courtesy of INAMED Health Corporation.)

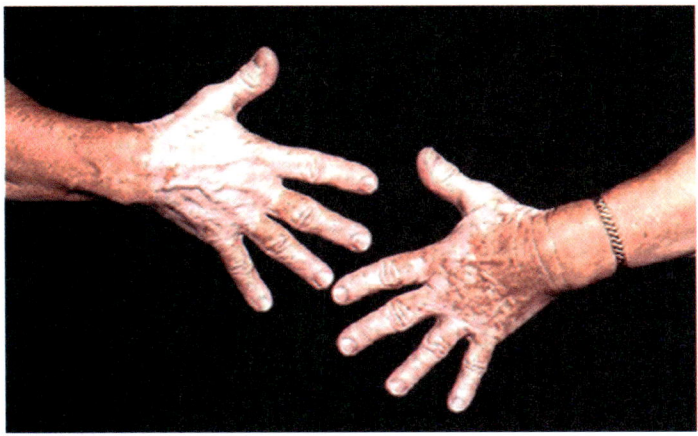

FIG. 22-1. Acral changes of growth hormone-secreting tumor excess: thickening of hands and fingers.

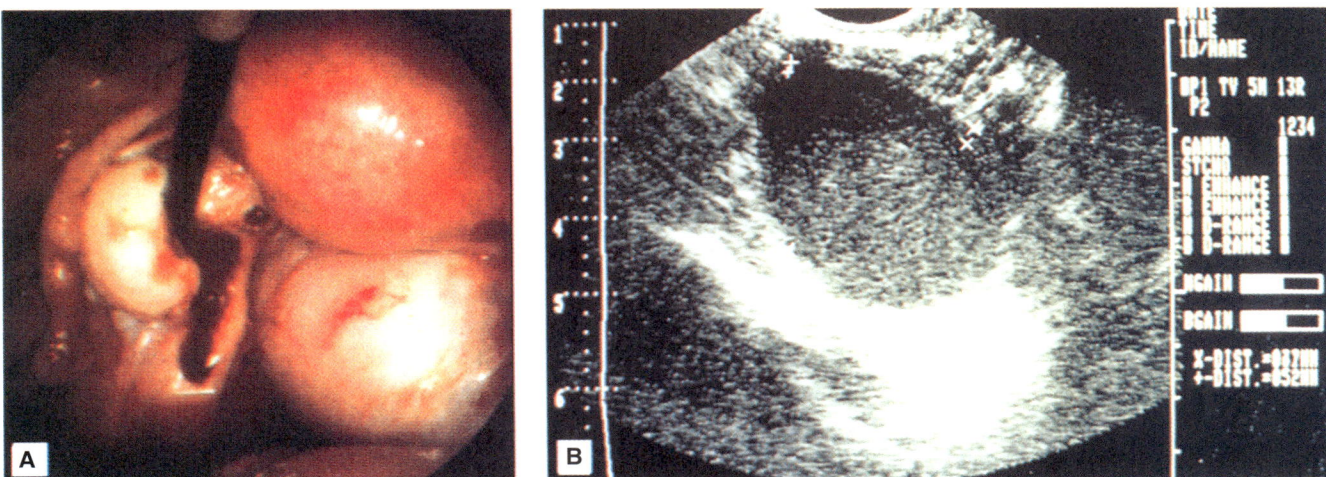

FIG. 29-1. Endometriomas. Ovarian endometriosis can be superficial or present as cystic masses called endometriomas. **A.** "Chocolate cyst." This term is applied to these ovarian masses because of the characteristic thick, dark brown fluid content (similar to chocolate syrup). **B.** Preoperative typical ultrasound appearance, with a concentric, half-moon layering effect of the fluid. (Stenchever MA, Mishell DR Jr. Atlas of clinical gynecology. Vol. III. Philadelphia [PA]: Appleton & Lange; 1999. p. 1.48.)

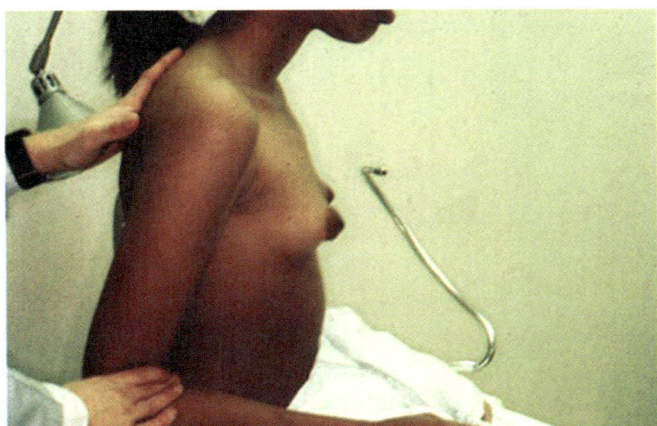

FIG. 33-1. An 18-year-old adolescent with tubular breasts resulting from inappropriate administration of high-dose oral estrogen (conjugated estrogens, 2.5 mg by mouth daily) to induce development of secondary sexual characteristics.

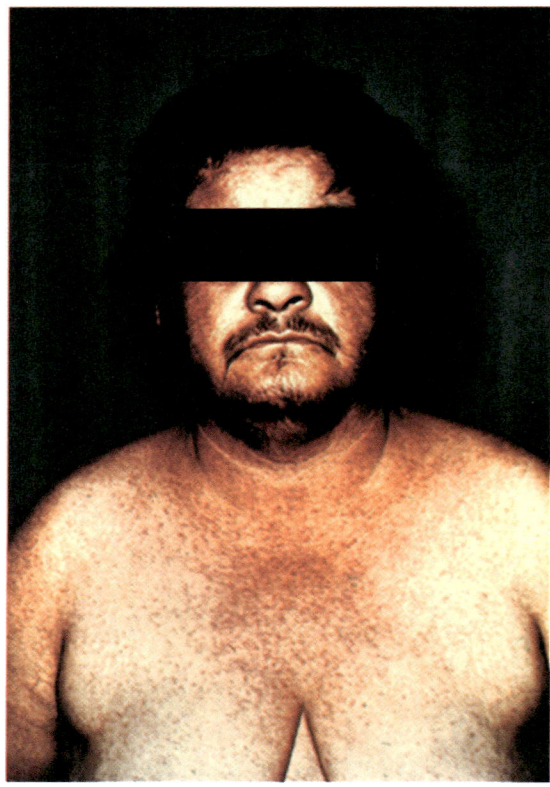

FIG. 45-1. A 57-year-old woman, 6 years postmenopause, with new onset hirsutism.

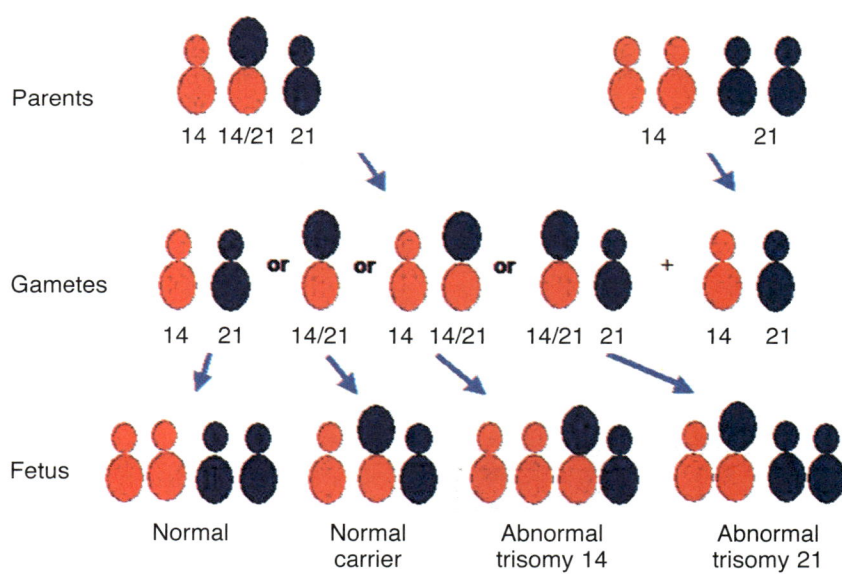

FIG. 46-1. Schematic representation of the segregation products within the gametes as well as the fertilization outcomes for a couple, one of whom harbors a *t(14q 21q)* Robertsonian chromosome translocation. Note that although 4 different gametes of equal occurrence after segregation of the translocation chromosomes would be expected, in actuality this does not happen. (Data from Simpson JL, Meyers CM, Martin AO, Elias S, Ober C. Translocations are infrequent among couples having repeated spontaneous abortion but no other abnormal pregnancies. Fertil Steril 1989;51:811–4.)

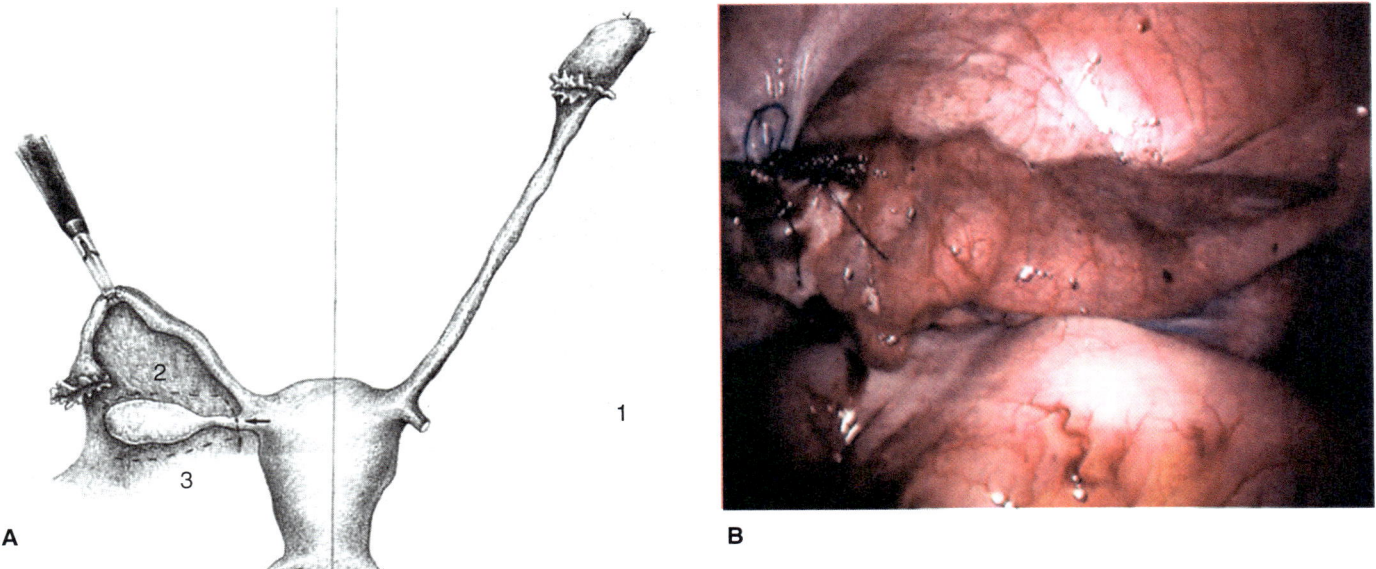

FIG. 55-1. Laparoscopic lateral ovarian transposition. **A.** The ovarian ligaments (1— see arrow) and mesovarium (2) are divided. If mobility is inadequate, a relaxing incision on the peritoneum inferior to the ovary (3) may be needed. The final location of the ovary is shown on the contralateral side. **B.** Photograph of a transposed ovary. (Reprinted from Fertility & Sterility, Vol 70, Tulandi T, Al-Took S, Laparoscopic ovarian suspension before irradiation, Copyright 1998, with permission from Elsevier.)

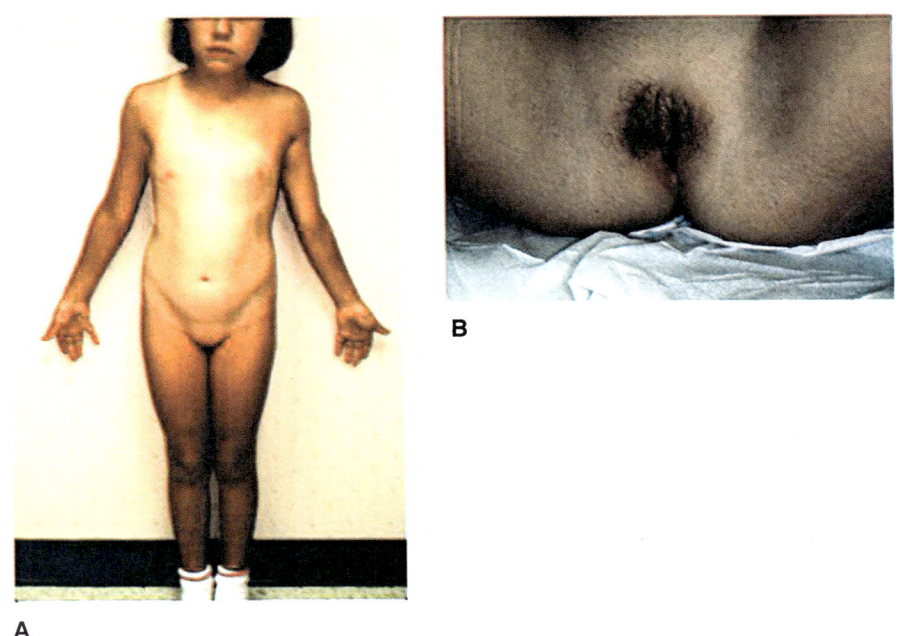

FIG. 59-1. A 7-year-old white girl with precocious adrenarche.

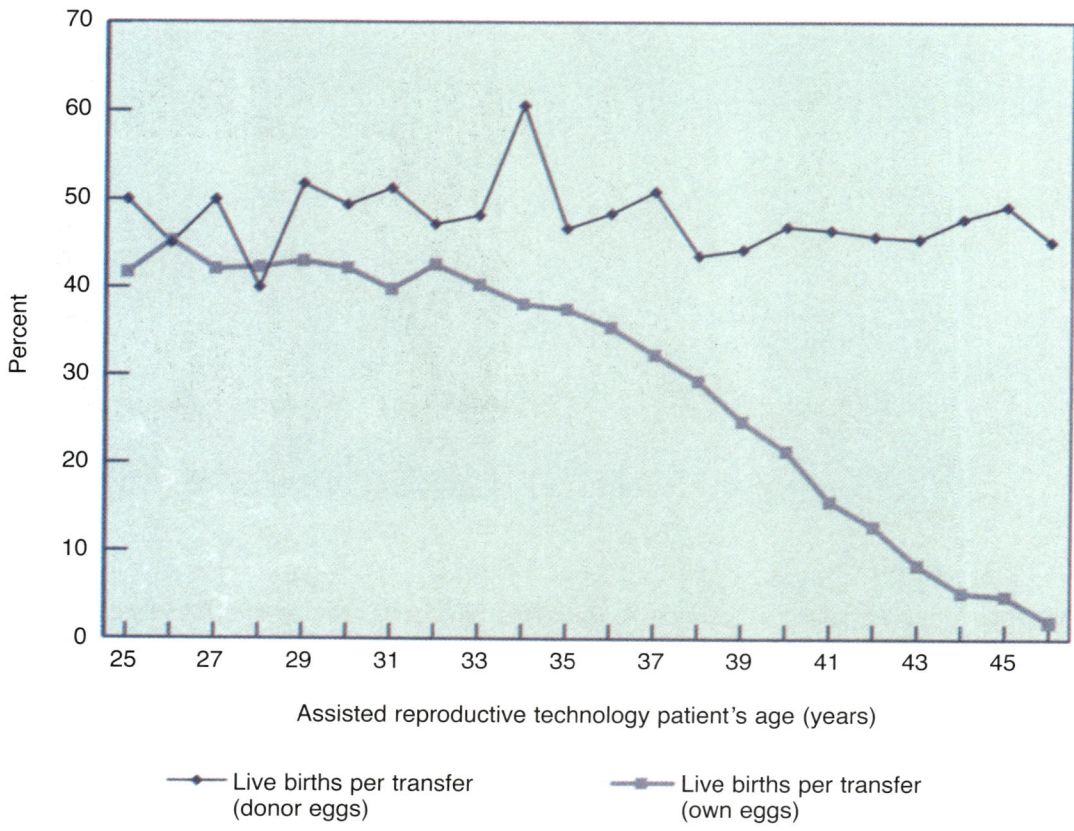

FIG. 63-2. Live births per transfer for assisted reproductive technology (ART) cycles using fresh embryos from own and donor eggs, by ART patient's age, 2001. (Centers for Disease Control and Prevention, Department of Health and Human Services. 2001 Assisted reproductive technology success rates. National summary and fertility clinic reports. Atlanta [GA]: Centers for Disease Control and Prevention; 2003. p. 47.)

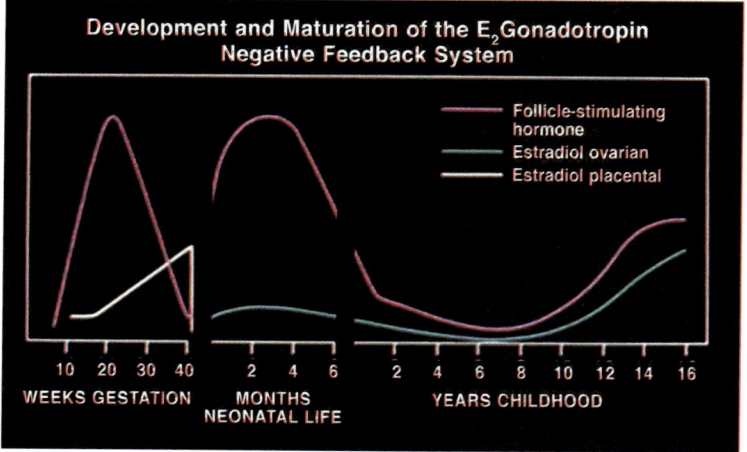

FIG. 75-2. Schematic curves for follicle-stimulating hormone and estradiol levels during fetal life, neonatal life, and childhood years in girls. Note the increase and decrease of gonadotropin levels during infancy, a time when only rarely is ovarian estrogen production sufficient to produce transient breast development. (Data from Faiman C, Winter JS, Reyes FI. Patterns of gonadotrophins and gonadal steroids throughout life. Clin Obstet Gynaecol 1976;3:467–83.)

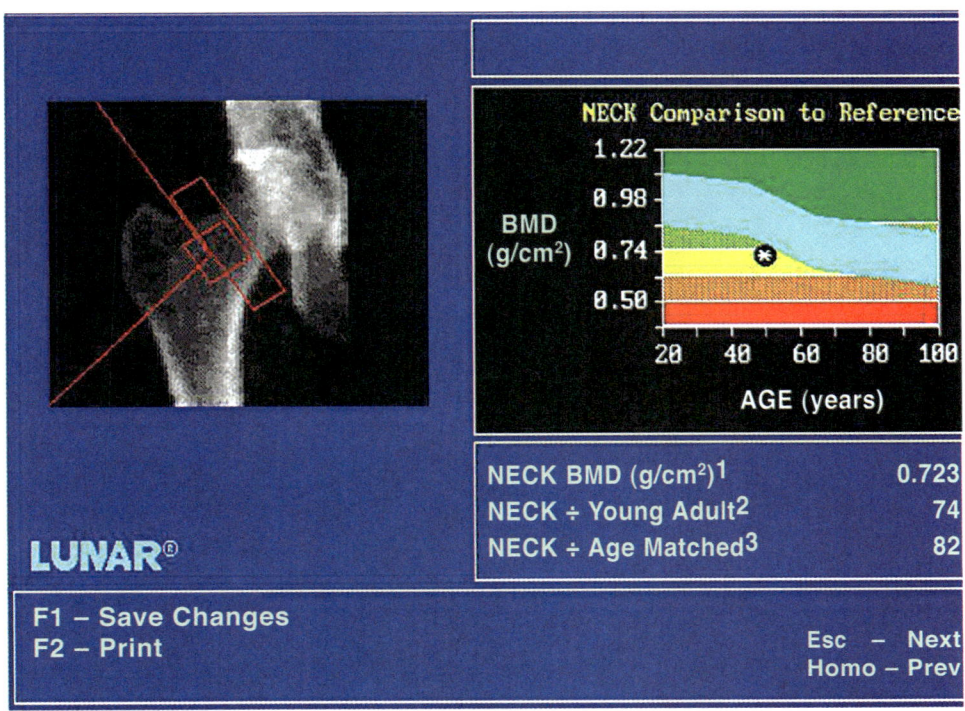

FIG. 102-1. A dual-energy X-ray absorptiometry scan of the femur of a 55-year-old postmenopausal woman.

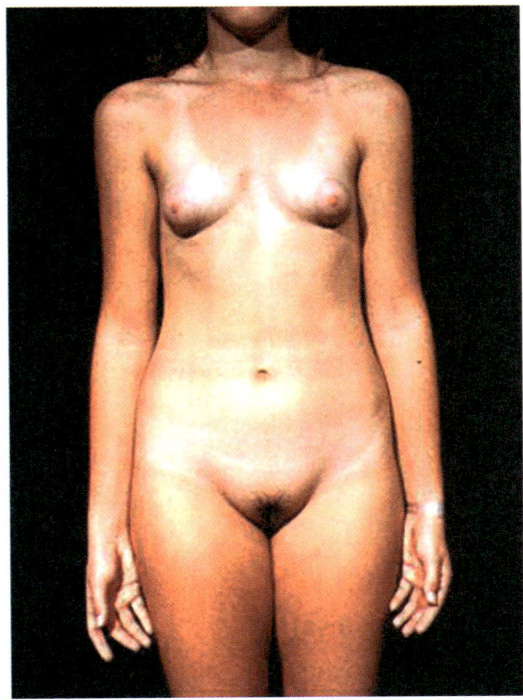

FIG. 103-1. A 16-year-old adolescent with a 46,XY karyotype, minimal pubic hair, and no axillary hair. Bilateral inguinal masses proved to be normal testes on surgery and were removed through a modified Pfannenstiel incision. (Reprinted from Rebar RW. Normal and abnormal sexual differentiation and development. In: Moore TR, Reiter RC, Rebar RW, Baker VV. Gynecology and obstetrics: a longitudinal approach. New York [NY]: Churchill Livingstone; 1993. p. 116. Copyright 1993, with permission from Elsevier.)

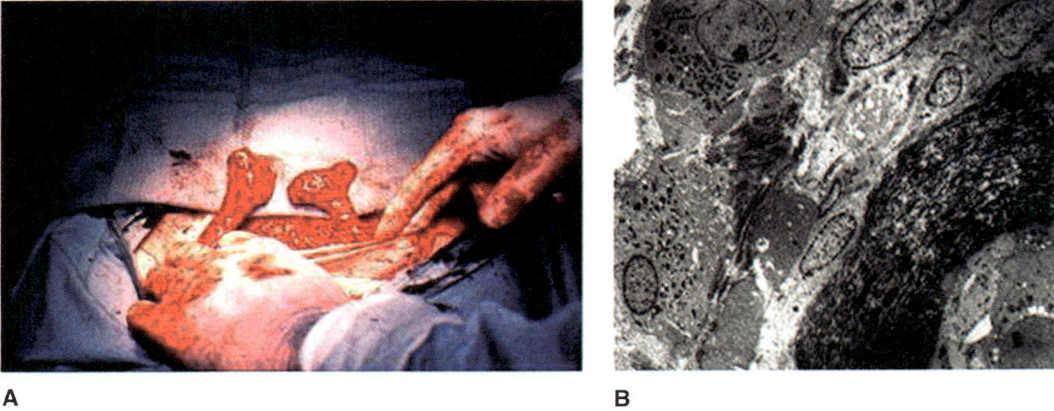

FIG. 103-2. A. Androgen sensitivity syndrome showing testes. **B.** Microscopic view of normal testes.

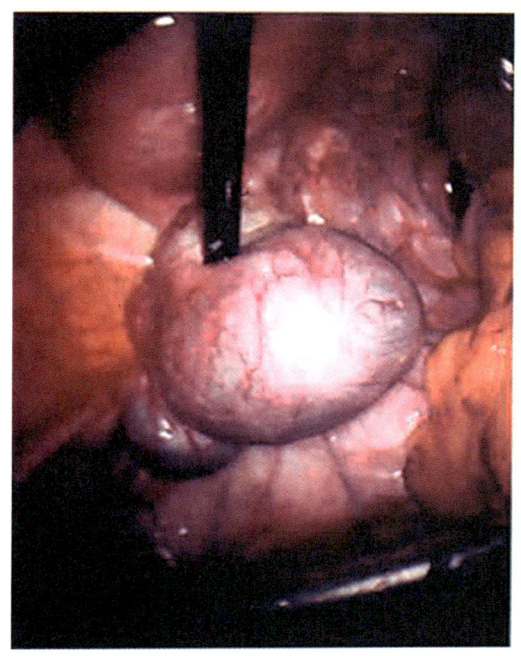

FIG. 107-1. Blunt probe elevates left recurrent hydrosalpinx.

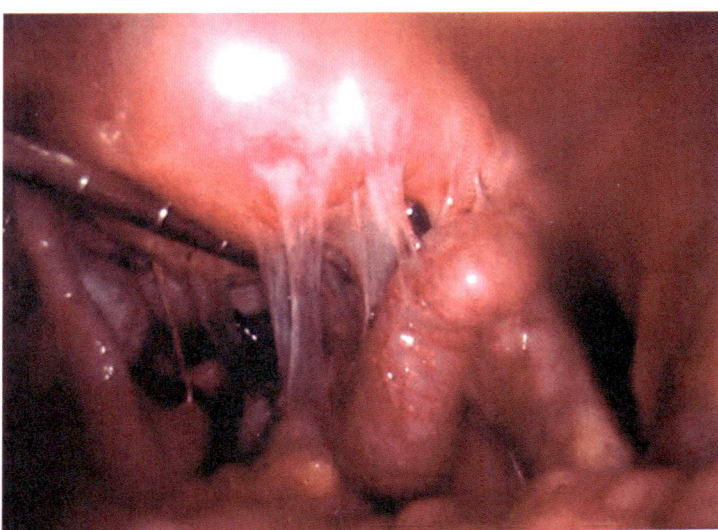

FIG. 107-2. Dense periadnexal adhesions encapsulate and obstruct right distal fallopian tube.

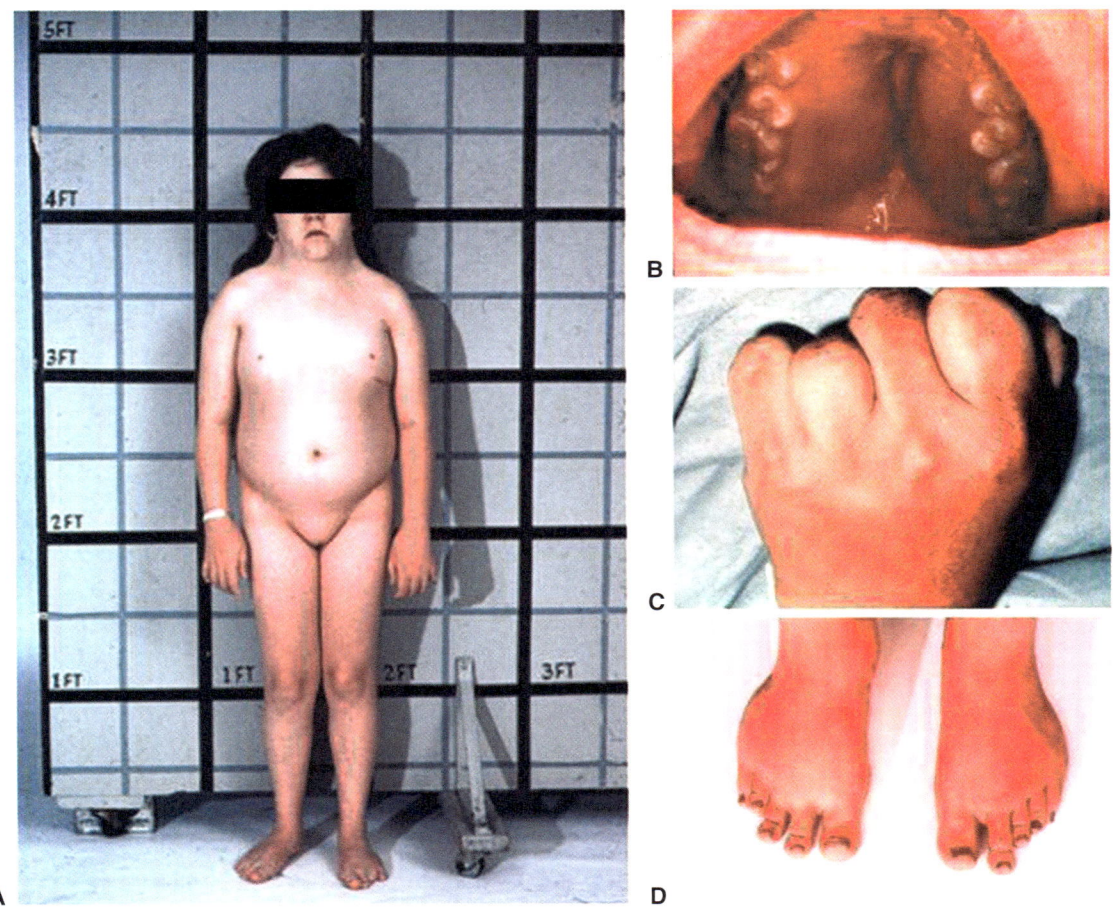

FIG. 117-1. A. A 16-year-old adolescent with 45,X gonadal dysgenesis and the stigmata of Turner's syndrome. A thoracotomy scar from the repair of her coarctation of the aorta at age 13 years is apparent. **B.** She has an abnormal high arched palate; **C.** the clenched fist shows a short fourth metacarpal; and **D.** short fourth metatarsals and dysplastic toenails are apparent on her feet. (Reprinted from Rebar RW. Normal and abnormal sexual differentiation and development. In: Moore TR, Reiter RC, Rebar RW, Baker VV. Gynecology and obstetrics: a longitudinal approach. New York [NY]: Churchill Livingstone; 1993. p. 102. Copyright 1993, with permission from Elsevier.)

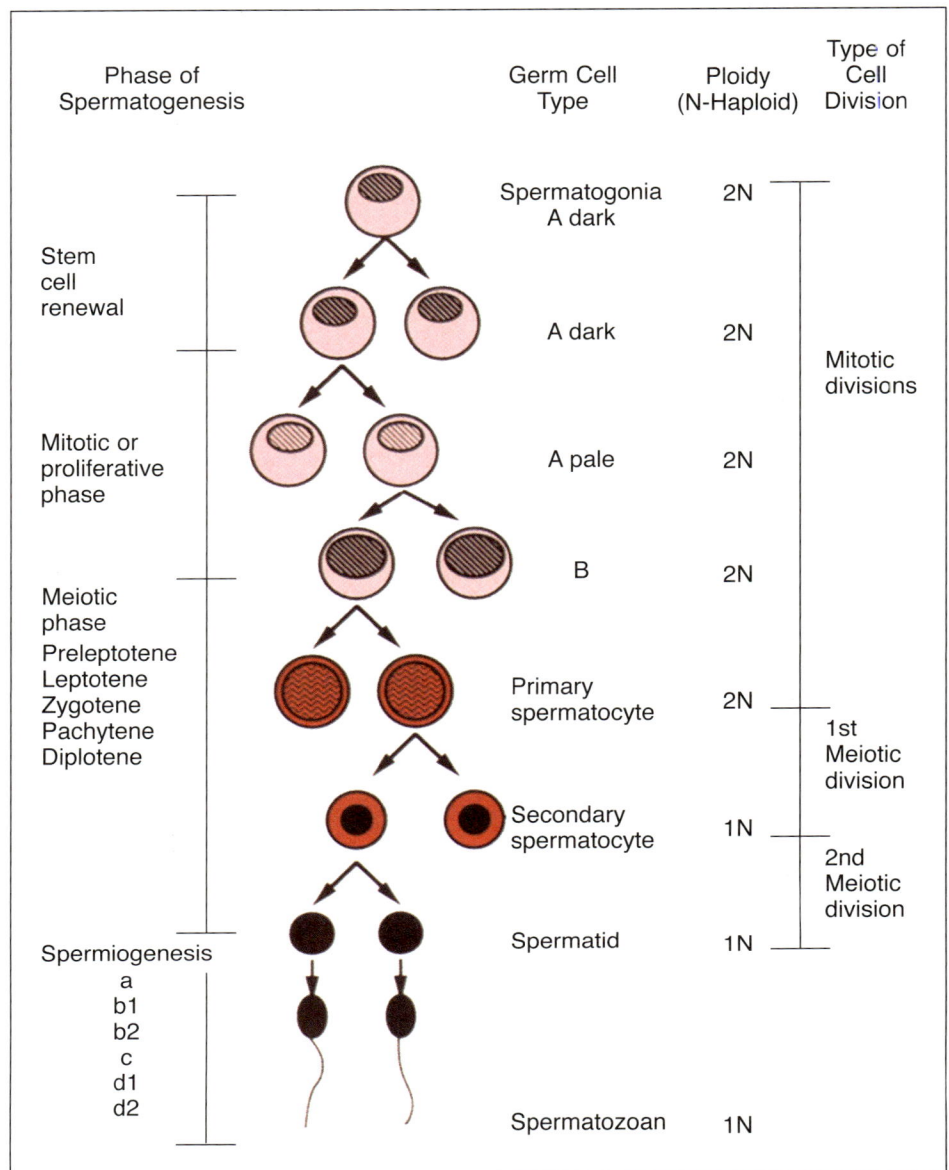

FIG. 129-1. Phases of spermatogenesis and the corresponding germ cell type, ploidy, and type of cell division. Each spermatogonium gives rise to 16 primary spermatocytes, each of which enters meiosis and gives rise to 4 spermatids and finally 4 spermatozoa. Therefore, each of the 3 million spermatogonia that begin spermatogenesis each day gives rise to 64 spermatids that undergo progressive maturation (spermiogenesis) involving 6 steps to form mature spermatozoa. (Adeshi EY, Rock JA, Rozenwaks Z, eds. Reproductive endocrinology, surgery, and technology. Vol. 2. Philadelphia [PA]: Lippincott-Raven; 1996. p. 365.)

PROLOG

Reproductive Endocrinology and Infertility

FIFTH EDITION

QUESTION BOOK

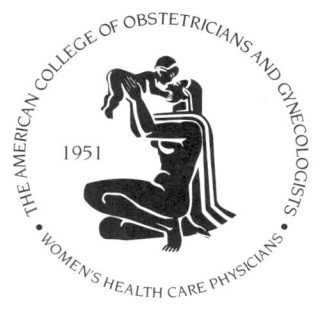

ISBN 1-932328-07-6

Copyright © 2005 by the American College of Obstetricians and Gynecologists. All rights reserved. No part of this publication may be reproduced, stored in a retrieval system, or transmitted, in any form or by any means, electronic, mechanical, photocopying, recording, or otherwise, without prior written permission of the publisher.

12345/98765

The American College of Obstetricians and Gynecologists
409 12th Street, SW
PO Box 96920
Washington, DC 20090-6920

Contributors

PROLOG Editorial and Advisory Committee

CHAIR
Ronald T. Burkman Jr, MD, Chair
   Chair, Department of Obstetrics and
     Gynecology
   Baystate Medical Center
   Springfield, Massachusetts
   Deputy Chair and Professor
   Department of Obstetrics and
     Gynecology
   Tufts University School of Medicine
   Boston, Massachusetts

MEMBERS
Peter E. Nielsen, MD, LTC, MC, USA
   OB/GYN Consultant to the US Surgeon
     General
   Division of Maternal–Fetal Medicine
   Department of Obstetrics and Gynecology
   Madigan Army Medical Center
   Tacoma, Washington
Louis Weinstein, MD
   Paula and Elloise B. Bowers Professor
     and Chair
   Department of Obstetrics and Gynecology
   Thomas Jefferson University
   Philadelphia, Pennsylvania
Sterling B. Williams, MD
   Vice President, Education
   The American College of
     Obstetricians and Gynecologists
   Washington, DC

PROLOG Task Force for *Reproductive Endocrinology and Infertility*, Fifth Edition

COCHAIRS
Robert W. Rebar, MD
   Executive Director
   American Society for Reproductive
     Medicine
   Volunteer Clinical Professor
   Department of Obstetrics and
     Gynecology
   University of Alabama, Birmingham
   Birmingham, Alabama
Craig A. Winkel, MD, MBA
   Professor
   Georgetown University
   School of Nursing
   Washington, DC

MEMBERS
John L. Frattarelli, MD
   Associate Residency Program Director
   Division Chief, Division of Reproductive
     Endocrinology and Infertility
   Department of Obstetrics and
     Gynecology
   Tripler Army Medical Center
   Honolulu, Hawaii
Daniel R. Grow, MD
   Associate Professor
   Chief, Division of Reproductive
     Endocrinology
   Department of Obstetrics and
     Gynecology
   Springfield, Massachusetts
Michael J. Heard, MD
   Reproductive Endocrinology and
     Infertility
   Pediatric/Adolescent Gynecology
   Servy Institute for Reproductive
     Endocrinology
   Augusta, Georgia

Continued on next page

PROLOG Task Force for *Reproductive Endocrinology and Infertility*, Fifth Edition *(continued)*

James H. Liu, MD
   Professor and Arthur H. Bill Chair
   Department of Reproductive Biology
   Case Western Reserve University
   Department of Obstetrics and
     Gynecology
   University Hospitals of Cleveland
   Cleveland, Ohio

Ricardo Loret de Mola, MD
   Chief, Division of Reproductive
     Endocrinology and Infertility
   Department of Reproductive Biology
   Case Western Reserve University
   Department of Obstetrics and
     Gynecology
   University Hospitals of Cleveland
   Cleveland, Ohio

William Meyer, MD
   Associate Professor
   Associate Residency Program Director
   Division of Reproductive
     Endocrinology and Infertility
   Department of Obstetrics and
     Gynecology
   University of North Carolina–Chapel
     Hill
   Chapel Hill, North Carolina

Steven T. Nakajima, MD
   Associate Professor
   Division of Reproductive
     Endocrinology and Infertility
   Department of Obstetrics, Gynecology,
     and Women's Health
   University of Iowa Hospitals
   Iowa City, Iowa

Richard H. Reindollar, MD
   Director
   Division of Reproductive Endocrinology
     and Infertility
   Department of Obstetrics, Gynecology,
     and Reproductive Biology
   Beth Israel Deaconess Medical Center
   Harvard Medical School
   Boston, Massachusetts

Valerie Montgomery Rice, MD
   Professor and Chair
   Department of Endocrinology and
     Infertility
   Department of Obstetrics and Gynecology
   Meharry Medical College
   Nashville, Tennessee

Estil Young Strawn Jr, MD
   Associate Professor
   Director, Division of Reproductive
     Endocrinology and Infertility
   Department of Obstetrics, Gynecology
   Medical College of Wisconsin
   Milwaukee, Wisconsin

ACOG STAFF

Sallye B. Brown, RN, MN
   Director, Educational Development
     and Testing
   Division of Education

Christopher T. George, MA
   Editor, PROLOG

Note: This PROLOG unit was developed under the direction of the PROLOG Advisory Committee and the Task Force for *Reproductive Endocrinology and Infertility,* Fifth Edition. PROLOG is planned and produced in accordance with the Standards for Enduring Materials of the Accreditation Council for Continuing Medical Education. Any discussion of unapproved uses of products is clearly cited.

    Current guidelines state that participants in continuing medical education (CME) activities should be made aware of any affiliation or financial interest by the contributors that may affect the development of the unit. The advisory committee and task force members declare that neither they nor any business associate nor any member of their immediate families has financial interest or other relationships with any manufacturer of any products or any providers of any of the services discussed in this publication except for **Craig A. Winkel, MD**, who is a consultant for and member of the TAP Pharmaceuticals Medical Advisory Board, is a consultant for Ortho-McNeil Pharmaceutical, is a principal in The North Group, is on the Wyeth Pharmaceuticals speakers bureau, and has been an investigator and volunteer intramural co-investigator on intramural studies for the National Institute of Child Health and Human Development (NICHD) and Ortho-McNeil Pharmaceutical; **Ronald T. Burkman Jr, MD**, who is a consultant for Pharmacea, has received lecture support from Ortho-McNeil Pharmaceutical, Wyeth Pharmaceuticals, Berlex Laboratories, Organon Pharmaceuticals USA Inc, and funding for research from NICHD and Ortho-McNeil Pharmaceutical; **Richard H. Reindollar, MD**, who has received research support and honoraria from Organon Pharmaceuticals USA Inc, Serono Laboratories, Wyeth Pharmaceuticals, Genzyme, and Columbia Laboratories; **Steven Nakajima, MD**, who has received research grants from Pfizer Pharmaceuticals and Warner Chilcott Laboratories; **James H. Liu, MD**, who is a member of the advisory boards of Merck US Human Health, Pfizer, Inc, Watson Pharmaceutical, Barr Laboratories, Novartis, and Solvay Pharmaceuticals and has received grants from the National Institutes of Health (NIH), Procter & Gamble Pharmaceuticals, Novartis Pharmaceuticals, Inc, Ortho—Personal Products, Organon Pharmaceuticals USA Inc, and Pfizer Pharmaceuticals; **William R. Meyer, MD**, who was a member of the Merck US Human Health 2003 speaker's bureau; **Valerie Montgomery Rice, MD**, who has received grants and research support from NIH, NICHD, Wyeth Pharmaceuticals, and Eli Lilly and Company; is a consultant for Wyeth Pharmaceuticals and the NICHD Committee; and is on the Advisory Boards of Novo Nordisk and the U.S. Food and Drug Administration Advisory Committee for Reproductive and Urological Health Drugs; **John L. Frattarelli, MD**, who is a speaker for TAP Pharmaceuticals; and **Daniel Grow, MD**, who is a consultant for TAP Pharmaceuticals.

Preface

Purpose

PROLOG (Personal Review of Learning in Obstetrics and Gynecology) is a voluntary, strictly confidential, self-evaluation program. It is designed to enable physicians to assess their current knowledge and to review current concepts within the specialty. The content is carefully selected and presented in multiple-choice questions that are clinically oriented. The questions are designed to stimulate and challenge physicians in areas of medical care that they confront in their practices or when they work as consultant obstetrician–gynecologists.

PROLOG provides the American College of Obstetricians and Gynecologists with a means of identifying the educational needs of the Fellowship. Individual scores are reported only to the participant; however, cumulative performance data obtained for each PROLOG unit help determine the direction for future educational programs offered by the College.

Continuing medical education credits may be earned by participation in the PROLOG self-evaluation process. In addition, PROLOG serves as a valuable study tool, reference guide, and means of attaining up-to-date knowledge in the specialty.

Process

PROLOG offers the most advanced knowledge available in 5 areas of the specialty: 1) obstetrics, 2) gynecology and surgery, 3) reproductive endocrinology and infertility, 4) gynecologic oncology and critical care, and 5) patient management in the office. A new PROLOG unit is produced annually, addressing 1 of those subject areas. *Reproductive Endocrinology and Infertility*, Fifth Edition, is the third unit in the fifth 5-year series of PROLOG.

Each unit of PROLOG represents the efforts of a special task force of subject experts under the supervision of an editorial and advisory committee. PROLOG sets forth current information as viewed by recognized authorities in the field of women's health. This educational resource does not define a standard of care, nor is it intended to dictate an exclusive course of management. It presents recognized methods and techniques of clinical practice for consideration by obstetrician–gynecologists for incorporation into their practices. Variations of practice that take into account the needs of the individual patient, resources, and the limitations that are special to the institution or type of practice may be appropriate.

Each unit of PROLOG is presented as a 2-part set. Performance information and cognate credit are available to those who choose to send their answer sheets for confidential scoring.

The first part of the PROLOG set is the Question Book, which contains educational objectives for the unit, multiple-choice questions, and a computer-scored answer sheet. Participants can work through the book at their own pace, choosing to use PROLOG as a closed- or open-book assessment. Return of the answer sheet for scoring is encouraged but voluntary.

The second part of PROLOG is the Critique Book, which reviews the educational objectives and questions set forth in the Question Book and contains a discussion, or critique, of each question. The critique provides the rationale for correct and incorrect options. Current, accessible references are listed for each question. ACOG Fellows may request additional literature searches as well as information about ACOG publications by contacting the Resource Center, PO Box 96920, Washington, DC 20090-6920, telephone (202) 863-2518.

Participants who return their answer sheets for credit will receive a Performance Report indicating their answers and their correct score percentage. A data package will be sent and will offer participants a means of comparing their scores with the scores of a sample group of other participants. *Please allow 1 month to process answer sheets.*

Fellows who submit their answer sheets for scoring will be credited automatically with 25 cognates of Formal Learning in the ACOG Program for Continuing Professional Development. For the Physician's Recognition Award of the American Medical Association, 25 category 1 credit hours may be reported.

Credit for PROLOG *Reproductive Endocrinology and Infertility*, Fifth Edition, is initially available through December 2007. During that year, the unit will be reevaluated. If it is determined that content in the unit remains current, credit will be extended for an additional 3 years. PROLOG is planned and produced in accordance with the Standards for Enduring Materials of the Accreditation Council for Continuing Medical Education.

Conclusion

PROLOG was developed specifically as a personal study resource for the practicing obstetrician–gynecologist. It is presented as a self-assessment mechanism that, with its accompanying performance information, should assist the physician in designing a personal, self-directed learning program. The many quality resources developed by the College, as detailed each year in the ACOG *Publications and Educational Materials Catalog*, are available to help fulfill the educational interests and needs that have been identified. PROLOG is not intended as a substitute for the certification or recertification programs of the American Board of Obstetrics and Gynecology.

PROLOG Objectives

PROLOG is a voluntary, strictly confidential, personal continuing education resource that is designed to be both stimulating and enjoyable. By participating in PROLOG, obstetrician–gynecologists will be able to do the following:

- Review and update clinical knowledge
- Recognize areas of knowledge and practice in which they excel, be stimulated to explore other areas of the specialty, and identify areas requiring further study
- Plan continuing education activities in light of identified strengths and deficiencies
- Compare and relate present knowledge and skills with those of other participants
- Obtain continuing medical education credit, if desired
- Have complete personal control of the setting and of the pace of the experience

The obstetrician–gynecologist who completes *Reproductive Endocrinology and Infertility*, Fifth Edition, will be able to do the following:

- Associate history as well as signs and symptoms with clinical diagnoses of specific gynecologic, obstetric, and general medical conditions
- Select appropriate laboratory tests and procedures and then analyze the results to make specific diagnoses
- Use an efficacious and cost-effective program of office management for each selected diagnosis
- Understand fundamental concepts of physiology and pathophysiology
- Apply epidemiologic principles to the health care of women
- Counsel patients regarding the extent of their medical problems, including benefits and risks of treatment as well as alternatives
- Apply professional medical ethics to the practice of obstetrics and gynecology
- Incorporate appropriate legal, risk management, and office management guidelines and techniques into clinical practice

Reproductive Endocrinology and Infertility, Fifth Edition, includes the following topics:

SCREENING AND DIAGNOSIS
Amenorrhea diagnosis
Biochemical hyperthyroidism and osteoporosis
Bone density studies
Bone markers for osteoporosis
Breast cancer in *BRCA*-positive patients
Chromosomal abnormalities in couples with recurrent abortion
Chronic labial agglutination
Chronic pelvic pain
Cushing's syndrome diagnosis
Ectopic pregnancy
Environmental toxicity and sperm counts
Evaluation of bleeding with hormone therapy
Fallopian tube occlusion
Gonadotropin-secreting tumors
Hereditary cancer syndromes
Hypogonadism as a cause of male infertility
Hypothyroidism diagnosis
Hysterosalpingogram versus sonohysterogram
Imperforate hymen versus transverse vaginal septum
Indicators for future fractures

Insulin resistance in polycystic ovary syndrome
Menopausal transition
Metabolic syndrome
Minimal endometriosis and infertility
Occlusion of the fallopian tubes
Oral contraceptives and venous thromboembolism
Osteoporosis markers
Ovarian androgen-secreting tumors
Ovarian hyperstimulation syndrome
Postpartum thyroiditis
Precocious thelarche
Premature ovarian failure
Prolactinemia
Salpingitis isthmica nodosa
Screening before hormone therapy
Secondary amenorrhea
Serum human chorionic gonadotropin levels
Sheehan's syndrome
Testing for thyroid dysfunction
Uterosacral ligament transection

MEDICAL MANAGEMENT
Abnormal uterine bleeding
Add-back therapy with analogs
Alternative therapies for the treatment of hot flushes
Androgen–estrogen use for increasing bone mineral density
Androgen insensitivity syndrome
Antiandrogen usage
Blastocysts and twinning
Bone loss with or following hormone therapy
Bulimia versus anorexia
Cardiovascular disease and hormone therapy
Chemotherapy, irradiation, and premature ovarian failure
Choice of agent in ovulation induction
Chronic labial agglutination
Contraception in menopausal transition
Craniopharyngioma
Depot medroxyprogesterone and abnormal bleeding
Depot medroxyprogesterone acetate and appetite
Dysmenorrhea
Emergency contraception
Fertility drugs and ovarian cancer
Fibroids in infertile women
Glucocorticoid-induced osteoporosis
Gonadotropin-releasing hormone agonist and antagonist
Hormonal contraception and weight gain
Hormonal contraceptive method choices
Hormone therapy and risk of breast cancer
Hyperprolactinemia
Hysterosalpingogram complications
Hyperthyroidism
Impotence
Intrauterine insemination complications
Late-onset adrenal hyperplasia and non-classic congenital adrenal hyperplasia
Levonorgestrel intrauterine system
Lipids and hormone therapy
Luteal phase support
Macroadenoma
Male infertility and hypergonadotropic hypogonadism
Male infertility and retrograde ejaculation
Management of delayed puberty
Metabolic syndrome
Mifepristone (Mifeprex) and pregnancy termination
Migraines and hormonal contraception
Oligospermic males and assisted reproductive technologies
Oral contraceptives and preexisting conditions
Ovarian cyst management during ovulation induction
Ovarian hyperstimulation syndrome
Ovulation induction selection of appropriate patients
Perimenopausal changes
Postpartum thyroiditis
Precocious adrenarche
Primary amenorrhea
Recurrent pregnancy loss
Risk of in vitro fertilization in Turner's syndrome
Selective estrogen receptor modulators and breast cancer
Selective estrogen receptor modulators in osteoporosis
Sheehan's syndrome
Transdermal patch versus vaginal ring
Treatment-related complications of uterine arterial embolization
Use of antiestrogens
Use of bisphosphonates and other agents in osteoporosis
Use of oral contraceptives to treat acne
Uterine and associated anomalies
Vaginoplasty versus Frank method for müllerian aplasia

SURGICAL MANAGEMENT
Bicornuate uterus
Bilateral tubal ligation and future fertility
Bowel injury during endoscopy
Chronic pelvic pain
Endometrial ablation complications
Endoscopic surgery risks
Hydrosalpinges and success of in vitro fertilization
Hysteroscopic endometrial ablation
In vitro fertilization versus surgery
Laser characteristics and safety
Management of weight reduction
Nonhysteroscopic endometrial ablation
Prevention of adhesions
Ruptured endometrioma
Septate uterus
Tubal anastamosis
Vascular injury with laparoscopy

PHYSIOLOGY AND PATHOPHYSIOLOGY
Diethylstilbestrol exposure
Hypothyroidism and hyperprolactinemia
Mechanism of action of oral contraceptives
Normal bone physiology
Normal pubertal development
Premature ovarian failure
Premature thelarche
Primary amenorrhea
Prolactin-secreting pituitary microadenoma
Sheehan's syndrome
Sperm physiology
Uterine and associated anomalies

COUNSELING
Achieving fertility with premature ovarian failure
Blastocysts and twinning
Bone loss with or following hormone therapy
Cardiovascular disease and hormone therapy
Congenital adrenal hyperplasia
Donor oocyte in the older patient
Hormone therapy and risk of breast cancer
Intracycloplastic sperm injection for male infertility
Lifestyle factors and fertility
Mifepristone (Mifeprex) and pregnancy termination
Risks of intracytoplasmic sperm injection

ETHICAL AND LEGAL ISSUES
Informed consent for donor eggs
Reproduction in individuals with acquired immunodeficiency disease syndrome (AIDS)
Use of donor sperm

A subject matter index appears at the end of the Critique Book.

Instructions

This book contains several types of questions. You will find special directions for each question type inside the book. Be sure that you understand the directions before answering any questions.

If you choose to participate in PROLOG for continuing medical education credit, your answers should be recorded on the separate answer sheet enclosed. Directions for recording your answers are included on the answer sheet. The registration code is printed on your answer sheet and is already encoded into the computer-readable grid. You do not need to fill out a registration code grid to identify your paper. The example below identifies PROLOG user #E20024.

PROLOG REGISTRATION

To ensure that your results are returned promptly, please complete your name and address on the answer sheet. We suggest that you keep a personal record of both your registration code and your answers so that you may check the individualized performance report that is returned to you.

The completed answer sheet should be submitted for scoring in the postage-paid return envelope enclosed with this package. *Please allow 1 month for score sheets to be processed.*

If you do not wish to submit your answers for scoring, you will not receive credit. The Critique Book enclosed in this package will, however, enable you to score your own test.

DIRECTIONS: Each of the questions or incomplete statements below is followed by suggested answers or completions. Select the ONE that is BEST in each case, and fill in the circle containing the corresponding letter on the answer sheet.

1

A 25-year-old woman received a diagnosis of premature ovarian failure. Her karyotype is 46,XX. Which of the following laboratory studies is most likely to be abnormal in this patient?

(A) Fasting glucose
(B) Calcium
(C) Cortisol
(D) Thyroid-stimulating hormone (TSH)
(E) Vitamin B_{12}

2

A 38-year-old multiparous woman with a history of 2 previous laparoscopic procedures for moderate to severe endometriosis desires long-term relief of symptoms. The most appropriate next surgical procedure is

(A) total abdominal hysterectomy and bilateral salpingo-oophorectomy
(B) laparoscopy and destruction of all identified lesions
(C) hysterectomy alone
(D) laparoscopic presacral neurectomy

Note: See Appendix A for a table of normal values for laboratory tests.

3

A 16-year-old adolescent (Fig. 3-1) is referred with primary amenorrhea. She has a normal cervix and vagina. The best explanation for these findings is

(A) androgen insensitivity
(B) pituitary insufficiency
(C) *DAX-1* gene mutation
(D) luteinizing hormone (LH) receptor gene mutation
(E) 21-hydroxylase deficiency

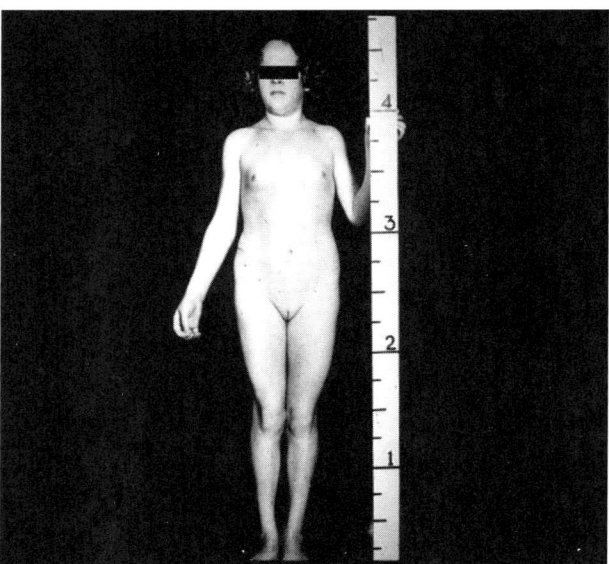

FIG. 3-1.

4

A 22-year-old woman who desires pregnancy presents with a 4-year history of amenorrhea. She is 1.6 m (5 ft 4 in.) tall and weighs 55.3 kg (122 lb). She lost 9.1 kg (20 lb) about the time her menses ceased. Her weight gradually increased with a total weight gain of more than 6.8 kg (15 lb) over the next 2 years, but menses did not resume. She admits to vomiting several times each week. The treatment most likely to effect resumption of menses is

(A) phenothiazine
(B) nutritional counseling
(C) selective serotonin reuptake inhibitors (SSRIs)
(D) cognitive–behavioral therapy
(E) monoamine oxidase inhibitors

5

A 53-year-old woman, para 2, presents with hot flushes, trouble concentrating, and problems sleeping. Her menstrual cycle length has increased from 32 days to more than 45 days, and her last menstrual period was approximately 2 months ago. Her physical examination is unremarkable. The results of a Pap test, thyroid-stimulating hormone test, and mammogram are normal. Her baseline lipid profile before starting hormone therapy shows total cholesterol level of 236 mg/dL, high density lipoprotein (HDL) cholesterol level of 35 mg/dL, low density lipoprotein (LDL) cholesterol level of 156 mg/dL, very LDL cholesterol level of 45 mg/dL, and triglyceride level of 378 mg/dL. She is started on cyclic micronized estradiol and medroxyprogesterone acetate. She returns 8 weeks later for follow-up. She reports relief of hot flushes and an improvement in her sleep pattern. She has noted intermittent "heartburn" 1–2 hours after she eats. The most appropriate next step in management is

(A) ultrasonography of the gallbladder
(B) liver function test
(C) repeat lipid profile
(D) stool hemoccult

6

A 48-year-old woman, gravida 1, para 0, underwent a simple mastectomy 5 years ago secondary to stage I breast cancer. She recently completed 5 years of tamoxifen citrate (Nolvadex) therapy for prevention of contralateral breast cancer. She has been amenorrheic for 6 months and is having occasional night sweats. She is interested in knowing whether she should consider taking raloxifene hydrochloride (Evista) to further decrease her risk of recurrent breast cancer and to reduce her vasomotor symptoms. You advise that at this time, the clinical indication for taking raloxifene is for

(A) cardiovascular disease
(B) endometrial hyperplasia
(C) recurrent breast cancer
(D) osteoporosis
(E) vasomotor symptoms

7

A 33-year-old nulliparous woman, who has regular menstrual periods, presents with a 1-year history of infertility. A recent workup, including hysterosalpingography, semen analysis, and prenatal laboratory values, was normal. She and her husband have been timing intercourse appropriately. Laparoscopy performed 2 years ago for suspected appendicitis showed minimal endometriosis, which was ablated. The next step in the management of this patient's infertility is

(A) laparoscopy for repeat coagulation of the endometriotic implants
(B) gonadotropin-releasing hormone (GnRH) agonist for 3 months
(C) empiric clomiphene citrate with intrauterine insemination (IUI)
(D) expectant management and stress reduction
(E) in vitro fertilization

8

Your patient's spouse is a 45-year-old male with a history of oligospermia who goes to the emergency room with chest pains. He is presently taking L-carnitine (Proxeed) and sildenafil citrate (Viagra) to help improve sperm quality as well as duration of erection and sexual response during timed intercourse. The medication that would most likely precipitate chest pains in the presence of sildenafil or other erection-enhancing drugs, such as tadalafil (Cialis) or vardenafil (Levitra), is

(A) tissue plasminogen activator
(B) nifedipine (Procardia)
(C) sublingual nitroglycerin
(D) lidocaine
(E) cimetidine (Tagamet)

9

A 7½-year-old African-American girl is referred for evaluation of precocious puberty. The appearance of pubic hair was noted at 6 years 11 months and breast budding 1 month ago. She is otherwise in excellent health and without any additional symptoms. Examination reveals Tanner stage III pubic hair and Tanner stage II breast development. Longitudinal growth has increased from the 55th to the 60th percentile. Her growth velocity chart demonstrates that she has moved from 4-cm to 5.5-cm growth per year. The most appropriate initial management is

(A) observation only
(B) bone age X-ray of the hand only
(C) magnetic resonance imaging (MRI) of the head only
(D) adrenocorticotropic hormone (ACTH) challenge test

10

A 21-year-old nulligravid college student comes to the student health center to request treatment for acne that significantly worsens the week before her menses and is associated with dysmenorrhea. The most cost-effective treatment for this patient is

- (A) depot medroxyprogesterone acetate
- (B) transdermal patch
- (C) levonorgestrel intrauterine system
- (D) monophasic combined oral contraceptive
- (E) progestin-only pill

11

A 29-year-old woman comes to your office with a history of unprotected intercourse within the past 24 hours. She requests emergency contraception therapy. The oral steroid hormone treatment that would provide her best option for emergency contraception is

- (A) ethinyl estradiol and norgestrel
- (B) mestranol
- (C) desogestrel
- (D) levonorgestrel
- (E) norgestimate

12

A 33-year-old nulligravid woman who is human immunodeficiency virus (HIV) negative requests information on how to eliminate her risks of becoming HIV positive when conceiving with sperm from her HIV-positive partner. They currently use condoms for all acts of sexual intercourse. You inform her that the only way to eliminate her risk is

- (A) in vitro fertilization with the partner's sperm
- (B) not to use her partner's sperm
- (C) intrauterine insemination with her partner's sperm
- (D) high-dose antiretroviral therapy for her partner
- (E) use of antiretroviral therapy by the patient

13

The occurrence of breast cancer in 2 first-degree relatives prompts genetic evaluation in a 38-year-old woman, gravida 2, para 2. Testing reveals the presence of a *BRCA1* gene mutation. The treatment option that would result in the lowest risk of breast cancer in this patient is

    (A) progestin-only contraceptive
    (B) a selective progesterone receptor modulator
    (C) bilateral mastectomy
    (D) bilateral oophorectomy
    (E) a selective estrogen receptor modulator

14

A 15-year-old adolescent comes in for evaluation. During corrective surgery for an imperforate anus identified at birth, she was found to have an ectopic kidney and anomalous ureters, which were repaired. She now experiences cyclic bloating and pain that has been labeled mittelschmerz, but she has amenorrhea. She has normal secondary sexual characteristics. A magnetic resonance imaging (MRI) study is suggestive of a bicornuate uterus. On examination under anesthesia, she is found to have a blind vaginal pouch and no evidence of a cervix. The study most likely to yield additional relevant clinical information about this patient is

    (A) X-ray of the spine
    (B) barium enema
    (C) molecular evaluation for fragile X syndrome
    (D) renal ultrasonography

15

A 65-year-old woman, who has had amenorrhea for 10 years and is not taking hormone therapy, comes in to discuss the results of her recent dual-energy X-ray absorptiometry (DXA) study. The DXA reveals decreases in the patient's lumbar and hip bone densities with T-scores of -2.7 and -2.4, respectively. You prescribe calcium, vitamin D, and a bisphosphonate and decide to check bone biomarkers after 3 months. The test result that would most likely represent evidence of compliance and drug efficacy is

    (A) a decrease in bone-specific serum alkaline phosphatase
    (B) an increase in urinary hydroxyproline
    (C) a decrease in urinary N-telopeptide
    (D) an increase in urinary deoxypyridinoline
    (E) a decrease in serum osteocalcin

16

Three months after she began taking low-dose oral contraceptives, a previously healthy 21-year-old woman has a "red, swollen, painful leg." Evaluation is consistent with deep vein thrombosis (DVT). Further evaluation is most likely to show which one of the following genetic abnormalities?

(A) Protein S deficiency
(B) Antithrombin III deficiency
(C) Protein C deficiency
(D) 20210A prothrombin mutation
(E) Factor V Leiden mutation

17

A 42-year-old woman, gravida 1, para 1, presents with severe hot flushes, trouble sleeping, fatigue, severe headaches, and increasing irritability for the past 2 months. One year ago, she received a diagnosis of breast cancer and was treated with wide local excision and chemotherapy. One lymph node was positive, and the tumor was estrogen and progestin receptor negative. After undergoing multiple courses of chemotherapy, her menstrual cycles became irregular. Her physical examination is unremarkable. Laboratory results showed normal thyroid stimulating hormone, elevated follicle-stimulating hormone, and low estradiol levels. Her complete blood count was within normal limits. The most appropriate next step in her management is

(A) clonidine
(B) progesterone
(C) selective serotonin reuptake inhibitor (SSRI)
(D) conjugated equine estrogen
(E) black cohosh

18

A 52-year-old woman, gravida 2, para 2, is referred for management of severe vasomotor symptoms. Her last regular menstrual period occurred 2 years ago. She has kept a diary and has documented more than 7 hot flushes per day and 4–5 periods of awakenings per night. On examination, she is of normal weight with a body mass index of 26 kg/m². She has an initial blood pressure reading of 140/90 mm Hg; however, following a rest period, her reading is 130/80 mm Hg. She occasionally exercises and smokes one half pack of cigarettes per day. Although she desires treatment for her vasomotor symptoms, she is concerned that taking hormone therapy (HT) may increase her risk for cardiovascular disease (CVD). In counseling her, you explain that the best intervention to decrease her risk for CVD is

(A) weight loss
(B) combination HT
(C) smoking cessation
(D) 30 minutes of exercise per day
(E) antihypertensive therapy

19

The patient in Fig. 19-1 (see color plate) presents with a 6-month history of amenorrhea, 9.1 kg (20 lb) weight gain, fatigue, and occasional headaches. Based on this patient's presentation, the best screening test for her condition is

(A) 24-hour urinary free cortisol excretion test
(B) high-dose dexamethasone (8 mg) suppression test
(C) overnight dexamethasone (1 mg) suppression test
(D) plasma adrenocorticotropic hormone (ACTH) concentration
(E) 4:00 PM serum cortisol concentration

20

A 37-year-old woman presents with menorrhagia. She has a history of chronic renal failure, type 1 diabetes mellitus, and controlled hypertension. Her hematocrit concentration is 30%. Management of her condition with cyclic progestins has caused weight gain, mastalgia, bloating, and depression. Endometrial biopsy demonstrates secretory endometrium and sonohysterography is normal. Her partner has had a vasectomy, and she has no interest in fertility. The next step in management is

(A) laparoscopically assisted vaginal hysterectomy
(B) nonhysteroscopic endometrial ablation
(C) hysteroscopically directed endometrial resection
(D) levonorgestrel intrauterine system

21

A 42-year-old obese woman, who is 1.63 m (5 ft 4 in.) tall, weighs 111 kg (245 lb), and has a body mass index (BMI) of 42 kg/m^2, comes in to be evaluated for bariatric surgery. She has a long-term history of obesity and is being treated for diabetes mellitus and hypertension. Her previous attempts at weight loss with diet, exercise, and medical therapy have failed. The most important criterion in recommending bariatric surgery is

- (A) medical co-morbidities
- (B) failed diet and exercise therapy
- (C) long-term obesity
- (D) BMI
- (E) age

22

A 32-year-old woman, gravida 2, para, 2, presents with amenorrhea of 1-year duration. Initial laboratory studies reveal follicle-stimulating hormone level of 3 mIU/mL, thyroid-stimulating hormone (TSH) level of 2.1 µU/mL, and serum prolactin level of 55 ng/mL. As you consider additional laboratory testing, you perform a directed physical examination to look specifically for

- (A) reduced body hair
- (B) increased generalized adiposity
- (C) skin hypopigmentation
- (D) acral changes
- (E) exophthalmos

23

A 41-year-old woman with symptoms of irregular vaginal bleeding, hot flushes, and dyspareunia is concerned about her risk for an unplanned pregnancy. She smokes 15 cigarettes per day and has a history of depression. She is self-conscious about her weight and is following a low-fat diet. The most convenient contraceptive method with the lowest failure rate for this woman is the

- (A) combination estrogen and progestin oral contraceptive
- (B) progestin-only oral contraceptives
- (C) intermittent injection of progestin, depot medroxyprogesterone acetate
- (D) progestin-releasing intrauterine device (IUD)
- (E) use of a diaphragm

24

A 38-year-old woman, gravida 2, comes in for evaluation. She has had 2 first-trimester pregnancy losses that occurred at 6 and 8 weeks of gestation. The patient's family history is negative for thromboembolic events and infertility. Her lupus anticoagulant and anticardiolipin test results are negative. A hysterosalpingogram performed after her last pregnancy loss is as shown (Fig. 24-1). You recommend a laparoscopy and possible hysteroscopy and inform her that if a bicornuate uterus is discovered, you will

(A) perform a hysterectomy
(B) perform a uterine unification procedure
(C) remove one of the uterine horns
(D) perform a laparoscopy only

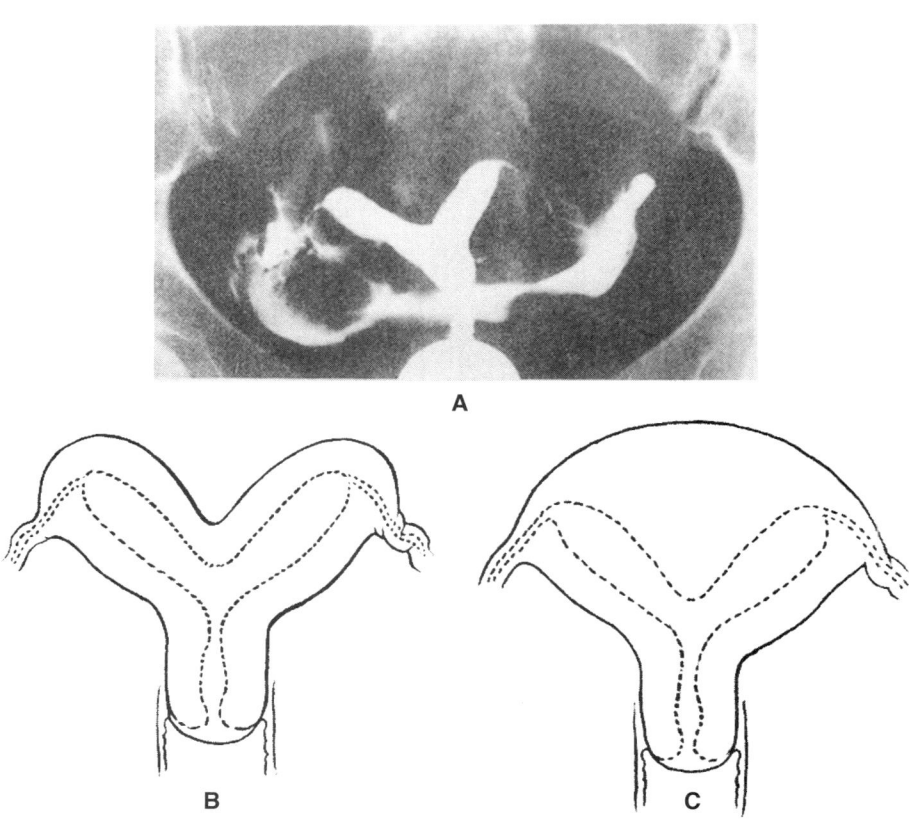

FIG. 24-1. (Adeshi EY, Rock JA, Rozenwaks Z, eds. Reproductive endocrinology, surgery, and technology. Vol. 2. Philadelphia [PA]: Lippincott-Raven; 1996. p. 2152.)

25

A 39-year-old woman undergoes uterine artery embolization for a 16-week gestation size uterus with intramural myomas. Several hours after the procedure, she develops severe pelvic pain, cramping, and a low-grade fever. The next best step in her management is

(A) blood cultures
(B) hospital observation with analgesia
(C) pelvic magnetic resonance imaging (MRI) study
(D) dilation and curettage
(E) total abdominal hysterectomy

26

A 33-year-old woman comes in for advice regarding her current oral contraceptive therapy. She has a medical history significant for type 2 diabetes mellitus, migraines with focal neurologic signs, hypertension, and menorrhagia. Recently, she had a breast biopsy, which revealed a fibroadenoma. She tells you that she has a family history of breast cancer. Her diabetes and hypertension are well controlled. Her physical examination is remarkable for a 14-week irregular uterus consistent with leiomyomata. In this patient's medical history, the most compelling reason to discontinue oral contraceptive use is

(A) diabetes mellitus
(B) migraine headaches with focal neurologic signs
(C) hypertension
(D) leiomyomata
(E) breast disease and family history of breast cancer

27

A 65-year-old woman comes in for her annual examination. She has vaginal dryness and burning during and after intercourse. Her pelvic examination shows a pale, pink, thinned vulva and absence of rugation of the vaginal mucosa. The remainder of her physical examination is normal. She had a normal mammogram and Pap test result 1 year ago. A cholesterol profile performed this year revealed a total cholesterol level of 236 mg/dL, high-density lipoprotein (HDL) cholesterol level of 35 mg/dL, low-density lipoprotein (LDL) cholesterol level of 156 mg/dL, very LDL cholesterol level of 45 mg/dL, and triglyceride level of 278 mg/dL. Her thyroid-stimulating hormone level was 3.3 µU/mL and thyroxine level was 9.8 mg/dL. A dual-energy X-ray absorptiometry (DXA) screening test showed T-scores of -1.2 at the spine and -1.3 at the hip. She takes a multivitamin, 1,500 mg of calcium, and 800 IU of vitamin D daily. The most appropriate management of this patient is

(A) vaginal lubricant
(B) alendronate sodium (Fosamax)
(C) oral estrogen-progestin therapy
(D) raloxifene hydrochloride (Evista)
(E) low-dose vaginal estrogen

28

A 19-year-old Hispanic woman with a history of hepatitis comes in for management of hirsutism present since puberty that has become more severe despite therapy with oral contraceptives. She has dark facial hair on the sides of her face, upper lip, and chin. She has neither acanthosis nigricans nor clitoromegaly. Her dehydroepiandrosterone sulfate (DHEAS), serum testosterone, and androstenedione levels are at the upper limits of normal. Thyroid-stimulating hormone and prolactin concentrations are normal. Her basal 17α-hydroxyprogesterone level is 230 ng/dL. Following administration of corticotropin, her 17α-hydroxyprogesterone level increases to 510 ng/dL. The next best step in management is to continue OCs and prescribe

(A) flutamide
(B) spironolactone
(C) finasteride
(D) gonadotropin-releasing hormone (GnRH) agonist

29

A 32-year-old nulligravid woman seeks consultation because of a 1-year history of progressively worsening pelvic pain. She refuses therapy with a gonadotropin-releasing hormone agonist. Pelvic examination reveals fullness in the right adnexa, a retroverted uterus, and cul-de-sac tenderness, particularly when palpating the uterosacral ligaments. An ultrasound examination is done and the findings are shown in Fig. 29-1 (see color plate). The best treatment for this patient is

(A) oophorectomy
(B) irrigation of the cyst cavity
(C) evacuation and cautery of the cyst
(D) excision of the endometrioma

30

A 25-year-old woman, gravida 3, para 0, with history of 2 previous miscarriages and unexplained secondary infertility, conceives after her second cycle of clomiphene citrate (Clomid, Serophene) with intrauterine insemination. The patient had an initial normal increase in her serum β-hCG levels and then a plateau at 2,500 mIU/mL at 6 weeks of gestation. She reports pelvic cramping and vaginal spotting. Which of the following ultrasound scans would be most consistent with this clinical scenario?

(A) 12-Week intrauterine pregnancy
(B) Pseudogestational sac with an adnexal mass
(C) Molar pregnancy
(D) Sonohysterogram demonstrating an endometrial polyp

31

A 29-year-old woman with a 4-year history of pelvic pain and severe dysmenorrhea is taken to the operating room for a laparoscopic procedure. At the time of the laparoscopy, lesions consistent with endometriosis are observed. Your assistant is a resident in training, and you discuss treatment options. The surgical procedure that will result in the greatest likelihood of pain relief in this patient is

(A) presacral neurectomy
(B) uterosacral nerve ablation
(C) simple destruction of lesions
(D) uterosacral nerve ablation and destruction of lesions

32

A 36-year-old woman, gravida 2, para 2, presents with amenorrhea for the past 6 years. Her medical history is significant for a diagnosis of paranoid schizophrenia, which is well controlled with medication. Her current medications include haloperidol decanoate (Haldol), benztropine mesylate (Cogentin), and lorazepam (Ativan). Her physical examination is unremarkable except for galactorrhea from the left breast. Laboratory studies are normal except for an elevated serum prolactin level of 142 ng/mL. A magnetic resonance imaging (MRI) scan of her pituitary shows no evidence of tumor. The most appropriate next step in her management is

(A) visual field
(B) reduce antipsychotic medications
(C) mammography
(D) dual-energy X-ray absorptiometry (DXA) scan

33

A 13-year-old adolescent comes in for evaluation of "lack of sexual development." The patient's medical history and family history are unremarkable. Vital signs are normal. Physical examination reveals a height of 142 cm (56 in.), Tanner stage I breast and pubic hair development (see Appendix D), webbed neck, high-arched palate, broad chest, small uterus, normal cervix, and nonpalpable ovaries. Bone age is 11.2 years. Laboratory analysis reveals a follicle-stimulating hormone level of 41 mIU/mL, a luteinizing hormone level of 24 mIU/mL, estradiol level of less than 10 pg/mL, and karyotype of 45,X. Appropriate initial management for this patient is

(A) thyroxine
(B) calcium
(C) recombinant human growth hormone
(D) medroxyprogesterone acetate

34

A 29-year-old nulligravid woman who recently immigrated from Asia to the United States undergoes a late luteal phase endometrial biopsy for infertility and amenorrhea. The biopsy results show lymphocytic infiltration, epithelioid tubercles, and several giant cells (Fig. 34-1). She has a history of oligomenorrhea, and her hysterosalpingogram is as shown (Fig. 34-2). The most frequent concurrent disease process in a patient with this presentation is

(A) pleuritis
(B) exudative salpingitis
(C) caseating cervicitis
(D) oophoritis
(E) myometritis

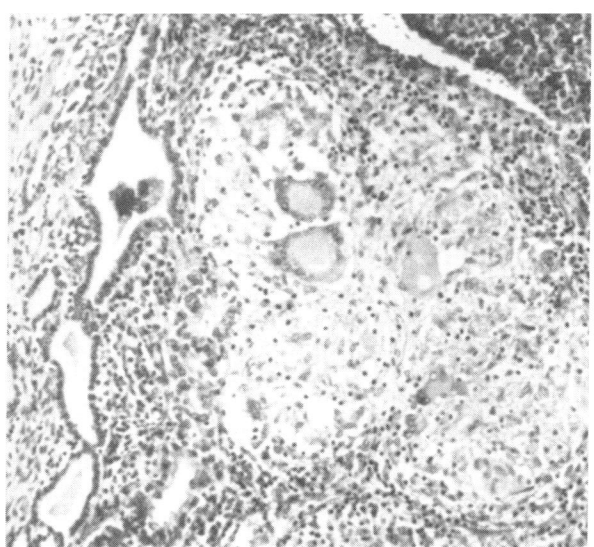

FIG. 34-1. (Kurman RJ, ed. Blaustein's pathology of the female genital tract. 5th ed. New York [NY]: Springer-Verlag; 2002. p. 429.)

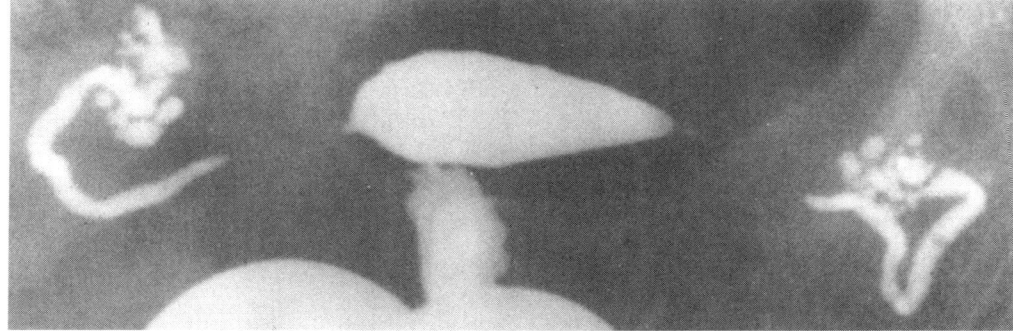

FIG. 34-2. (Reprinted from Wallach EE, Zacur HA. Reproductive medicine and surgery. 1st ed. St. Louis [MO]: Mosby; Copyright 1995, with permission from Elsevier.)

35

A 28-year-old nulliparous woman developed premature ovarian failure at age 22 years and, subsequently, 46,XX premature ovarian failure was diagnosed. Her older sister developed the same condition at age 31 years. At laparoscopy for pelvic pain, she was found to have very small round ovaries measuring 1 cm bilaterally. Before considering her youngest sister as an oocyte donor, the patient should be screened for which one of the following causes of familial ovarian failure?

(A) Swyer syndrome
(B) Galactosemia
(C) Fragile X premutation
(D) Follicle-stimulating hormone (FSH) receptor gene mutation
(E) 17α-Hydroxylase deficiency

36

A 28-year-old nulligravid woman with primary infertility has been treated with clomiphene citrate (Clomid, Serophene) for superovulation for the past 2 months. She presents on day 3 of her menstrual cycle with right lower quadrant pain and the ultrasonogram taken at that time is shown (Fig. 36-1). The most appropriate management is

(A) continue the clomiphene citrate
(B) combined oral contraceptives
(C) ovarian cystectomy
(D) expectant management
(E) transvaginal cyst aspiration

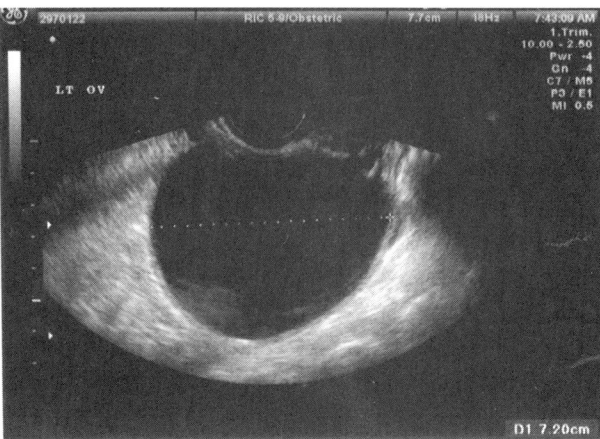

FIG. 36-1.

37

A 33-year-old nulligravid woman undergoes a laparoscopic resection of deep endometriosis that primarily involves the right uterosacral ligament. The patient comes to the emergency department 4 days later with nausea, bloating, and inability to pass gas or have a bowel movement. Physical examination is unremarkable except for hypoactive bowel sounds. A flat plate and upright film of the abdomen and complete blood count are all normal. The next best diagnostic study is

(A) computerized axial tomography (CAT) scan
(B) upper gastrointestinal series with small bowel follow-through
(C) pelvic and abdominal ultrasonography
(D) repeat flat plate and upright film in 24 hours
(E) blood urea nitrogen (BUN) and creatinine

38

A 46-year-old woman presents with a 9-month history of irregular menstrual periods with unpredictable onset. She has noticed associated periodic hot flushes with profuse perspiration, which have caused her to awaken from sleep. Pelvic examination demonstrates a normal uterine size, without palpable adnexal masses. The most appropriate way to diagnose the menopausal transition in this patient is

(A) serum follicle-stimulating hormone (FSH)
(B) serum luteinizing hormone (LH)
(C) serum estradiol
(D) menstrual history and symptoms
(E) basal body temperature chart

39

A 4-year-old child is referred for evaluation of precocious thelarche associated with a serum estradiol level of 382 pg/mL. The patient has Tanner stage III breast development and Tanner stage I pubic hair. Her longitudinal growth is in the 75th percentile, an increase from the 50th percentile of the previous years. The most appropriate next step in management is

(A) observation for 6 months
(B) gonadotropin-releasing hormone (GnRH) challenge test
(C) pelvic ultrasound examination
(D) magnetic resonance imaging (MRI) of the head

40

A 13-year-old adolescent comes in for evaluation and treatment of rapid weight gain and irregular menstrual cycles. She has a family history of obesity and diabetes mellitus in her father and endometriosis in her aunt. On physical examination, she is morbidly obese and has evidence of acanthosis nigricans. Her waist circumference is 90 cm, her fasting blood glucose level is 175 mg/dL, and her total cholesterol level is 300 mg/dL. The most common pathophysiologic basis for her disorder is

(A) hyperlipidemia
(B) hypothalamic dysfunction
(C) hyperandrogenemia
(D) insulin resistance
(E) leptin gene mutation

41

A 35-year-old African-American woman undergoes a dual-energy X-ray absorptiometry study. Her T-score at the hip is -2.8. She has eumenorrhea and a history of systemic lupus erythematosus. Her medications include daily prednisone (20 mg) for immunosuppression, a thiazide and ace inhibitor for hypertension, and Coumadin as prophylaxis. She also takes supplemental vitamin D and calcium. At this time, it would be most appropriate to

(A) discontinue thiazide
(B) add bisphosphonate
(C) change Coumadin to heparin
(D) add raloxifene
(E) add calcitonin

42

A 24-year-old woman with a history of ectopic pregnancy and left total salpingectomy presents with findings consistent with a right tubal pregnancy. She underwent a tubal sterilization reversal 4 months ago. A laparoscopy is performed for worsening pain and anemia. A leaking ectopic pregnancy approximately 5 cm in size is visualized at the site of the tubal reversal in the isthmic portion of the fallopian tube, and she has distal peritubal adhesions. The remainder of the tube on either side of the ectopic pregnancy has a normal appearance. The most appropriate next step in the surgical management of this patient is

(A) right salpingectomy
(B) hysterectomy
(C) salpingostomy with removal of ectopic pregnancy
(D) partial salpingectomy to remove ectopic pregnancy
(E) partial salpingectomy with immediate tubal anastomosis

43

A 28-year-old woman, gravida 1, para 1, was admitted to labor and delivery with a retained placenta following a planned home delivery. The patient was managed with intravenous fluid therapy and manual removal of the placenta under anesthesia. Postoperatively, her hematocrit concentration was 19%. She was given 3 units of whole blood and her posttransfusion hematocrit concentration is now 32% and stable. She has experienced orthostatic symptoms and fatigue for the past 2 days but refuses further blood transfusions. She has no milk production and is concerned that her infant will become dehydrated. On examination, she appears tired and sleepy. In the supine position, her blood pressure level is 76/40 mm Hg and her pulse rate is 105 beats per minute. Her blood pressure level decreases to 60/30 mm Hg and pulse increases to 130 beats per minute 2 minutes after shifting into the sitting position. The most appropriate next step in her management is

(A) blood transfusion
(B) intravenous glucose
(C) corticosteroid therapy
(D) toxicology screen

44

In a 25-year-old woman, gravida 2, para 2, with a 9-month history of dysmenorrhea and dyspareunia, the diagnosis that would most likely be confirmed by laparoscopy only is

(A) endometriosis
(B) interstitial cystitis
(C) irritable bowel syndrome
(D) musculoskeletal disease

45

A 57-year-old woman (Fig. 45-1; see color plate), 6 years postmenopausal, presents with new onset hirsutism and increased sensitivity and size of the clitoris. Physical examination shows normal blood pressure level and increased muscle mass but is negative for hypertension, acanthosis nigricans, adnexal mass, or striae. Pelvic ultrasonography reveals normal appearing ovaries, and computed tomography (CT) scan shows normal adrenal glands. Her serum testosterone level is 300 ng/dL. The most likely diagnosis is

(A) adult onset congenital adrenal hyperplasia
(B) adrenal tumor
(C) hilus cell tumor
(D) Cushing's syndrome
(E) hyperinsulinemia and hyperthecosis

Reproductive Endocrinology and Infertility

46

Five couples come in for further evaluation for recurrent pregnancy loss. Of the following pregnancy histories, the couple most likely to have a parental balanced chromosome translocation as the cause for their loss(es) has

(A) 6 spontaneous abortions
(B) 2 spontaneous abortions
(C) 3 spontaneous abortions, each separated by a healthy term infant
(D) 1 spontaneous abortion, 2 term infants (1 with unbalanced translocation)
(E) 1 term infant followed by 3 spontaneous abortions

47

A 26-year-old woman, weighing 92 kg (205 lb), has a 6 cm × 7 cm persistent complex left adnexal mass. She is scheduled to have a laparoscopy and left ovarian cystectomy. After placing the laparoscope, you unsuccessfully attempt to transilluminate the deep inferior epigastric vessels before insertion of the accessory trocars. The best strategy to avoid damage to the deep inferior epigastric vessels during placement of secondary trocars is to

(A) place the trocars 2 cm lateral to and 2 cm above the iliac crest
(B) identify the umbilical ligaments
(C) use only a single suprapubic midline trocar
(D) insert the trocars 5 cm medial to the iliac crest

48

A 45-year-old woman, gravida 1, para 1, presents with abnormal uterine bleeding and is given a diagnosis of endometrial cancer. She tells you that colorectal cancer was diagnosed in her brother, her only sibling, at age 45 years, and her mother developed ovarian cancer at age 62 years. The mutation that is most likely to test positive in this woman is

(A) *BRCA1*
(B) *MSH2*
(C) *APC*
(D) *TP53*
(E) *MEN1*

49

A 40-year-old woman, gravida 3, para 3, requests contraception. Her past medical history is significant for chronic hypertension, which is currently controlled with a diuretic and a β-blocker. Which of the following methods of contraception would be the most cost-effective for this patient?

(A) Combined oral contraceptive
(B) Transdermal patch
(C) Progestin-only pill
(D) Intrauterine device (IUD)
(E) Laparoscopic bilateral tubal ligation

50

A 23-year-old woman comes to the emergency department following a minor motor vehicle accident. A skull film (Fig. 50-1) demonstrates a large lesion in the intrasellar and suprasellar spaces, with scattered areas of calcification throughout. On further questioning, the patient states that although she initiated pubertal development, she has never had a menstrual period. On physical examination, she has Tanner stage I breast development, confused by a very chubby chest, and Tanner stage IV pubic hair. Laboratory evaluation reveals a follicle-stimulating hormone level of less than 2 mIU/mL, luteinizing hormone level of less than 2 mIU/mL, serum prolactin level of 800 ng/mL, and thyroid-stimulating hormone level of 0.1 µU/ml. The most appropriate next step in treatment is

(A) observation
(B) transfrontal surgical removal
(C) dopamine agonist therapy followed by transsphenoidal resection
(D) transsphenoidal resection
(E) dopamine agonist therapy alone

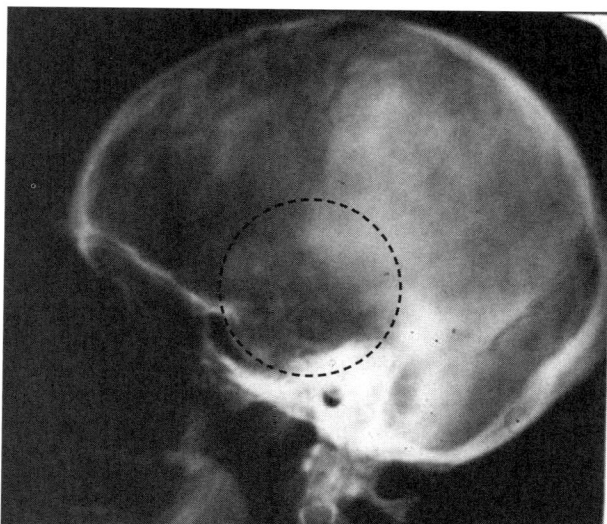

FIG. 50-1.

51

A tobacco farmer is concerned that his occupation may be contributing to his documented oligoasthenospermia (ie, reduced sperm count with low motility). He admits to occasional use of marijuana. The factor that is most likely to be responsible for his increased risk of asthenospermia is

(A) polychlorinated biphenyl hydrocarbons (PCBs)
(B) lead
(C) tetrahydrocannabinol
(D) ionizing radiation
(E) nicotine

52

A 36-year-old nulligravid woman and her husband come in for consultation regarding the best method for them to achieve a pregnancy. The husband has undergone 2 semen analyses, which have documented sperm concentrations of 1–2 million sperm per mL, sperm motilities of 10–15%, and normal sperm morphologies of 10–15%. His urologist has documented a small nonpalpable varicocele on ultrasonography. The woman has an ovulatory menstrual history and no history suspicious for pelvic adhesions. The most cost-effective means of achieving a pregnancy in this couple not concerned about paternity is

(A) varicocele repair for the husband
(B) clomiphene citrate (Clomid, Serophene) for the husband
(C) in vitro fertilization with intracytoplasmic sperm injection (ICSI)
(D) donor insemination
(E) intrauterine inseminations with the husband's sperm

53

A 43-year-old multiparous woman presents with unpredictably heavy menstrual bleeding for the past 2 years. Her medical history and review of systems are unremarkable, and she is using no medications. The physical examination is unremarkable, and the uterus is felt to be of normal size. No adnexal masses are palpated. The Pap test and endometrial biopsy results are normal. Ultrasonography is done (Fig. 53-1). She refuses all forms of medical therapy as well as hysterectomy. Her best option for therapy will be

(A) balloon ablation
(B) radiofrequency ablation
(C) hot circulating saline ablation
(D) hysteroscopic ablation
(E) hysteroscopic resection

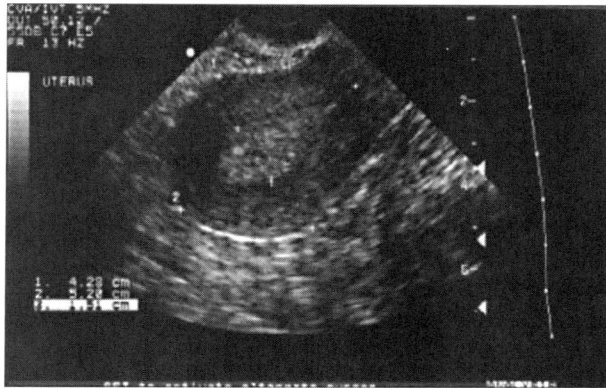

FIG. 53-1.

54

A 27-year-old woman presents with a history of irregular menstrual cycles for the past 8 months. Menses are unpredictable and occur at 27–60-day intervals punctuated by vaginal spotting or full flow. She has gained approximately 7.3 kg (16 lb) during the past year. Menarche occurred at age 11 years, and she had regular cycles of 26–29 days' duration until age 19 years. She was started on oral contraceptives and remained on them until age 26 years when she discontinued them to attempt pregnancy. She denies having headaches, hot flushes, or visual disturbances and is not taking any medications. There have been no changes in her diet or exercise pattern. On examination, her thyroid gland is not enlarged, and her breasts have no masses or discharge. Her thyroid-stimulating hormone (TSH), total thyroxine, and follicle-stimulating hormone levels are normal. Two basal serum prolactin values are elevated at 57 ng/mL and 65 ng/mL. A magnetic resonance imaging (MRI) scan with contrast of the pituitary region shows an isolated nodule 2.5 mm in diameter in the left lateral anterior pituitary. The most appropriate next step in her management is

(A) observation
(B) exogenous gonadotropins
(C) dopamine receptor agonist
(D) clomiphene citrate (Clomid, Serophene)

55

A 25-year-old single woman in whom stage III Hodgkin's disease was recently diagnosed is scheduled to begin systemic chemotherapy and pelvic irradiation. She is referred to you to discuss how to preserve her ovarian function and future fertility. On the basis of available data, the most effective proven treatment is

(A) gonadotropin-releasing hormone (GnRH) agonist during therapy
(B) combination oral contraceptive during therapy
(C) collection of oocytes for cryopreservation
(D) laparoscopic transposition of the ovaries
(E) removal and cryopreservation of ovarian tissue strips

56

A 52-year-old woman comes to your office to discuss her options regarding her hormone therapy (HT) regimen in view of the results of the Women's Health Initiative trial. The patient had her last menstrual period approximately 5 years ago and has been taking combination HT for the past 2 years for treatment of vasomotor symptoms. The patient believes this regimen has helped control her hot flushes and insomnia. She is concerned that remaining on HT may increase her risk for breast cancer, although she has no family history of this disease. You counsel her that

(A) combination HT does not increase her risk of breast cancer
(B) the progestin protects her from developing cancer
(C) only medroxyprogesterone acetate is associated with an increased risk of breast cancer
(D) only conjugated estrogen is associated with an increased risk of breast cancer
(E) there appears to be some increased risk of breast cancer with any combination HT

57

A 24-year-old woman, gravida 2, presents for contraceptive management. She has been using depot medroxyprogesterone acetate for contraception for the past 3 years and reports that her weight has increased by more than 22.7 kg (50 lb). She reports no menstrual bleeding over the past 18 months. Physical examination reveals a blood pressure level of 136/87 mm Hg, a plump facies, a small fat pad in the posterior neck, and scattered white stretch marks near the hips and buttocks. Laboratory evaluations show normal levels of thyroid-stimulating hormone (TSH), human chorionic gonadotropin, serum prolactin, and follicle-stimulating hormone. Her serum cortisol level is less than 5 µg/dL after an overnight dexamethasone suppression test. The factor that has most likely contributed to her current weight gain is

(A) Cushing's syndrome
(B) depot medroxyprogesterone acetate
(C) polycystic ovary syndrome
(D) acromegaly

58

A 7-year-old girl presents with findings of chronic labial agglutination. Her mother reports that the labia are adherent periodically, but there is no redness or problems with urinating. Her symptoms recur despite repeated application of estrogen cream. On physical examination, the child exhibits Tanner stage I breast development and Tanner stage I pubic hair (see Appendix D). The labia are adherent in the midline with minimal erythema without bleeding or discharge. The urethra is patent and unobstructed. The most appropriate next step in management is

(A) surgery for failed medical therapy
(B) vulvar biopsy to determine the etiology of the chronic symptoms
(C) reassurance and discontinuation of use of estrogen therapy
(D) corticosteroid cream
(E) office adhesiolysis under local anesthesia

59

A 7-year-old white girl (Fig. 59-1; see color plate) presents with pubic hair growth, oily skin, and body odor. She has no signs of masculinization. Her blood pressure level is 90/60 mm Hg. Her longitudinal height and weight charts are shown in Fig. 59-2. The most likely pathophysiologic process responsible for these signs is

(A) hyperprolactinemia
(B) 11β-hydroxysteroid dehydrogenase deficiency
(C) impaired insulin sensitivity
(D) 5α-reductase deficiency
(E) adrenal tumor

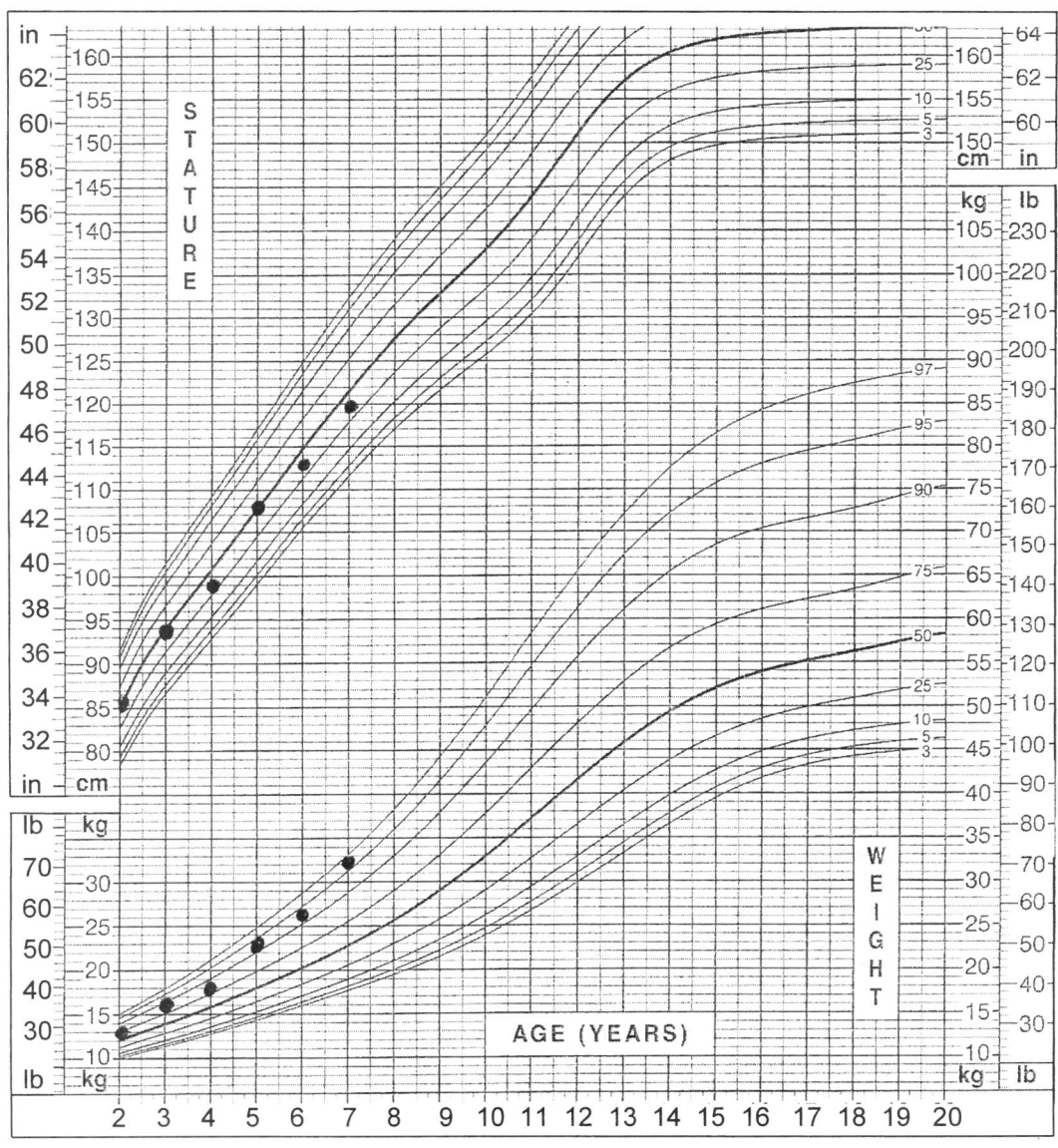

FIG. 59-2.

60

A 28-year-old nulligravid woman has polycystic ovary syndrome (PCOS). She undergoes controlled ovarian hyperstimulation using recombinant follicle-stimulating hormone for a cycle of intrauterine insemination with a peak estradiol level of 1,800 pg/mL on the day of human chorionic gonadotropin (hCG) stimulation. Four days after the insemination, she comes to the emergency department with abdominal distention, weight gain, generalized abdominal pain, and nausea. The most likely explanation for her symptoms is

(A) ectopic pregnancy
(B) acute appendicitis
(C) ovarian cyst
(D) ovarian hyperstimulation syndrome
(E) ovarian torsion

61

A patient with longstanding infertility undergoes hysterosalpingography, which shows bilateral proximal tubal occlusion (Fig. 61-1). In the proximal tube, there is a honeycomb pattern of contrast that seems to enter the tubal wall. Subsequent laparoscopy shows multiple 1–2 cm nodules in the isthmus of one fallopian tube. The most likely diagnosis is

(A) chronic chlamydial salpingitis
(B) tuberculous salpingitis
(C) salpingitis isthmica nodosa
(D) prenatal exposure to diethylstilbestrol
(E) ectopic pregnancy

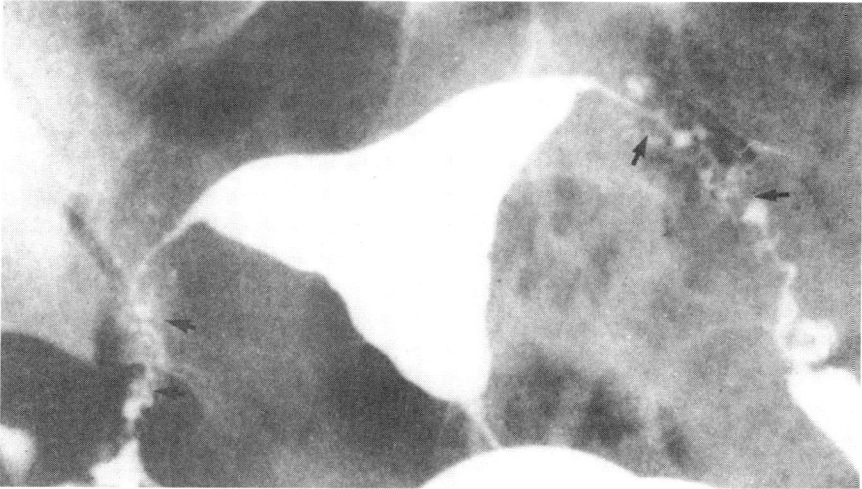

FIG. 61-1. (Reprinted from Wallach EE, Zacur HA. Reproductive medicine and surgery. St. Louis [MO]: Mosby; 1995. p. 501. Copyright 1995, with permission from Elsevier.)

62

A 14-year-old adolescent is referred from the local emergency department for recurrent severe pelvic–abdominal pain. A midline pelvic mass was palpated on rectal examination and a pelvic ultrasonogram suggests a hematocolpometra. Although less than optimal, a vaginal examination suggests that the upper vagina ends blindly. On repeat rectal examination, the bulging mass is found to extend cephalad from the top of the blind vagina. The next best step in management for this patient is

(A) renal ultrasonography
(B) bone malformation assessment
(C) imaging of the vagina, cervix, and uterus
(D) examination under anesthesia
(E) aspiration of the bulging mass

63

A 43-year-old woman, gravida 4, para 1, comes in for infertility evaluation. She had a 5-year-old son who died in an accident, and she has a history of 3 early pregnancy losses since age 40 years. She and her husband have normal peripheral karyotypes. She has a normal pelvic ultrasonogram, hysterosalpingogram, glucose tolerance test result, serum thyroid-stimulating hormone level, lupus anticoagulant level, anticardiolipin antibody level, antinuclear antibody level, mammogram, and prenatal laboratory test result. A clomiphene citrate (Clomid, Serophene) challenge test shows a day 10 follicle-stimulating hormone level of 15 mIU/L. The therapy that will result in the greatest probability of a term pregnancy in this patient is

(A) in vitro fertilization (IVF)
(B) gestational surrogacy with the patient's eggs
(C) donor oocyte IVF
(D) superovulation and intrauterine insemination
(E) intravenous immunoglobulin

64

A 41-year-old woman and her husband have decided to try in vitro fertilization (IVF) in an attempt to conceive. The woman has had both fallopian tubes removed as treatment for ruptured ectopic pregnancies. The couple is concerned about the risks and complications associated with IVF techniques. They have heard about assisted reproductive technology (ART) that involves blastocyst culture and transfer. In counseling this couple, the most accurate statement based on current data is that blastocyst culture, compared with day 3 transfer, is associated with

(A) reduced incidence of cycle cancellation
(B) similar pregnancy rates
(C) reduced incidence of twin pregnancy
(D) higher pregnancy rates in women older than 40 years

65

A 34-year-old woman, gravida 1, para 1, has a history of pelvic pain secondary to endometriosis. Over the past 8 years, she has been treated with multiple 6-month courses of gonadotropin-releasing hormone (GnRH) agonist for recurrent pelvic pain. With each GnRH agonist treatment, she had good pain relief. Within 3–4 months, however, her pain had returned. Laparoscopy 1 year ago showed stage II pelvic endometriosis. Dual-energy X-ray absorptiometry indicates a T-score of −2.6 at the spine and −2.1 at the hip. She desires conservation of her reproductive function. With respect to her bone health, the most appropriate medical management of this patient is

(A) alendronate sodium (Fosamax)
(B) salmon calcitonin (Miacalcin)
(C) raloxifene hydrochloride (Evista)
(D) human parathyroid hormone 1-34 (Forteo)
(E) oral contraceptives

66

A 70-year-old woman who has been taking combination hormone therapy (HT) for 15 years decides to discontinue therapy after hearing the results of the Women's Health Initiative study. Her baseline bone mineral density (BMD) showed T-scores of −2 in the lumbar vertebrae and −0.8 in her proximal femur. Dual-energy X-ray absorptiometry (DXA) 2 years ago showed improved T-scores for both the lumbar vertebrae and proximal femur. In discussing expectations for maintaining bone health and preventing fractures in this patient, you tell her that following discontinuation of therapy she will experience the most rapid bone loss in

(A) year 1
(B) year 3
(C) year 5
(D) year 10

67

An 18-year-old woman with acute myelogenous leukemia is scheduled to undergo high-dose chemotherapy and total body irradiation for a bone marrow transplant in 5 days. Her hematologist requests advice regarding the best approach to conserve ovarian function and to reduce the likelihood of vaginal bleeding during the anticipated chemotherapy-induced pancytopenia. The patient has regular menstrual cycles, and her last menstrual period began 6 days ago. She is not using contraceptives. The most appropriate treatment regimen for this patient is

(A) gonadotropin-releasing hormone (GnRH) agonist
(B) depot medroxyprogesterone acetate
(C) combination oral contraceptives
(D) gonadotropin-releasing hormone antagonist
(E) transposition of the ovaries

68

A 25-year-old woman, gravida 3, para 0, with history of polycystic ovary syndrome, comes in for evaluation of recurrent miscarriages. The patient reports a history of irregular menstrual cycles ranging in length from 35 to 90 days. She undergoes hysterosalpingography (HSG) on day 8 of her cycle to evaluate the uterine cavity after 3 days of light flow. After injection of dye, an intrauterine filling defect is noted as shown (Fig. 68-1). A pregnancy test result is positive. The most important complication to discuss with the patient is

(A) spontaneous abortion
(B) fetal anomalies from radiation
(C) pelvic infection
(D) hemorrhage
(E) intrauterine adhesions

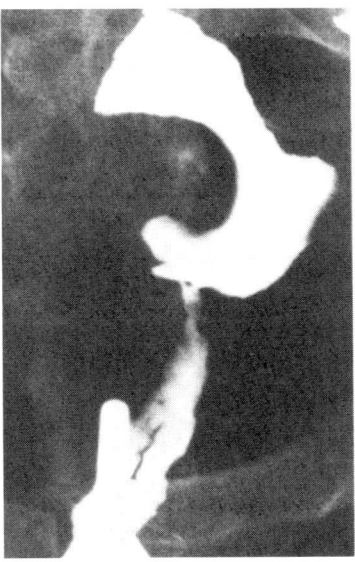

FIG. 68-1. (Justesen P, Rasmussen F, Anderson PE. Inadvertently performed hysterosalpingography during early pregnancy. Acta Radiol Diagn [Stockh] 1986;27:712.)

69

A 25-year-old man with azoospermia receives a diagnosis of Klinefelter's syndrome and is found to have immature spermatozoa on testicular biopsy. In vitro fertilization (IVF) with intracytoplasmic sperm injection (ICSI) is performed, and his wife becomes pregnant. A 16-week amniocentesis is most likely to find a fetus with which one of the following karyotypes?

(A) 47,XXY
(B) 45,X
(C) Normal karyotype
(D) 47,XYY
(E) Trisomy 21

70

A 27-year-old woman presents with a 5-month history of daily headaches, irregular vaginal bleeding, and pelvic pain. She had been taking low-dose combination oral contraceptives for 3 years and stopped them 6 months ago. Vaginal ultrasonography reveals bilateral multicystic ovaries, with the right ovary measuring 69 mm × 43 mm (Fig. 70-1) and the left ovary measuring 56 mm × 51 mm. She has a basal serum follicle-stimulating hormone (FSH) level of 10 mIU/mL, prolactin level of 8 ng/mL, and thyroid-stimulating hormone (TSH) level of 1.6 µU/mL. Her serum estradiol level is 840 pg/mL. The next step in the management of this patient is

(A) ultrasound-guided aspiration of the cysts
(B) surgical excision of the cysts
(C) magnetic resonance imaging (MRI) of the sella turcica
(D) thyrotropin-releasing hormone (TRH) stimulation test
(E) administration of combination oral contraceptives

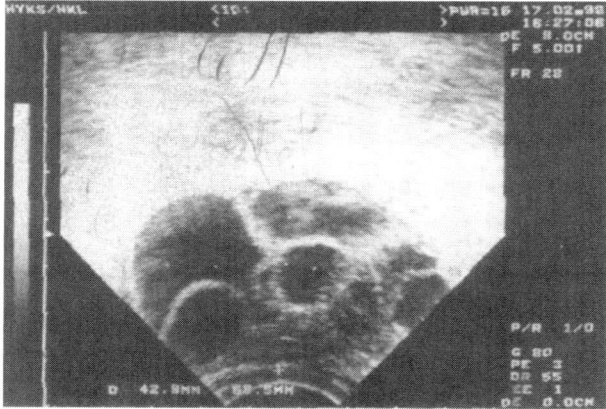

FIG. 70-1. (Välimäki MJ, Tiitinen A, Alfthan H, Paetau A, Poranen A, Sane T, et al. Ovarian hyperstimulation caused by gonadotroph adenoma secreting follicle-stimulating hormone in 28-year-old woman. J Clin Endocrinol Metab 1999;84:4205.)

71

A 25-year-old nulligravid woman presents with lethargy, constipation, cold intolerance, and breast discharge. On physical examination, her pulse rate is 55 beats per minute, and she has spontaneous bilateral galactorrhea. Her prolactin level is 67 ng/mL, and she has a thyroid-stimulating hormone (TSH) level of 15 µU/mL. The hormone responsible for prolactin elevations and galactorrhea in this patient is

(A) insulinlike growth factor-I
(B) thyrotropin-releasing hormone (TRH)
(C) free thyroxine (T_4)
(D) TSH
(E) vasopressin

Reproductive Endocrinology and Infertility

72

A 44-year-old Chinese-American woman is considering using an oocyte donor because of her age. The preferable age of the donor is

(A) 17 years
(B) 20 years
(C) 26 years
(D) 35 years
(E) 38 years

73

A 28-year-old woman, gravida 1, para 1, gave birth 1 year ago after conceiving in her fifth cycle of clomiphene citrate (Clomid, Serophene). She currently is breastfeeding. She does not have a family history of ovarian cancer but remains concerned about an increased risk of ovarian cancer because of her use of clomiphene. The best next step is annual

(A) serum CA 125 level testing
(B) pelvic examination
(C) transvaginal ultrasonography
(D) pulsed Doppler study of the ovaries

74

A 28-year-old woman whose spouse has long-term diabetes mellitus wishes to undergo donor sperm insemination because of male factor infertility. The couple requested the use of a known sperm donor. The spouse's medical history is negative except for smoking, and he has fathered 2 children in the past. The couple has requested processing of fresh sperm for insemination rather than freezing sperm to increase the chance for pregnancy and overall success. The most commonly recommended test for screening candidates for donor insemination is

(A) genetic testing for inheritable disease
(B) screening for sexually transmitted diseases (STDs)
(C) psychologic testing
(D) urine drug screen

75

A 20-month-old child is referred for evaluation of premature breast development. Physical examination demonstrates Tanner stage II–III breast development (Fig. 75-1), absent pubic hair, and prepubertal genitalia. She is in the 65th percentile for height and weight measurements. The most appropriate next step in management is

(A) bone age imaging of the hand and wrist
(B) observation and follow-up in 6 months
(C) gonadotropin-releasing hormone (GnRH) challenge test
(D) magnetic resonance imaging (MRI) of the head

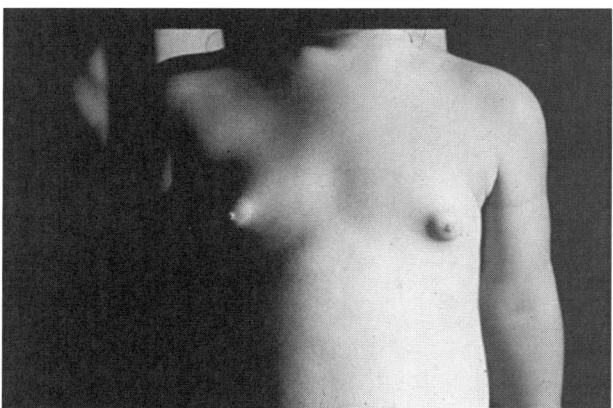

FIG 75-1.

76

A 29-year-old pregnant woman, 5 weeks from her last menstrual period, documented on her calendar, presents with sharp abdominal pain. She undergoes a left ovarian cystectomy for a bleeding corpus luteum. The woman begins progesterone therapy immediately after the laparoscopy. To reduce the likelihood of a spontaneous abortion, progesterone supplementation should be continued through which week of gestation?

(A) 6
(B) 10
(C) 14
(D) 18
(E) 22

77

An 18-year-old woman requests information about the creation of a functional vagina. An ultrasonogram has documented absence of a uterus, cervix, and vagina. Physical examination reveals mature Tanner stage V breast and pubic hair development and a blind vagina with 3 cm depth. The least invasive approach that has the greatest likelihood for creating a functional vagina for this patient is

(A) use of a split thickness skin graft around a vaginal mold in the potential space
(B) coitus every other day
(C) laparoscopic placement of a vaginal expander
(D) use of a firm dilator by the patient over several months

78

A 33-year-old woman comes in for evaluation of primary infertility. She is in good health with normal menstrual cycles. The initial evaluation reveals that follicle-stimulating hormone and luteinizing hormone concentrations are normal. Her serum prolactin level is 31 ng/mL. Her thyroid-stimulating hormone (TSH) level is 4 µU/mL and free thyroxine (T_4) level is 1.1 ng/dL. The most appropriate next diagnostic test for this patient is

(A) triiodothyronine (T_3) concentration
(B) repeat TSH concentration
(C) thyrotropin-releasing hormone (TRH) stimulation test
(D) pituitary magnetic resonance imaging (MRI)
(E) thyroid ultrasonography

79

A 48-year-old Asian woman, gravida 2, para 2, comes in for her annual examination. Over the past 2 years, her menstrual cycles have decreased from every 28–30 days to every 21–23 days. A decade ago, Hashimoto's thyroiditis was diagnosed, and her thyroid gland was ablated by radioactive iodine. Since then, she has used levothyroxine sodium (Synthroid), and her only symptom has been low back pain. On physical examination, her height has decreased by 0.05 m (2 in.) to 1.6 m (5 ft 2 in.), her weight is 56.7 kg (125 lb), blood pressure level is 122/74 mm Hg, and pulse rate is 88 beats per minute. She appears to be clinically euthyroid, and the remainder of her physical examination is unremarkable. Laboratory studies show a thyroid-stimulating hormone (TSH) level of 0.04 µU/mL and total thyroxine (T_4) level of 14 µg/dL. In addition to the Pap test and mammography, the most appropriate step in her management would be

(A) day 3 follicle-stimulating hormone (FSH) level test
(B) estradiol level test
(C) dual-energy X-ray (DXA) scan
(D) thyroid antibodies screen

80

A 45-year-old woman nonsmoker presents with menorrhagia over the past 6 menstrual cycles; however, last month she skipped a cycle. A pregnancy test result is negative, and endometrial biopsy shows a proliferative endometrium. The patient also has occasional hot flushes, night sweats, and irritability. She requests hormonal intervention to manage her hot flushes and control her bleeding. Of the following therapies, the most appropriate method to manage the patient's signs and symptoms is

(A) combined hormone therapy
(B) sequential hormone therapy
(C) low-dose combination oral contraceptives
(D) monthly 10-day course of medroxyprogesterone acetate
(E) transdermal estradiol patch

81

A healthy 20-year-old woman has a 2-year history of dysmenorrhea with pain that is moderately severe the first 3 days of her 5-day menses. Ibuprofen provides some relief. Her menstrual cycles are regular but with heavy flow. Pelvic ultrasonography is negative. She would like to attempt pregnancy in 6 months but requests treatment to decrease the number of bleeding days, relieve pain during menses, and provide reliable contraception with few side effects. The best therapy for her is

(A) cyclic oral contraceptives
(B) continuous oral contraceptives
(C) gonadotropin-releasing hormone (GnRH) agonist
(D) depot medroxyprogesterone acetate
(E) progestin-only pill

82

A 28-year-old woman, gravida 2, comes in for evaluation of oligomenorrhea. She had a normal uncomplicated vaginal delivery 10 months ago and continues to bottle-feed her infant. Her laboratory results include a serum human chorionic gonadotropin (hCG) level of 48 mIU/mL and normal thyroid-stimulating hormone and prolactin levels. Repeat hCG tests 3 and 10 days later show levels of 52 mIU/mL and 49 mIU/mL, respectively. Urine pregnancy test results remain negative. The most likely diagnosis is

(A) hydatidiform mole
(B) choriocarcinoma
(C) "phantom" hCG
(D) ectopic gestation
(E) intrauterine gestation

83

In counseling patients on the use of donor oocytes, it is important to inform them of a substantially increased risk of maternal death during pregnancy if their ovarian failure is associated with

(A) premature menopause at age 35 years
(B) natural menopause at age 50 years
(C) bilateral oophorectomy for stage IV endometriosis
(D) Turner's syndrome
(E) fragile X gene premutation

84

A 37-year-old woman, gravida 1, para 1, presents with amenorrhea and galactorrhea of 2 years' duration. She reports that she has experienced increasingly severe frontal headaches over this period. Initial laboratory studies reveal serum follicle-stimulating hormone (FSH) level of 21 mIU/mL, prolactin level of 46 ng/mL, and thyroid-stimulating hormone (TSH) level of 2.6 µU/mL. The best next step in the management is

(A) pituitary function testing
(B) formal visual field testing
(C) pelvic ultrasonography
(D) magnetic resonance imaging (MRI) of the sella turcica
(E) treatment with a dopamine agonist

85

A sedentary 32-year-old woman with body mass index of 28 kg/m^2 consumes daily 1 glass of wine and 3 cups of coffee; she smokes 1 pack of cigarettes per day. She requests your advice regarding the lifestyle modification that would most improve her success with in vitro fertilization (IVF). The change in lifestyle that would likely lead to the highest success rate in her use of IVF would be to

(A) initiate an exercise program
(B) reduce caffeine intake
(C) initiate a low-fat diet
(D) stop smoking
(E) reduce alcohol consumption

86

A 25-year-old woman presents with marked weakness and fatigue. Her last pregnancy 8 months ago was complicated by a postpartum hemorrhage with a blood loss of 2,000 mL, and she required a transfusion of 4 units of blood. She also experienced profound hypotension as a result of the blood loss. She has amenorrhea despite the discontinuation of oral contraceptives 3 months ago. In this clinical scenario, the hormone that is most likely preserved is

(A) prolactin
(B) follicle-stimulating hormone (FSH)
(C) vasopressin
(D) adrenocorticotropic hormone (ACTH)
(E) thyroid-stimulating hormone (TSH)

87

In the anovulatory woman, the principal site of action for clomiphene citrate (Clomid, Serophene) is the

(A) uterus
(B) ovary
(C) anterior pituitary gland
(D) posterior pituitary gland
(E) hypothalamus

88

A 23-year-old woman, gravida 1, para 1, with type 1 diabetes mellitus, presents with fatigue, palpitations, and dizziness at 3 months postpartum. On examination, she has a resting pulse rate of 90 beats per minute and a slightly enlarged tender thyroid gland. Laboratory studies reveal a serum thyroid-stimulating hormone (TSH) level less than 0.1 µU/mL and a free thyroxine level of 2.6 ng/dL. The most likely explanation for this woman's symptoms is

(A) depression
(B) multinodular goiter
(C) thyroiditis
(D) Graves' disease
(E) thyroid papillary carcinoma

Reproductive Endocrinology and Infertility

89

A 34-year-old woman had a spontaneous vaginal delivery 5 months ago and now requests a reliable method of contraception as soon as possible. Her pregnancy was complicated by severe preeclampsia. She is currently bottle-feeding her infant. Physical examination is unremarkable except for a blood pressure reading of 150/100 mm Hg. She is not compliant in taking her antihypertensive medications. The method of long-term reversible contraception that would be most cost-effective for this patient is

(A) combined oral contraceptives
(B) transdermal patch
(C) vaginal ring
(D) intrauterine device (IUD)
(E) progestin-only pill

90

A 44-year-old woman, who smokes 1 pack of 20 cigarettes per day, has a history of heavy menstrual periods. Her menstrual periods are regular, last 8 days, and are heavy for 5 days with intermittent passage of small clots. Evaluation to date has included saline infusion ultrasonography, which shows slightly enlarged anterior–posterior diameter and a normal endometrial cavity. Pap test and cervical culture results are negative. Endometrial biopsy showed secretory endometrium. She has no immediate interest in fertility. The most appropriate treatment for this patient is

(A) cyclic oral contraceptives (OCs)
(B) leuprolide acetate (Lupron) for 3–6 months
(C) depot medroxyprogesterone acetate
(D) levonorgestrel intrauterine system

91

A 33-year-old woman comes to the emergency department with intermittent severe cramping abdominal pain with associated nausea 72 hours after an operative laparoscopy for removal of an 8 cm × 8 cm right ovarian dermoid cyst. She is afebrile, and her abdomen is distended and tender precluding a satisfactory examination. The best way to evaluate her for bowel injury is

(A) colonoscopy
(B) computerized axial tomography (CAT) scan of the abdomen
(C) flat plate and upright abdominal X-ray
(D) upper gastrointestinal series with small bowel follow-through

92

A 29-year-old woman, gravida 1, para 1, gave birth 18 months ago and breastfed her infant for 16 months. For the past 8 weeks, she has attempted to wean the infant, but her breasts continue to engorge and leak. She mentions that she has not slept well during breastfeeding and has "pressure-type" headaches that are relieved with ibuprofen. She has had amenorrhea since the delivery. Physical examination is significant for bilateral galactorrhea, decreased rugation of the vaginal mucosa, and normal visual fields by confrontation. Laboratory studies indicate a prolactin level of 240 ng/mL, thyroid-stimulating hormone (TSH) level of 2.3 µU/mL, follicle-stimulating hormone (FSH) level of 2.4 mIU/mL, thyroxine (T_4) level of 9.2 µg/dL, and growth hormone (GH) level of less than 1 ng/mL. A computed tomography (CT) scan of the pituitary with contrast reveals a 19-mm lesion in the left anterior pituitary gland without distortion of the optic chiasm. The most appropriate next step in the management of this patient is

(A) observation
(B) bromocriptine mesylate (Parlodel)
(C) oral contraceptives
(D) pituitary irradiation
(E) transsphenoidal hypophysectomy

93

A 28-year-old nulligravid woman comes in for evaluation of an enlarged uterus and inability to conceive. She has a normal bleeding pattern and has documented that she is ovulatory by ovulation kits. Her husband has a normal semen analysis. A recent ultrasound examination documented the presence of 3 uterine leiomyomata. Her primary care physician told her that she would require further evaluation to determine if the fibroids will interfere with her ability to conceive. The next step in evaluation is

(A) sonohysterography
(B) laparoscopy
(C) hysteroscopy
(D) hysterosalpingography (HSG)

94

A 38-year-old woman is in her first trimester of pregnancy after her first in vitro fertilization cycle for unexplained infertility. She has been treated for Hashimoto's thyroiditis for 3 years. Her thyroid-stimulating hormone (TSH) levels have varied between 0.75 µU/mL and 1.5 µU/mL during the past 2 years with a maintenance dose of 50 µg of levothyroxine. A repeat TSH level obtained at the 6-week visit is 3.75 µU/mL. The most appropriate management plan for this patient is to

(A) maintain the current dosage of levothyroxine through pregnancy and repeat TSH test after delivery
(B) increase the levothyroxine dosage and repeat the TSH test in 6 weeks
(C) maintain the current dosage of levothyroxine and repeat the TSH test in the mid-second trimester
(D) decrease the levothyroxine dosage and repeat the TSH test in 6 weeks
(E) discontinue thyroid therapy and repeat the TSH test in the mid-second trimester

95

A healthy 29-year-old woman, 6 weeks past her last menstrual period, has been treated for medical termination of pregnancy. On her first treatment visit, she received mifepristone (Mifeprex), and 2 days later she received misoprostol. Her bleeding had been heavy for 5 days, and now, 10 days after she received mifepristone, she reports that she continues to experience bleeding at a rate similar to a normal menstrual period, with no clotting blood but with the need to change pads every 4 hours. Office ultrasonography reveals no sac present but a 1.2-cm hyperechoic area consistent with tissue and blood. Her hematocrit concentration is 37%, her pulse rate is 90 beats per minute, and she shows no orthostatic changes with standing. The next step in management is

(A) reassurance
(B) dilation and curettage
(C) repeat misoprostol
(D) measurement of human chorionic gonadotropin (hCG) level

96

A newborn term infant is evaluated for ambiguous genitalia. A brief physical examination reveals no palpable mass in the labioscrotal folds. The infant has a phallic structure and evidence of internal müllerian structures. Based on these findings the most likely diagnosis is

(A) mixed gonadal dysgenesis
(B) congenital adrenal hyperplasia (CAH)
(C) androgen insensitivity
(D) male pseudohermaphroditism

97

A 32-year-old woman, gravida 1, para 1, wants a second opinion for secondary infertility. She conceived easily 3 years ago and had a normal term vaginal delivery. After breastfeeding for 14 months, she did not resume regular menstrual cycles. Her menstrual cycles are now at 21–42-day intervals. She reports heavy menses or vaginal spotting and occasional hot flushes. Laboratory test results show a serum prolactin level of 14 ng/mL, thyroid-stimulating hormone (TSH) level of 2.1 µU/mL, day 3 follicle-stimulating hormone (FSH) level of 32 mIU/mL, and estradiol level of 32 pg/mL. After 5 days of clomiphene citrate (Clomid, Serophene) at a dose of 100 mg per day (clomiphene challenge test), she has a day 10 FSH level of 41 mIU/mL and an estradiol level of 54 pg/mL. Her mother had natural menopause at age 45 years, and her 39-year-old sister continues to menstruate. The approach that would provide the best chance for this patient to achieve pregnancy would be

(A) human menopausal gonadotropin (hMG)
(B) clomiphene citrate
(C) donor oocytes with assisted reproductive technology (ART)
(D) gonadotropin-releasing hormone (GnRH) agonist flare with hMG
(E) clomiphene citrate with hMG

98

A 22-year-old nulligravid woman presents with a history of severe dysmenorrhea for the past 6 months. On physical examination, you find a markedly retroverted, fixed uterus with significant nodularity on the uterosacral ligaments and bilateral adnexal fullness. You perform operative laparoscopy for extensive endometriosis with severe peritoneal adhesions, complete obliteration of the cul-de-sac, and bilateral endometriomas. The best method to prevent postoperative adhesions in this patient is

(A) intraperitoneal dexamethasone
(B) lactated Ringer's solution with heparin
(C) oxidized regenerated cellulose (Interceed)
(D) oral indomethacin (Indocin)
(E) 32% dextran 70 (Hyskon)

99

A 42-year-old woman, gravida 2, para 2, with congestive heart failure and iron deficiency anemia has severe menorrhagia from a 3 cm submucosal myoma. A hysteroscopic resection and endometrial ablation is scheduled. The optimal intraoperative management would involve which type of electrosurgical resectoscope and distention medium?

	Electrosurgical resectoscope	Distention medium
(A)	bipolar	normal saline
(B)	bipolar	1.5% glycine
(C)	monopolar	normal saline
(D)	monopolar	1.5% glycine
(E)	monopolar	3% sorbitol

100

A 32-year-old man with normal gonadotropin levels has severe oligospermia on multiple semen analyses. He and his wife request information about intracytoplasmic sperm injection. You counsel the couple that with the following condition 100% of male children will be affected.

(A) Y chromosome microdeletion
(B) Mutation in the cystic fibrosis transmembrane conductance regulator gene
(C) Premature testicular failure
(D) Congenital bilateral absence of the vas deferens

101

A 25-year-old nulligravid woman seeks nonsurgical management of her pelvic pain. She describes the pain as persistent lower abdominal pain that increases in severity immediately preceding and following menses. She has been treated in the past with antibiotics, cyclic oral contraceptives, and nonsteroidal antiinflammatory drugs (NSAIDs); however, none has resolved her pain. You suspect she has endometriosis, and you have chosen not to perform laparoscopy. Based on your clinical suspicion of endometriosis and her desire to avoid surgery, the best medication to prescribe to relieve her pelvic pain is

(A) gonadotropin-releasing hormone (GnRH) agonist
(B) danazol (Danocrine)
(C) continuous oral contraceptives
(D) depot medroxyprogesterone acetate

102

A 55-year-old postmenopausal woman has a lateral chest X-ray that shows 2 prior vertebral crush fractures. She is 1.68 m (5 ft 6 in.) tall, weighs 41 kg (110 lb), and smokes 8 cigarettes per day. A dual-energy X-ray absorptiometry scan of her femur shows a bone mineral density (BMD) of 0.723 mg/cm^2 (T score -1.3, Z score -0.4) (Fig. 102-1; see color plate). Her mother died at age 70 years, 3 months after a hip fracture. Given this patient's history, her greatest risk factor for a future fracture is

(A) low bone mass
(B) previous vertebral fractures
(C) smoking history
(D) weight
(E) family history

103

A 16-year-old adolescent with no history of sexual activity is being evaluated for primary amenorrhea. On physical examination, she has Tanner stage IV breast development, Tanner stage II pubic hair, a 2 cm vaginal pouch, no visible cervix, and no palpable uterus or ovaries. Laboratory analysis reveals a follicle-stimulating hormone level of 8.3 mIU/mL, testosterone level of 811 ng/dL, and a 46,XY karyotype. The next step in management for this patient is

(A) breast augmentation
(B) estrogen therapy
(C) vaginoplasty
(D) psychologic counseling

104

An infertile couple is contemplating in vitro fertilization (IVF) after previous failed therapies. They have heard about the use of intracytoplasmic sperm injection (ICSI) in assisted reproductive technology (ART) but do not know if it is indicated in their case. The most appropriate indication for use of ICSI during IVF is

(A) sperm count of 5 million per mL
(B) sperm motility of 50%
(C) semen volume of 0.5 cc
(D) strict morphology of 8% normal sperm

105

A 25-year-old woman requests depot medroxyprogesterone acetate contraception. She is most interested in the convenience of this method because she lives close to a health center, which could provide the injections. She is concerned about rumors she has heard about bleeding problems associated with depot medroxyprogesterone acetate. The medical intervention that is likely to enhance continued use of this method is

(A) intermittent estrogen
(B) monthly depot medroxyprogesterone acetate injections
(C) ibuprofen
(D) pretreatment counseling
(E) raloxifene

106

A 24-year-old woman with a longstanding history of oligomenorrhea, facial hirsutism, and acanthosis nigricans has recently received a diagnosis of insulin-resistant polycystic ovary syndrome (PCOS). Her oral glucose tolerance test (OGTT) revealed a glucose level of 156 mg/dL at 2 hours. The diagnosis was confirmed by a fasting plasma glucose level of 115 mg/dL and a serum insulin level of 30 µU/mL. The patient is confused about her diagnosis and wants to know why she is not considered to have diabetes at this point. You inform the patient that the criterion for a diagnosis of diabetes mellitus is

(A) a 2-hour plasma glucose level of at least 150 mg/dL
(B) a random plasma glucose level greater than or equal to 126 mg/dL
(C) an elevated fasting glucose to insulin ratio
(D) a fasting plasma glucose level greater than or equal to 126 mg/dL
(E) an elevated 2-hour insulin level

107

A 28-year-old nulligravid woman undergoes laparoscopy for persistent infertility and pelvic pain. Two years ago she had a bilateral neosalpingostomy. Based on the intraoperative findings (Figs. 107-1 and 107-2; see color plates), you perform a bilateral salpingectomy in preparation for future in vitro fertilization (IVF). The effect that the presence of hydrosalpinges during IVF would have is to

(A) significantly increase the risk of pelvic infection after oocyte retrieval
(B) decrease oocyte recruitment
(C) decrease the rate of embryo implantation
(D) retard in vitro embryonic cleavage rates

108

A 17-year-old adolescent requests advice on different contraceptive methods. She currently uses an oral contraceptive (OC) with 20 µg ethinyl estradiol. She is unhappy with her current method because of a 4.5 kg (10 lb) weight gain. She desires reliable contraception. The most appropriate recommendation for contraception in this patient is to

(A) continue use of current OC and begin counseling about diet and exercise
(B) change to depot medroxyprogesterone acetate
(C) change to a progestin-releasing intrauterine device (IUD)
(D) change to a progestin-only OC
(E) change to partner's use of latex condoms

109

A 15-year-old adolescent presents with primary amenorrhea. There is no family history for developmental anomalies or delayed puberty. On physical examination, she is 1.73 m (5 ft 8 in.) tall, her arm span is 1.78 m (5 ft 10 in.), and she weighs 56.9 kg (127 lb). Her breasts are at Tanner stage I development, there is fine axillary hair, she has Tanner stage II pubic hair and a virginal introitus with small cervix, and the uterus is not palpable. Laboratory studies show normal thyroid-stimulating hormone and prolactin levels while follicle-stimulating hormone (FSH) and estradiol levels are low. She appears to have a normal sense of smell. The best next step in management is to obtain

(A) a pituitary stimulation test
(B) insulinlike growth factor (IGF)-1 level
(C) growth hormone (GH) level
(D) an X-ray of her wrist
(E) karyotype

110

A 23-year-old nulligravid student requests a new contraceptive method. She wants something that has more predictable bleeding than an oral contraceptive because she is sometimes troubled by breakthrough bleeding. Her schedule is hectic, and she occasionally forgets to take her oral contraceptive but cannot always explain why she has spotting or delayed menses. She has contact dermatitis and a prior history of positive gonorrhea and chlamydia cultures. The contraceptive that you recommend is

(A) copper intrauterine device (IUD)
(B) vaginal contraceptive ring (NuvaRing)
(C) transdermal contraceptive patch (Ortho Evra)
(D) levonorgestrel intrauterine system

111

A 28-year-old woman presents with a history of infrequent menstrual periods. Her last period was 4 months ago. Physical examination reveals a body mass index (BMI) of 26 kg/m^2 and galactorrhea bilaterally. Laboratory results show a negative β-hCG level, a normal thyroid-stimulating hormone (TSH) level, a dehydroepiandrosterone sulfate (DHEAS) level of 180 μg/dL, and a fasting prolactin level of 75 ng/mL. A repeat prolactin test confirms the prior elevated level. A magnetic resonance imaging (MRI) study of her pituitary gland is normal. The most appropriate next step in management is

(A) clomiphene citrate (Clomid, Serophene)
(B) dexamethasone (Decadron)
(C) weight reduction
(D) metformin (Glucophage)
(E) bromocriptine mesylate (Parlodel)

112

A couple with tubal factor infertility undergoes a treatment cycle with in vitro fertilization and transfer of one embryo on day 5 at the blastocyst stage. The transfer results in a twin pregnancy. The most likely explanation for this pregnancy outcome is

(A) embryology laboratory error
(B) spontaneous conception
(C) dizygotic twinning
(D) monozygotic twinning

113

A 29-year-old woman with type 1 diabetes mellitus has developed secondary amenorrhea as a result of premature ovarian failure. She is considering using an oocyte donor for in vitro fertilization. The donor who is most suitable for this patient is a

(A) 17-year-old nulligravid sister with irregular menses
(B) 24-year-old nulligravid half-sister with irregular menses
(C) 27-year-old, gravida 1, para 1, unrelated woman with regular menses
(D) 22-year-old nulligravid unrelated woman with regular menses after chemotherapy
(E) 33-year-old, gravida 3, para 3, unrelated woman with regular menses after tubal ligation

114

A 28-year-old woman with history of recurrent abortion undergoes a diagnostic laparoscopy and subsequent operative hysteroscopy to incise a small uterine septum that occupies less than 50% of the uterine cavity. The procedure is uncomplicated, and there is no evidence of uterine perforation or damage to the surrounding endometrium. The most important next step in the clinical management of this patient in the postoperative period is

(A) an intrauterine device (IUD)
(B) oral estrogen for 2 weeks postoperatively
(C) oral contraceptives
(D) hysterosalpingography (HSG)

115

A 43-year-old nulligravid woman requests a second opinion regarding treatment for osteoporosis. Osteoporosis has been diagnosed by dual-energy X-ray absorptiometry (DXA), and she has begun to take alendronate at her physician's recommendation. She takes calcium supplements, 1,500 mg per day, with vitamin D, 400 IU per day. She runs approximately 16 km (10 mile) per week and bikes 80.5 km (50 mile) every weekend. On physical examination, she is 1.7 m (5 ft 8 in.) tall, she weighs 57.2 kg (126 lb), her blood pressure level is 96/60 mm Hg, and pulse rate is 64 beats per minute. The remainder of her examination is unremarkable. Laboratory studies, including thyroid-stimulating hormone, estradiol, follicle-stimulating hormone, and serum prolactin levels, are normal. In addition, her electrolyte, human parathyroid hormone, serum calcium, and 24-hour urinary free calcium levels obtained while she is off calcium supplementation also are normal. To monitor her response to alendronate, the most appropriate next step in her management is

(A) repeat DXA scan
(B) urinary N-telopeptide level
(C) lateral X-ray of spine
(D) urinary calcium excretion rate
(E) ultrasonography of calcaneus

116

A 38-year-old woman, gravida 3, para 3, in a new relationship with a 32-year-old man, comes in for a fertility evaluation after a failed tubal ligation reversal that was done 18 months ago. The patient had a day 3 follicle-stimulating hormone (FSH) level of 5 mIU/mL. She has a normal hysterosalpingogram. Her partner has a semen analysis with normal parameters. The patient is interested in the in vitro fertilization (IVF) success rate in her particular case with a history of tubal factor infertility. The factor most likely to predict IVF success is

(A) age of patient
(B) failed tubal anastomosis
(C) age of spouse
(D) FSH level

117

A 16-year-old adolescent comes in for evaluation of primary amenorrhea and lack of breast development. She denies being sexually active and has no history of vaginal bleeding. Her height is 134.6 cm (53 in.). She has Tanner stage I breast development and Tanner stage I pubic hair (Appendix D). She has a normal vaginal length, visible cervix, small palpable uterus, and no palpable ovaries. Initial laboratory evaluation reveals a negative serum pregnancy test result and normal levels of prolactin and thyroid-stimulating hormone (TSH). The serum measurement that would provide the most information to make the diagnosis is

(A) follicle-stimulating hormone (FSH)
(B) estradiol
(C) testosterone
(D) dehydroepiandrosterone sulfate (DHEAS)
(E) 17-hydroxyprogesterone

118

A 27-year-old woman, gravida 4, para 0, is referred to you with a history of recurrent first-trimester pregnancy loss and a normal hysterosalpingogram. Her records from 2 months ago indicate normal endocrine parameters, positive anticardiolipin immunoglobulin (Ig) G, and normal parental karyotypes. A repeat anticardiolipin IgG is elevated. The most effective therapy is

(A) clomiphene citrate (Clomid, Serophene)
(B) progesterone
(C) heparin and low-dose aspirin
(D) initiation of intravenous immune globulin

119

A 29-year-old woman comes in for intrauterine insemination (IUI) with her husband's washed semen sample. The couple has unexplained infertility, and they have just completed their fourth IUI with the co-administration of clomiphene citrate (Clomid, Serophene). Before her initial procedure, her cervical cultures were negative for gonorrhea and chlamydia. The most common side effect associated with an IUI is

(A) acute salpingitis
(B) anaphylactoid reaction to components in the media used to prepare the semen
(C) formation of antisperm antibodies
(D) uterine contractions
(E) transmission of viruses into the uterine cavity

120

A 23-year-old nulligravid woman recently received a diagnosis of midline pelvic pain secondary to endometriosis. A laparoscopy performed 8 months ago demonstrated stage I disease with endometriosis implants localized to the cul-de-sac and bilateral ovarian fossae. Her implants were ablated. Postoperatively, she was managed with continuous oral contraceptives for 4 months, but they were discontinued because of irregular bleeding and recurrent pelvic pain. She was subsequently placed on leuprolide acetate (Lupron) at a dose of 3.75 mg per month. On this new regimen, her pain has improved, but she reports dyspareunia and severe vasomotor symptoms. In addition to prescribing a gonadotropin-releasing hormone (GnRH) agonist, the most appropriate daily management will be

(A) norethindrone acetate, 10 mg
(B) combination oral contraceptives
(C) 0.625 mg of conjugated estrogens
(D) 0.625 mg of conjugated estrogens and 5 mg of norethindrone acetate
(E) 10 mg of medroxyprogesterone acetate

121

A 23-year-old woman comes in for contraception and management of her migraines. She is in a monogamous relationship. She currently takes a β-blocker, which has reduced the number and severity of her migraines. She denies a history of neurologic prodromes associated with her migraines and states that her headaches are worse during her menses. She inquires whether hormonal contraception will further ameliorate her migraines. She does not smoke and does not have a history of sexually transmitted diseases or abnormal Pap test results. Physical examination and vital signs are normal. The most appropriate contraceptive for this patient is

* (A) continuous low-dose monophasic oral contraceptives (OCs)
* (B) triphasic low-dose OCs
* (C) progestin-only OCs
* (D) progestin-containing intrauterine device (IUD)
* (E) copper-containing IUD

122

A 68-year-old woman comes in for her annual examination with no specific symptoms. She is 1.6 m (5 ft 4 in.) tall, weighs 82 kg (181 lb), has a body mass index (BMI) of 31 kg/m², and a waist circumference of 99 cm (39 in.). She has a blood pressure reading of 129/83 mm Hg. She walks 30 minutes per day, 3 times per week. She smoked one half a pack of cigarettes per day until 4 years ago. She takes no medications. Two sisters are overweight and one has taken metformin hydrochloride (Glucophage) for 2 years for type 2 diabetes mellitus. Her mother died from a heart attack at age 69 years. Her fasting laboratory results are as follows: glucose level of 121 mg/dL, total cholesterol level of 230 mg/dL, triglyceride level of 240 mg/dL, high-density lipoprotein (HDL) cholesterol level of 38 mg/dL, and low-density lipoprotein (LDL) cholesterol level of 134 mg/dL. You make a diagnosis of metabolic syndrome and recommend that she make therapeutic lifestyle changes with regard to diet, weight loss, and increased exercise. In addition to an increased risk of type 2 diabetes mellitus, this patient has an increased risk of

* (A) hypertension
* (B) hyperthyroidism
* (C) pancreatic cancer
* (D) hepatic failure
* (E) renal disease

Reproductive Endocrinology and Infertility

123

A 29-year-old woman requests alternatives to oral contraceptives to treat her long-standing abnormal facial hair growth. She has used oral contraceptives for control of acne and facial hair growth for the past 9 years but is not satisfied with the results. You recommend for treatment of her hirsutism

(A) gonadotropin-releasing hormone agonist (Lupron)
(B) flutamide
(C) ketoconazole (Nizoral)
(D) spironolactone

124

A 32-year-old woman underwent bilateral oophorectomy with uterine preservation 5 years ago for severe endometriosis. Since then she has experienced decreased libido. Vasomotor symptoms persist despite an increase in the daily dose of conjugated estrogens and medroxyprogesterone acetate. Results of dual-energy X-ray absorptiometry are consistent with osteoporosis. Secondary causes of osteoporosis have been excluded. Her lipid profile is normal. The medication most likely to manage her symptoms and address her bone mineral density (BMD) is

(A) methyltestosterone
(B) venlafaxine hydrochloride (Effexor)
(C) clonidine (Catapres-TTS)
(D) black cohosh (*Cimicifuga racemosa*) (Remifemin)
(E) yohimbine

125

A 35-year-old woman, gravida 1, para 1, presents with occasional palpitations and fatigue. She is 2 months postpartum after an uncomplicated vaginal delivery. She is breastfeeding exclusively. Her medical history and antenatal history are unremarkable. Vital signs reveal a resting pulse rate of 102 beats per minute and a blood pressure reading of 110/72 mm Hg. The physical examination is normal with the exception of a mildly enlarged thyroid gland. She has a normal complete blood count and free thyroxine (T_4) level of 2.1 ng/dL. Her thyroid-stimulating hormone (TSH) level is 0.15 µU/mL. The most appropriate immediate management for this patient is

(A) levothyroxine
(B) methimazole
(C) radioactive iodine
(D) thyroidectomy
(E) β-blocker

126

The method of hormonal contraception associated with the lowest failure rate at 1 year of use is

(A) combined oral contraceptives
(B) transdermal patch
(C) vaginal ring
(D) levonorgestrel intrauterine system
(E) progestin-only pill

127

A 39-year-old man with a 10-year history of type 1 diabetes mellitus is referred for evaluation of an abnormal semen analysis. He and his wife have a 3-year history of infertility. The referring physician has completed an infertility workup on the couple. The wife's evaluation and history are unremarkable. The man has had 3 semen analyses in the past year, each after 48–72 hours of abstinence, which demonstrated a volume of 0.1–0.3 mL, sperm concentration of 1–2 million per mL, normal motility, and normal morphology. He denies a history of dysuria, urethral discharge, radiation, or testicular trauma. You explain to the couple that the next step in his evaluation is

(A) repeat semen analysis after a longer period of abstinence
(B) collect a postejaculate urine sample
(C) testicular ultrasonography
(D) testicular biopsy
(E) gonadotropin-releasing hormone (GnRH) stimulation test

128

A 69-year-old woman used diethylstilbestrol (DES) during 2 pregnancies. She has never smoked cigarettes or consumed alcohol. Based on current information, compared with women of a similar age, this patient is at increased risk for cancer of the

(A) endometrium
(B) cervix
(C) lung
(D) breast
(E) colon

129

A couple is referred to your office for evaluation of primary infertility. The 34-year-old woman has a normal history, workup, and examination. The 36-year-old man has a history of testicular cancer and recently completed alkylating chemotherapy. His semen analysis demonstrates a volume of 3.2 mL, sperm concentration of 3.7 million sperm per mL, sperm motility of 25%, and normal sperm morphology of 35%. The cell type most affected by the chemotherapy in this patient is the

(A) spermatogonium
(B) primary spermatocyte
(C) secondary spermatocyte
(D) spermatid
(E) spermatozoa

130

A 59-year-old woman with severe osteoarthritis and recent multiple lumbar vertebral fractures comes in for a bone mineral density (BMD) study. The patient is a smoker, and her mother has severe osteoporosis. Four years ago, a dual-energy X-ray absorptiometry (DXA) scan showed a spine T-score of -2. She has taken a bisphosphonate for 4 years. Based on her history, the best next step in evaluation is a

(A) ultrasonography of the calcaneus
(B) lateral spine X-ray
(C) peripheral DXA of the wrist
(D) central DXA of the spine
(E) quantitative computed tomography scan

131

A 30-year-old woman with primary infertility of 1-year duration undergoes hysterosalpingography (HSG), which reveals a normal uterine cavity but bilateral proximal tubal occlusion at the uterotubal junction. The patient has no history of previous abdominal surgery, sexually transmitted diseases, pelvic pain, or dysmenorrhea. She would prefer not to undergo surgery or anesthesia at this time. An appropriate next step for examination of the fallopian tubes is

(A) 3-dimensional ultrasonography
(B) repeat HSG
(C) sonohysterography
(D) office hysteroscopy

DIRECTIONS: Each of the questions below consists of lettered headings followed by a list of numbered words or statements. For each numbered word or statement, select the ONE lettered heading that is associated most closely with it and fill in the circle containing the corresponding letter on the answer sheet. Each lettered heading or lettered component may be selected once, more than once, or not at all.

132–135

For each of the following clinical scenarios (132–135), match the most appropriate diagnostic tools (A–D).

(A) Hysterosalpingography (HSG)
(B) Sonohysterography
(C) Hysteroscopy
(D) Transvaginal ultrasonography

132. A 32-year-old woman comes in for follow-up 6 months after a tubal ligation reversal.

133. A 30-year-old woman presents with continuous vaginal bleeding refractory to medical therapy for 4 months. Her pelvic examination in the office is normal.

134. A 25-year-old woman presents with a history of pelvic inflammatory disease and infertility.

135. A 33-year-old woman presents with a positive pregnancy test result and pelvic pain.

136–138

For each postmenopausal woman taking hormone therapy (HT) referred for evaluation of uterine bleeding (136–138), select the most appropriate management (A–D).

(A) Sonohysterography
(B) Endometrial biopsy
(C) Dilation and curettage
(D) Observation

136. A 52-year-old symptomatic woman, gravida 3, para 3, started taking combination HT 6 weeks ago. She has experienced episodic daily spotting for the past 2 weeks, requiring sanitary protection. Her gynecologic medical history is unremarkable.

137. A 37-year old nulliparous woman began taking combination HT after a bilateral oophorectomy 3 years ago for endometriomas. She experienced no bleeding for the first 2 years of HT but has bled for 3–4 days on 4 occasions in the past 8 months.

138. A 62-year-old nulliparous woman has undergone multiple dilation and curettage procedures for uterine polyps before menopause. She has been taking HT for more than 10 years and has had 2 recent 1-day episodes of bleeding.

Reproductive Endocrinology and Infertility

139–141

Match the following clinical scenarios (139–141) with the most appropriate uterine anomaly (A–D).

(A) Unicornuate uterus
(B) Obstructed hemivagina
(C) Rudimentary uterine horn
(D) Uterine septum

139. A 31-year-old woman with history of preterm delivery has an irregular shaped uterus and one fallopian tube seen at cesarean delivery.

140. A 13-year-old adolescent with pelvic pain has irregular menstrual cycles, an absent right kidney, and a right pelvic mass.

141. 25-year-old woman with secondary infertility and recurrent miscarriage has an abnormal hysterosalpingogram and normal uterine fundus noted on laparoscopy.

142–145

For each of the following types of gynecologic surgery (142–145), select the laser (A–D) that has the most appropriate characteristics and safety history.

(A) Carbon-dioxide laser
(B) Argon laser
(C) KTP laser
(D) Neodymium:yttrium-aluminum-garnet (nd:YAG) laser

142. Standard glass lenses (eg, those commonly used in reading glasses) are sufficient to defuse laser energy and prevent eye injury.

143. When used in the noncontact mode, laser energy has a depth of tissue penetration of 3–7 mm.

144. The wavelength of energy produced is highly absorbed by the water within cells and, thus, has minimal tissue penetration.

145. The wavelength of the energy produced is altered during passage through a crystal before traveling to the surgical handpiece.

146–149

Select the most appropriate associated clinical scenario (146–149) based on current understanding of normal physiology of müllerian development (A–D).

(A) Absence of *bcl-2* protein
(B) Failure of bi-directional resorption
(C) Defects in pericentric region of chromosome 8
(D) X-linked laterality sequence

146. A normal female fetus at 18 weeks of gestation with normal uterus and no uterine septum.

147. A 16-year-old adolescent with a blind ending vagina, mild mental retardation, and facial asymmetry.

148. A 26-year-old woman with a single uterus, complete uterine septum, cervical duplication, and complete longitudinal vaginal septum.

149. A 38-year-old woman with uterine septum and hypertelorism has 2 daughters with uterine septa and hypertelorism.

150–151

Select the steroid hormone (150–151) found in the combination oral contraceptive that results in the mechanism of action (A–E).

(A) Increases free testosterone
(B) Increases follicle-stimulating hormone (FSH) secretion
(C) Increases luteinizing hormone (LH) secretion
(D) Inhibits LH secretion
(E) Increases sex hormone-binding globulin

150. Ethinyl estradiol

151. Norethindrone

152–154

For each woman (152–154) who presents with severe vasomotor symptoms, and who has had a recent normal mammogram, a normal lipid profile 2 years previously, and a last menstrual cycle at least 12 months ago, select the most appropriate test for screening before beginning hormone therapy (HT) (A–E).

(A) Dual-energy X-ray absorptiometry (DXA) bone density study
(B) Lipid profile
(C) Fasting glucose and insulin levels
(D) *BRCA1*
(E) Follicle-stimulating hormone (FSH) test

152. A 54-year-old Hispanic woman, gravida 3, para 3, with type 2 diabetes mellitus is mildly obese and smokes 1–2 packs of cigarettes daily.

153. A 48-year-old Caucasian nulliparous woman exercises regularly and has never smoked. Breast cancer was diagnosed in her mother and maternal aunt at age 45 years.

154. A 50-year-old African-American woman, gravida 2, para 2, has a history of asthma and requires periodic steroid treatment.

155–158

For each of the following patients with infertility (155–158), select the most appropriate treatment option to help achieve pregnancy (A–E).

(A) In vitro fertilization (IVF) with intracytoplasmic sperm injection (ICSI)
(B) Bilateral salpingectomy followed by IVF
(C) IVF alone
(D) Bilateral neosalpingostomy
(E) Bilateral tubal reversal

155. A 34-year-old woman has bilateral hydrosalpinges greater than 3 cm confirmed on ultrasonography. Her husband has 44 million sperm per cc on multiple semen analysis.

156. A 35-year-old woman has a history of severe dysmenorrhea, stage III endometriosis, and severe pelvic adhesive disease. Her husband has 66 million sperm per cc.

157. A 29-year-old woman with a history of chlamydial salpingitis, has bilateral proximal tubal occlusion confirmed on hysterosalpingography. Her husband has 2 million sperm per cc.

158. A 27-year-old woman with Hulka clip tubal sterilization is newly married and desires 2 more children. Her husband has 34 million sperm per cc.

159–162

For each patient (159–162) who presents with a history of secondary amenorrhea, negative β-hCG level, and a partial evaluation at referral, select the most appropriate next test (A–G).

(A) Vaginal smear
(B) Karyotype
(C) Echocardiography
(D) Antithyroid antibodies
(E) Thyroid-stimulating hormone (TSH)
(F) Serum prolactin
(G) Imaging study of the head

159. An 18-year-old adolescent presents with amenorrhea of 8 months' duration. She experienced menarche at age 16 years followed by 3 menses at approximately 2-month intervals before the onset of amenorrhea.

160. A 32-year-old woman with a 10-year history of irregular menses and amenorrhea for the past 6 months was referred with a negative progestin challenge test result and a follicle-stimulating hormone (FSH) level of 110 mIU/mL.

161. A 15-year-old adolescent is referred with amenorrhea of 7 months' duration. Her first menses occurred at age 13 years and was followed by 1½ years of bleeding twice monthly. Evaluation by her primary care physician reveals an FSH level of 160 mIU/mL, TSH level of 1.5 μU/mL, normal intravenous pyelogram, and chromosome analysis of 45,X/47,XXX.

162. A 16-year-old adolescent is referred for evaluation of secondary amenorrhea of 18 months' duration. Menarche occurred at age 12½ years and was followed with monthly menses until the sudden cessation of bleeding reported to her primary care physician. Her vaginal mucosa was atrophic and cervical mucus was absent. Prior evaluation included FSH level of 3 mIU/mL, prolactin level of 5 ng/mL, and TSH level of 1.8 μU/mL.

163–166

For each of the patients (163–166) who comes in for tubal ligation, select the potential complications (A–E) that must be considered during laparoscopy.

(A) Decreased cardiac output resulting in cardiovascular collapse
(B) Alveolar rupture resulting in permanent lung injury
(C) Atrioventricular dissociation resulting in severe hypotension
(D) Postoperative atelectasis resulting in severe hypoxemia
(E) Pulmonary hypertension leading to pulmonary edema

163. A 29-year-old obese woman with a history of cardiomyopathy of pregnancy.

164. A 37-year-old woman with a history of extensive pulmonary fibrosis secondary to asbestos exposure.

165. A 33-year-old woman with a history of recurrent vasovagal reaction to the placement of an intrauterine device.

166. A 42-year-old woman with a history of neck cancer treated surgically followed by irradiation, who has an elevated hemidiaphragm.

167–170

For each man who presents with azoospermia (167–170), select the most likely differential diagnosis (A–G).

(A) Klinefelter's syndrome
(B) Laurence-Moon syndrome
(C) Idiopathic hypogonadotropic hypogonadism
(D) Kallmann syndrome
(E) Gonadotropin-releasing hormone (GnRH) receptor gene mutation
(F) *DAX-1* gene mutation
(G) Follicle-stimulating hormone (FSH) receptor gene mutation

167. A 29-year-old man diagnosed with adrenal insufficiency at age 2 years and with hypogonadism at age 15 years despite corticoid therapy.

168. An otherwise healthy 32-year-old man with complete pubertal development and FSH level of 4 mIU/mL, luteinizing hormone level of 2 mIU/mL, and testosterone level of 60 ng/dL.

169. A 28-year-old man who is taller than predicted mid-parental height with reduced lean body mass and scanty pubic hair. Laboratory evaluation included FSH level of 24 mIU/mL, testosterone level of 98 ng/dL, and fasting blood glucose level of 145 mg/dL.

170. A 32-year-old man of Scandinavian descent with a normal physical examination except for reduced testicular size. A sister received a diagnosis with ovarian failure at age 19 years and a brother was evaluated for infertility and found to have a low sperm count.

Appendix A

Table of Normal Values for Laboratory Tests*

Analyte	Conventional Units
Alanine aminotransferase, serum	8–35 U/L
Alkaline phosphatase, serum	15–120 U/L
Menopause	
Amniotic fluid index	3–30 mL
Amylase	20–300 U/L
>60 years old	21–160 U/L
Aspartate aminotransferase, serum	15–30 U/L
Bicarbonate	
Arterial blood	21–27 mEq/L
Venous plasma	23–29 mEq/L
Bilirubin	
Total	0.3–1 mg/dL
Conjugated (direct)	0.1–0.4 mg/dL
Newborn, total	1–10 mg/dL
Blood gases (arterial) and pulmonary function	
Base deficit	<3 mEq/L
Base excess, arterial blood, calculated	–2 to +3 mEq/L
Forced expiratory volume	3.5–5 L
	>80% of predicted value
Forced vital capacity	3.5–5 L
Oxygen saturation (So_2)	95% or higher
Pao_2	≥80 mm Hg
Pco_2	35–45 mm Hg
Po_2	80–95 mm Hg
Peak expiratory flow rate	approximately 450 L/min
pH	7.35–7.45
Pvo_2	30–40 mm Hg
Blood urea nitrogen	
Adult	7–18 mg/dL
>60 years old	8–20 mg/dL
CA 125	<34 U/mL
Calcium	
Ionized	4.6–5.3 mg/dL
Serum	8.6–10 mg/dL
Chloride	98–106 mEq/L
Cholesterol	
Total	
Desirable	140–199 mg/dL
Borderline high	200–239 mg/dL
High	≥240 mg/dL
High-density lipoprotein	40–85 mg/dL
Low-density lipoprotein	
Desirable	<130 mg/dL
Borderline high	140–159 mg/dL
High	>160 mg/dL
Total cholesterol-to-high-density lipoprotein ratio	
Desirable	<3
Borderline high	3–5
High	>5
Triglycerides	<150 mg/dL
<20 years old	35–135 mg/dL

*Values listed are specific for adults or women, if relevant, unless otherwise differentiated.

(continued)

Table of Normal Values for Laboratory Tests* *(continued)*

Analyte	Conventional Units
Cortisol, plasma	
8 AM	5–23 µg/dL
4 PM	3–15 µg/dL
10 PM	<50% of 8 AM value
Creatinine, serum	0.6–1.2 mg/dL
Dehydroepiandrosterone sulfate	60–340 µg/dL
Erythrocyte	
Count	3,800,000–5,100,000/mm^3
Distribution width	10±1.5%
Sedimentation rate	
Wintrobe method	0–15 mm/h
Westergren method	0–20 mm/h
Estradiol-17β	
Follicular phase	30–100 pg/mL
Ovulatory phase	200–400 pg/mL
Luteal phase	50–140 pg/mL
Child	0.8–56 pg/mL
Ferritin, serum	18–160 µg/L
Fibrinogen	150–400 mg/dL
Follicle-stimulating hormone	
Premenopause	2.8–17.2 mIU/mL
Midcycle peak	15–35 mIU/mL
Postmenopause	24–170 mIU/mL
Child	0.1–7 mIU/mL
Glucose	
Fasting	70–105 mg/dL
2-hour postprandial	<120 mg/dL
Random blood	65–110 mg/dL
Hematocrit	36–48%
Hemoglobin	12–16 g/dL
Fetal	<1% of total
Hemoglobin A$_{1c}$ (nondiabetic)	5.5–8.5%
Human chorionic gonadotropin	0–5 mIU/mL
Pregnant	>5 mIU/mL
17α-Hydroxyprogesterone	
Adult	50–300 ng/dL
Child	32–63 ng/dL
25-Hydroxyvitamin D	10–55 ng/mL
Iron, serum	65–165 µg/dL
Binding capacity total	240–450 µg/dL
Lactate dehydrogenase, serum	313–618 U/L
Leukocytes	
Total	5,000–10,000/mm^3
Differential counts	
Basophils	0–1%
Eosinophils	1–3%
Lymphocytes	25–33%
Monocytes	3–7%
Myelocytes	0%
Band neutrophils	3–5%
Segmented neutrophils	54–62%
Lipase	10–140 U/L
>60 years old	18–180 U/L
Luteinizing hormone	
Follicular phase	3.6–29.4 mIU/mL
Midcycle peak	58–204 mIU/mL
Postmenopause	35–129 mIU/mL
Child	0.5–10.3 mIU/mL

*Values listed are specific for adults or women, if relevant, unless otherwise differentiated.

(continued)

Table of Normal Values for Laboratory Tests* *(continued)*

Analyte	Conventional Units
Magnesium	
Adult	1.6–2.6 mg/dL
Child	1.7–2.1 mg/dL
Newborn	1.5–2.2 mg/dL
Mean corpuscular	
Hemoglobin	27–33 pg
Hemoglobin concentration	33–37 g/dL
Volume	80–100 µm^3
Partial thromboplastin time	30–45 s
Activated	21–35 s
Phosphate, inorganic phosphorus	2.5–4.5 mg/dL
Platelet count	140,000–400,000/mm^3
Potassium	3.5–5.3 mEq/L
Progesterone	
Follicular phase	<3 ng/mL
Luteal phase	2.5–30 ng/mL
On oral contraceptives	0.1–0.3 ng/mL
>60 years old	0–0.2 ng/mL
1st trimester	9–47 ng/mL
2nd trimester	16.8–146 ng/mL
3rd trimester	55–255 ng/mL
Prolactin	0–17 ng/mL
Pregnant	34–386 ng/mL by 3rd trimester
Prothrombin time	10–13 s
Reticulocyte count	Absolute: 25,000–85,000 mm^3
	0.5–2.5% of erythrocytes
Semen analysis, spermatozoa	
Antisperm antibody	% of sperm binding by immunobead technique: >20% = decreased fertility; normal is <20% with adherent particles
Count	≥20 million/mL
Motility	≥60%
Morphology	≥60% normal forms
Sodium	135–145 mEq/L
Testosterone, female	
Total	6–86 ng/dL
Pregnant	3–4 × normal
Postmenopause	1/2 of normal
Free	
20–29 years old	0.9–3.2 pg/mL
30–39 years old	0.8–3 pg/mL
40–49 years old	0.6–2.5 pg/mL
50–59 years old	0.3–2.7 pg/mL
>60 years old	0.2–2.2 pg/mL
Thyroid-stimulating hormone	0.3–3 µU/mL
Thyroxine	
Serum free	0.9–2.3 ng/dL
Total	1.5–4.5 µg/dL
Triiodothyronine uptake	25–35%
Urea nitrogen, blood	
Adult	7–18 mg/dL
>60 years of age	8–20 mg/dL
Uric acid, serum	2.6–6 mg/dL
Urinalysis	
Epithelial cells	0–3/HPF
Erythrocytes	0–3/HPF
Leukocytes	0–4/HPF

*Values listed are specific for adults or women, if relevant, unless otherwise differentiated.

(continued)

Table of Normal Values for Laboratory Tests* *(continued)*

Analyte	Conventional Units
Urinalysis *(continued)*	
Protein (albumin)	
Qualitative	none detected
Quantitative	10–100 mg/24 hours
Specific gravity	
Normal hydration and volume	1.005–1.03
Concentrated	1.025–1.03
Diluted	1.001–1.01

*Values listed are specific for adults or women, if relevant, unless otherwise differentiated.

Appendix D

A
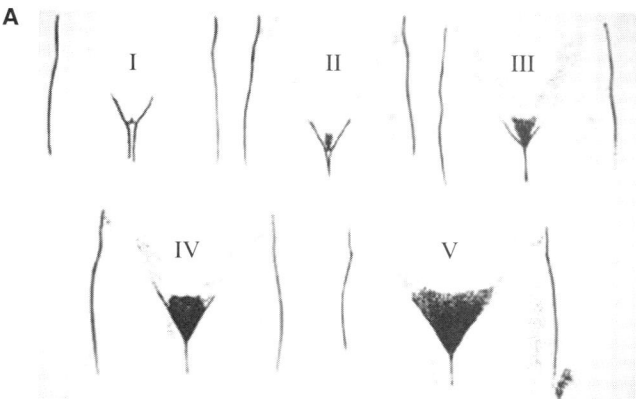

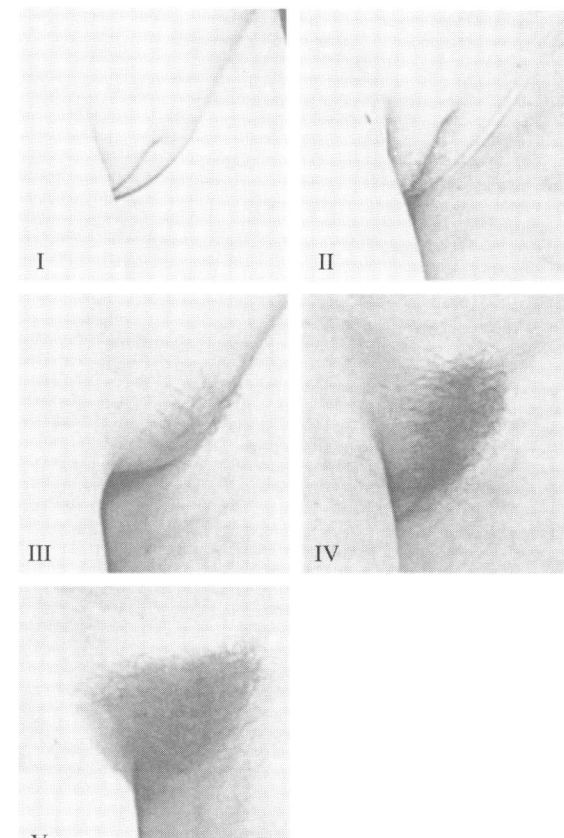

A. Tanner staging of pubic hair development. (Modified from Ross GT, Vandewiele RL, Frantz AG. The ovaries and the breasts. In: Williams RH [ed]. Textbook of endocrinology. 6th ed. Philadelphia [PA]: WB Saunders; 1981, p. 355, as modified from Marshall WA, Tanner JM. Variations in patterns of pubertal changes in girls. Arch Dis Child 1969;44:291–303. Copyright 1981, with permission from Elsevier. Yen SS, Jaffe RB, Barbieri RL, Reproductive endocrinology: physiology, pathophysiology, and clinical management. 4th ed. Baltimore [MD]: Lippincott Williams & Wilkins; 1999. p. 393.)

(continued)

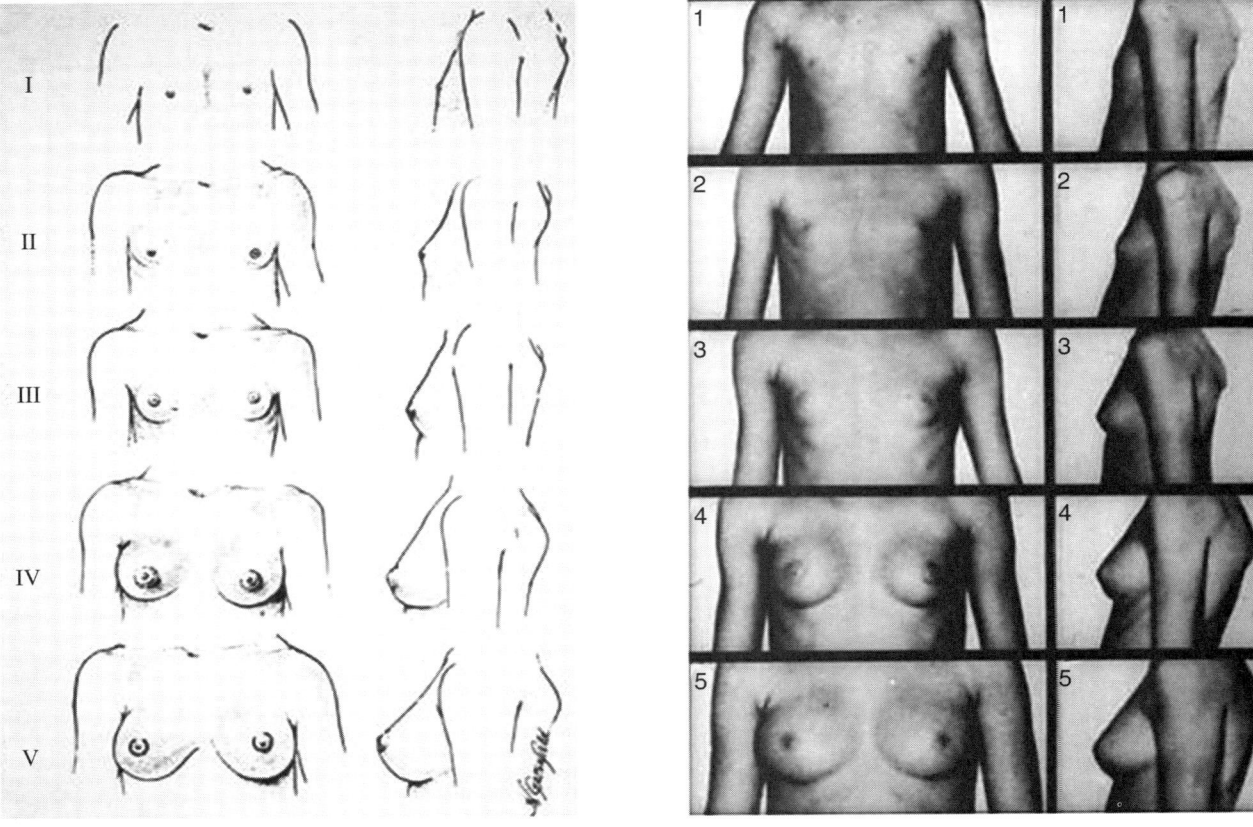

B. Tanner staging of breast development. (Reprinted from Ross GT, Vandewiele RL, Frantz AG. The ovaries and the breasts. In: Williams RH [ed]. Textbook of endocrinology. 6th ed. Philadelphia [PA]: WB Saunders; 1981, p. 355, as modified from Marshall WA, Tanner JM. Variations in patterns of pubertal changes in girls. Arch Dis Child 1969;44:291–303. Copyright 1981, with permission from Elsevier.)

PROLOG USER DEMOGRAPHICS AND PROLOG EVALUATION

To obtain a profile of the group of Fellows choosing to use self-assessment as a continuing medical education tool, the Education Division would appreciate the following information. This is for education program planning only and will not be associated with score reports in any way.

Part I. Demographics

171. Which of the following best describes the focus of your practice?

    (A) General obstetrics and gynecology
    (B) Oncology
    (C) Maternal–fetal medicine
    (D) Endocrinology
    (E) Urogynecology
    (F) Other

172. Are you board certified in obstetrics and gynecology?

    (A) Yes
    (B) No

173. Do you have subspecialty certification?

    (A) Yes
    (B) No

174. Have you been recertified?

    (A) Yes
    (B) No

175. How many years have you been in practice?

    (A) 10 years or less
    (B) 11–20 years
    (C) More than 20 years

Part II. PROLOG Evaluation

For each of the reasons listed (176–179), indicate the degree of importance to you for selecting PROLOG as a means of professional development, using the scale below:

    4 = Very important
    3 = Somewhat important
    2 = Not very important
    1 = Not important at all

176. Update my knowledge

177. Verify my current practice

178. Earn continuing medical education credits

179. Use as a home study program

For questions 180–183, indicate whether you are using this unit of PROLOG to prepare for the following:

180. The in-training examination of the Council on Residency Education in Obstetrics and Gynecology (CREOG)

181. The written board examination of the American Board of Obstetrics and Gynecology (ABOG)

182. The oral board examination of ABOG

183. The 6-year recertification examination of ABOG

184. In your estimation, what percentage of the content in PROLOG is new information to you?

   (A) Less than 10%
   (B) 10–20%
   (C) 21–50%
   (D) 51–75%
   (E) More than 75%

For each of the statements below (185–189), indicate the degree to which you agree, using the following scale:

   4 = Strongly agree
   3 = Somewhat agree
   2 = Somewhat disagree
   1 = Strongly disagree

185. The items in PROLOG closely relate to my clinical practice.

186. PROLOG is helpful in assessing my knowledge.

187. I have made 1 or more changes in patient management after reading PROLOG.

188. The critiques are useful.

189. The references accompanying each answer are useful.

Indicate how you would rate the following in preference for obtaining professional development (190–199), using the following scale:

   4 = Highest preference
   3 = Somewhat high
   2 = Somewhat low
   1 = Lowest preference

190. Postgraduate courses

191. ACOG district annual meeting

192. ACOG Annual Clinical Meeting

193. PROLOG self-assessment

194. PROLOG Dialogue audiotape programs

195. Videotape programs

196. CME programs offered by hospital departments

197. CME programs offered by other organizations

198. CD ROM

199. Internet

200. Was experimental or unlabeled use of products clearly reflected in the critiques?

   (A) Yes
   (B) No

201. Was there evidence of "conflict of interest" disclosures by task force members?

   (A) Yes
   (B) No

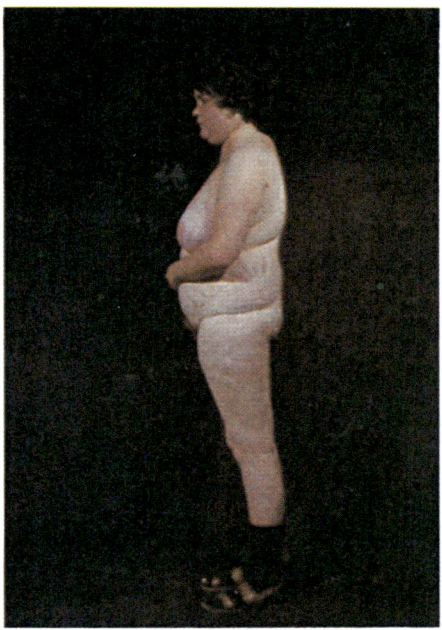

FIG. 19-1. (Yen SS, Jaffe RB, Barbieri RL, Reproductive endocrinology: physiology, pathophysiology, and clinical management. 4th ed. Baltimore [MD]: Williams & Wilkins. p. 529.)

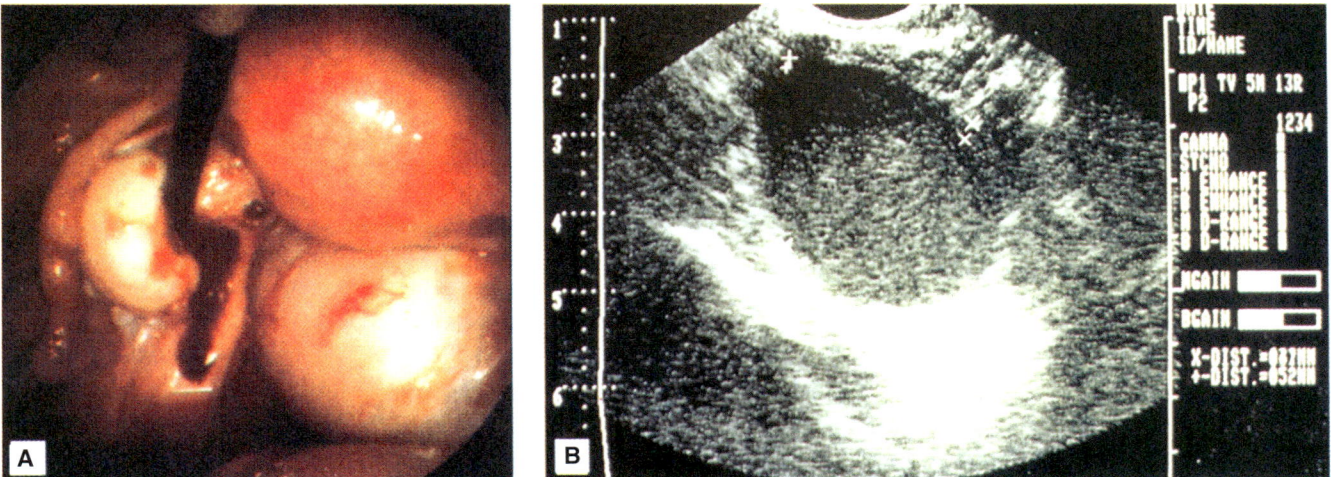

FIG. 29-1. (Stenchever MA, Mishell DR Jr. Atlas of clinical gynecology. Vol. III. Philadelphia [PA]: Appleton & Lange; 1999. p. 1.48.)

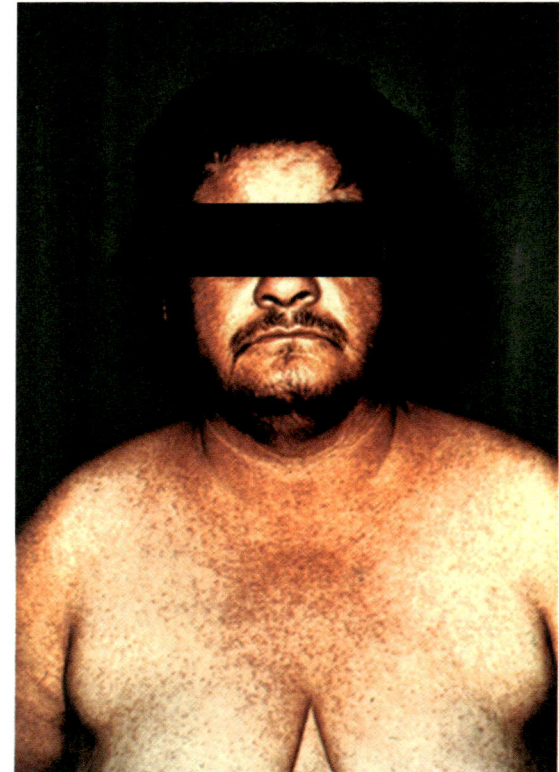

FIG. 45-1.

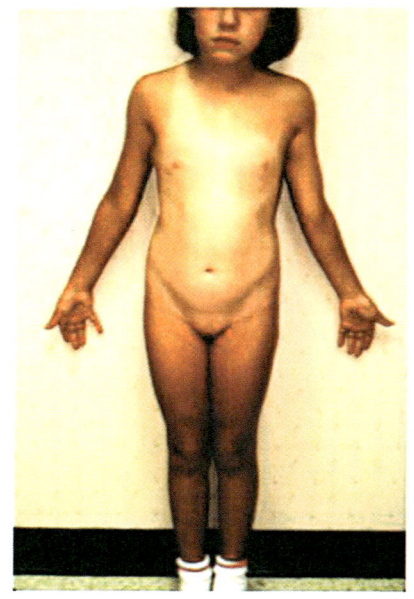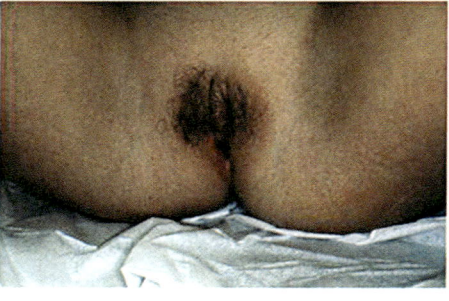

A

B

FIG. 59-1.

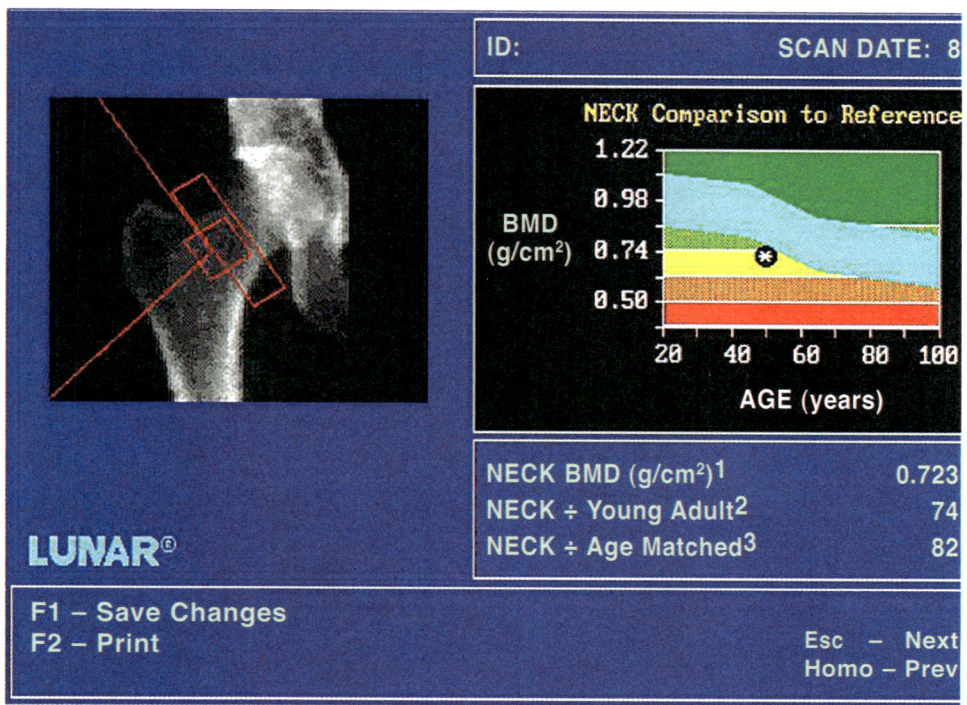

FIG. 102-1.

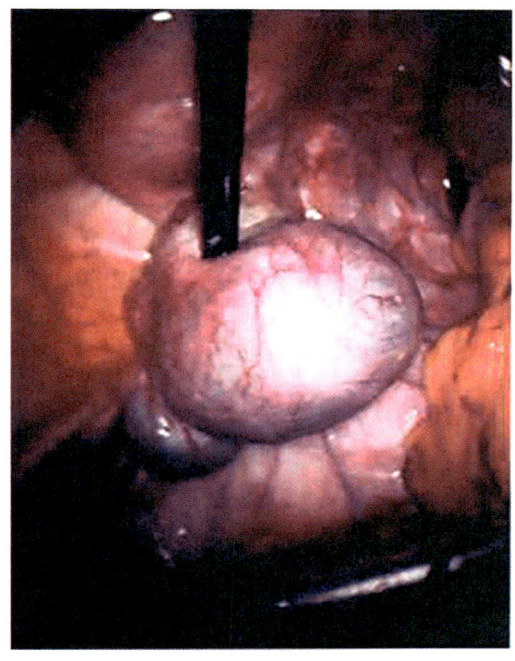

FIG. 107-1.

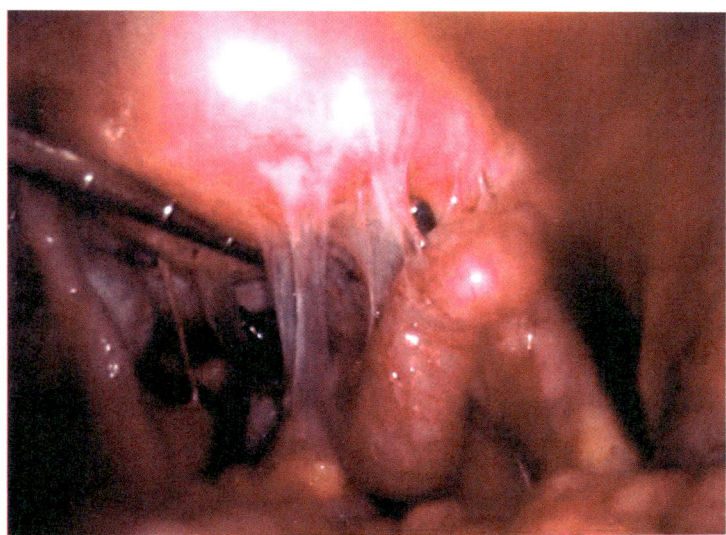

FIG. 107-2.